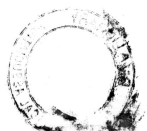

Commissioning Editor: Pauline Graham
Development Editor: Helen Leng
Project Manager: Glenys Norquay, Elouise Ball
Designer/Design Direction: Charles Gray
Illustration Manager: Gillian Richards

GYNAECOLOGY ILLUSTRATED

Catrina Bain MBChB MRCOG

Consultant Obstetrician and Gynaecologist
Glasgow Royal Infirmary
Glasgow, UK

Kevin Burton MD MRCOG

Consultant Gynaecological Oncologist
Glasgow Royal Infirmary
Glasgow, UK

C Jay McGavigan MD MRCOG FRANZCOG

Consultant Obstetrician
Head Fetal-Maternal Medicine
Flinders Medical Centre
South Australia

Illustrations by

Robin Callander FFPh FMAA AIMBI

Medical Illustrator, Formerly Director of Medical Illustrations, University of Glasgow,
Glasgow, UK

Ian Ramsden

Head of Medical Illustration Unit, University of Glasgow,
Glasgow, UK

SIXTH EDITION

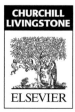

CHURCHILL LIVINGSTONE

ELSEVIER

Edinburgh   London   New York   Oxford   Philadelphia   St Louis   Sydney   Toronto   2011

CHURCHILL
LIVINGSTONE
ELSEVIER

First edition 1972
Second edition 1978
Third edition 1985
Fourth edition 1993
Fifth edition 2000
Sixth edition 2011

ISBN 9780702030673

International ISBN 9780702030772

British Library Cataloguing in Publication Data
A catalogue record for this book is available from the British Library

Library of Congress Cataloging in Publication Data
A catalogue record for this book is available from the Library of Congress

ELSEVIER

your source for books,
journals and multimedia
in the health sciences

www.elsevierhealth.com

Working together to grow
libraries in developing countries

www.elsevier.com | www.bookaid.org | www.sabre.org

ELSEVIER   BOOK AID International   Sabre Foundation

The Publisher's policy is to use **paper manufactured from sustainable forests**

Printed in China

PREFACE

This is the 6th edition of *Gynaecology Illustrated*, a textbook that owes its long-standing popularity to the clarity of its line-drawn illustrations and of the accompanying text. The latest edition has been extensively revised and updated by three new authors who have complementary specialist interests. The structure of the text has been reorganised to place particular emphasis upon clinical areas of clinical relevance. Despite the extensive revisions the authors have remained true to the original objectives of their predecessors and *Gynaecology Illustrated* continues to offer an up-to-date and focused visual learning experience in this practical specialty.

Catrina Bain
Kevin Burton
Jay McGavigan

CONTENTS

1. Embryology of the Reproductive Tract   1

Development of the Ovary   2–4
Development of Uterus and Fallopian Tubes   5, 6
Development of External Genitalia   7, 8
Development of Male External Genitalia   9

2. Anatomy of the Reproductive Tract   11

The Perineum   12
The Vulva   13, 14
Bartholin's Gland   15
Muscles of the Perineum   16
The Urogenital Diaphragm   17
Ischiorectal Fossa   18
Muscles of the Pelvis   19
Pelvic Diaphragm   20
Pelvic Fascia   21
The Vagina   22–24
Uterus   25–31
Fallopian Tube   32
Broad Ligament   33
Ovary   34–37
Changes in the Genital Tract with Age   38
Blood Supply of the Pelvis   39–41
Lymphatic Drainage of the Genital Tract   42
Nerves of the Pelvis   43
Autonomic Nerve Supply of the Pelvis   44

3. Physiology of the Reproductive Tract   45

Ovulation   46–50
Cyclical Ovarian Hormonal Changes   51
Action of Ovarian Hormones   52
Effects of Ovarian Hormones   53
Puberty   54
The Menopause   55

4. Disorders of Sex Development   57

Maturation of Germ Cells: Meiosis   58
Genetic Abnormalities   59–61
Congenital Abnormalities   62, 63
Abnormalities of Ovary and Tube   64
Abnormalities of the Uterus   65, 66
Abnormalities of the Vagina   67
Abnormalities of the Vulva   68

5. History and Examination   69

Taking the History   70, 71
Pelvic Pain   72, 73
Other Gynaecolgical Symptoms   74
Abdominal Examination   75–77
Examination of the Vulva   78
Bimanual Pelvic Examination   79
Speculum Examination   80, 81
Examination of the Breasts   82
Laparoscopy   83–85

6. Abnormalities of Menstruation   87

Normal and Physiological Changes in the Menstrual Cycle   88
Physiological Amenorrhoea   89
Uterine and Lower Genital Tract Disorders   90, 91
Ovarian Disorders   92–96
Pituitary Disorders   97–100
Hypothalamic Disorders   101
Investigation of Amenorrhoea   102–104
Hirsutism   105
Virilisation   106
Management of Hirsutism   107, 108
Menstrual Disorder   109
Dysfunctional Uterine Bleeding   110
Investigation of the Endometrium   111, 112
Investigations of Endometrium - Complications   113
Management of Heavy Menstrual Bleeding   114–119
Dysmenorrhoea   120, 121

Adenomyosis 122
Endometriosis 123–128
Premenstrual Syndrome 129, 130

7. Gynaecological Infections 131

Inflammation in the Lower
   Gynaecological Tract 132
Vulval Inflammation 133
Vaginal Discharge and Infection 134
Complaints of Vaginal Discharge 135
Vaginal Discharge 136–138
Vaginitis 139
Genital Herpes 140
Genital Warts 141
Bacterial Infections 142
Tropical Sexually Transmitted
   Infections 143
Gonorrhoea 144
Syphilis 145–147
Physiological Variation of the Cervix 148
Pelvic Inflammatory Disease 149, 150
Genital Tuberculosis 151, 152
Human Immunodeficiency Virus 153, 154

8. Diseases of the Vulva 155

Vulval Dermatoses 156, 157
Benign Tumours of the Vulva 158
Vulval Intraepithelial Neoplasia 159
Carcinoma of the Vulva 160–164
Diseases of the Urethra 165

9. Diseases of the Vagina 167

Benign Vaginal Disease 168
Malignant and Premalignant Disease 169
Carcinoma of the Vagina 170, 171
Plastic Surgery of the Vagina 172

10. Diseases of the Cervix 173

Normal Cervical Epithelium 174
The Role of Human Papilloma Virus
   in Cervical Disease 175
Screening for Cervical Cancer 176
Cervical Smears 177

Premalignant and Malignant Cervical
   Disease 178
Colposcopy 179
Treatment of Cervical Intraepithelial
   Neoplasia 180–182
Carcinoma of the Cervix 183–185
Diagnosis of Cervical Carcinoma 186
Staging of Cervical
   Carcinoma 187, 188
Radiotherapy and Chemotherapy in
   Cervical Carcinoma 189
Surgery for Cervical Carcinoma 190–193

11. Diseases of the Uterus 195

Uterine Polyps 196
Fibroids 197–200
Endometrial Hyperplasia 201, 202
Carcinoma of the Endometrium 203, 204
Staging of Endometrial Carcinoma 205
Spread of Endometrial Carcinoma 206
Aetiological Factors in Endometrial
   Carcinoma 207
Prognosis of Endometrial Carcinoma 208
Treatment of Endometrial Carcinoma 209
Recurrence of Endometrial
   Carcinoma 210
Sarcoma of the Uterus 211, 212

12. Prolapse and Urogynaecology 213

Retroversion of the Uterus 214, 215
Uterovaginal Prolapse 216, 217
Vaginal Prolapse 218, 219
Clinical Features of Prolapse 220
Differential Diagnosis of Prolapse 221
Pessary Treatment 222
Anterior Colporrhaphy
   (and Repair of Cystocele) 223, 224
Manchester Repair 225, 226
Posterior Colpoperineorrhaphy
   (Including Repair of Rectocele) 227
Repair of Enterocele 228
Vaginal Hysterectomy 229, 230
Urogynaecology 231, 232
Blood Supply of the Ureter 233

Physiology of Micturition 234, 235
Mechanism of Voiding 236
Detrusor Instability 237
Genuine Stress Incontinence 238
Other Incontinence Mechanisms 239
The Urethral Syndrome 240
Investigation of Incontinence 241
Urodynamic Investigation of Bladder
    Function 242
Indications for Urodynamic
    Assessment 243
Treatment of Stress Incontinence 244
Surgical Treatment of Stress
    Incontinence 245
Marshall–Marchetti–Krantz
    Urethropexy 246
Burch's Colposuspension
    Operation 247
Sling Procedures 248
Treatment of Detrusor Instability 249

**13. Diseases of the Ovary and
Fallopian Tube**   **251**

Clinical Features of Ovarian
    Tumours 252–254
Differential Diagnosis 255–258
Ovarian Cyst Accidents 259–261
Benign and Malignant Ovarian
    Tumours 262, 263
Risk Factors of Ovarian Cancer 264
Epithelial Ovarian Tumours 265, 266
Germ Cell Ovarian Tumours 267–270
Hormone-Producing Tumours 271–274
Other Hormone-Producing
    Tumours 275
Surgical Treatment of Ovarian
    Tumours 276
Treatment of Ovarian
    Cancer 277, 278
Staging of Ovarian Cancer 279, 280
Principles of Chemotherapy 281
Chemotherapeutic Agents in Ovarian
    Cancer 282
Broad Ligament Cysts 283, 284
Carcinoma of Fallopian Tubes 285

**14. Complications of
Gynaecological Surgery**   **287**

Urinary Tract Injuries 288
Injury to the Ureter 289
Management of Ureteric Injury 290, 291
Fistula Formation 292, 293
Lymphoedema and Lymphocyst 294
Venous Thrombosis 295–297
Clinical Features of Deep Venous
    Thrombosis 298
Investigations for Deep Venous
    Thrombosis 299
Methods of Thromboprophylaxis 300, 301
Pulmonary Embolism 302–304
Treatment of Pulmonary Embolus 305
Mortality 306

15. Early Pregnancy   **307**

Miscarriage 308, 309
Management 310–313
Recurrent Miscarriage 314–316
Termination of Pregnancy 317–319
Ectopic Pregnancy 320
Diagnosis of Tubal Pregnancy 321, 322
Sites of Implantation 323
Treatment of Tubal Pregnancy 324
Gestational Trophoblastic
    Disease 325–330

16. Sexuality and Contraception   **331**

Physiology of Coitus 332, 333
Dyspareunia 334
Sexual Problems Affecting the Male 335
Treatment Options for Erectile
    Dysfunction 336
Medico-Legal Problems 337
Methods of Contraception 338, 339
Hormonal Contraception 340, 341
Minor Side Effects of OCs 342
Oral Contraception: Risks 343–345
Intrauterine Devices (IUDs) 346, 347
Complications of Intrauterine Devices 348
Diaphragms and Caps 349
Condoms 350

Contraception Based on Time of
   Ovulation   351
Postcoital Contraception   352
Irreversible Methods   353, 354
Laparoscopic Sterilisation   355
Vasectomy   356

17. Infertility   **357**

Infertility   358, 359
Investigations   360
Evidence of Ovulation   361–363
Seminal Analysis   364
Sperm Production Tests   365
Abnormalities in Sperm Production 366
Sperm Function Tests   367
Tests of Tubal Patency   368, 369

Assisted Conception   370
Fertility Drugs   371, 372
Tubal Surgery   373
Assisted Conception Techniques 374–379
Assisted Conception   380

18. The Menopause   **381**

The Menopause   382, 383
The Greene Climacteric Scale 384
Changes in the Genital Tract 385
Osteoporosis   386–388
Cardiovascular Disease and the
   Menopause   389, 390
Hormone Replacement Therapy 391–393

Index   395

CHAPTER 1

EMBRYOLOGY OF THE REPRODUCTIVE TRACT

Development of the Ovary   2
Development of Uterus and Fallopian Tubes   5
Development of External Genitalia   7
Development of Male External Genitalia   9

DEVELOPMENT OF THE OVARY

The germ cells, which will eventually inhabit the gonads, originate from the primitive hind gut. They appear around the 25th day.

By 30 days, the gut, complete with its mesentery, is formed. The germ cells now migrate from the gut to the root of the mesentery. Of the original 6 or 7 million, only 1–2 million are present at birth and this number is reduced to 300,000 at puberty. A smaller number of these cells may be a factor that leads to premature menopause.

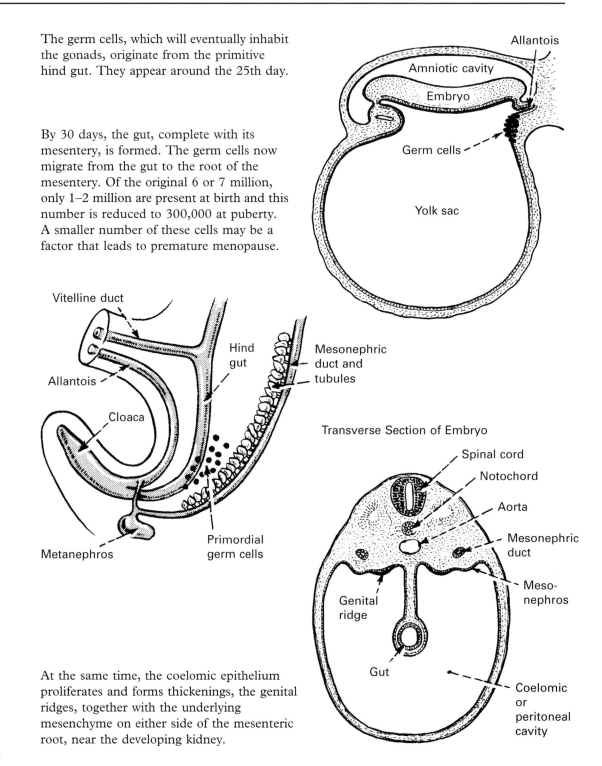

Transverse Section of Embryo

At the same time, the coelomic epithelium proliferates and forms thickenings, the genital ridges, together with the underlying mesenchyme on either side of the mesenteric root, near the developing kidney.

DEVELOPMENT OF THE OVARY

At this stage, the primitive gonad (genital ridge) consists of a mesoderm (coelomic epithelium plus mesenchyme) covered by the coelomic epithelium. The germ cells now migrate from the root of the mesentery to the genital ridge.

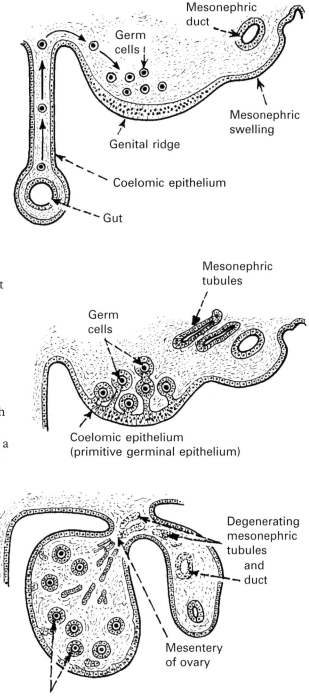

The coelomic epithelium, growing into the genital ridge, forms the so-called sex cords, which enclose each germ cell.

Until this time, that is, around the 7th week, the gonad is of an indifferent type, the male being indistinguishable from the female.

The germ cells and most of the sex cord cells remain in the superficial part, which is the future cortex of the ovary. The cords then lose contact with the surface epithelium and form small groups of cells, each with its germ cell, a primitive follicle. Some of the sex cord cells grow into the medulla. These tend to regress and form rudimentary tubules, the rete.

As the ovary grows, it projects increasingly into the peritoneal (coelomic) cavity, thus forming a mesentery.

DEVELOPMENT OF THE OVARY

Simultaneously, the ovary descends extraperitoneally within the abdominal cavity. Two ligaments develop and these may help to control its descent, guiding it to its final position and preventing its complete descent through the inguinal ring, in contrast to the testes. The first structure is the suspensory ligament attached to the anterior (cephalic) pole of the ovary which connects it with its site of origin, the genital ridge.

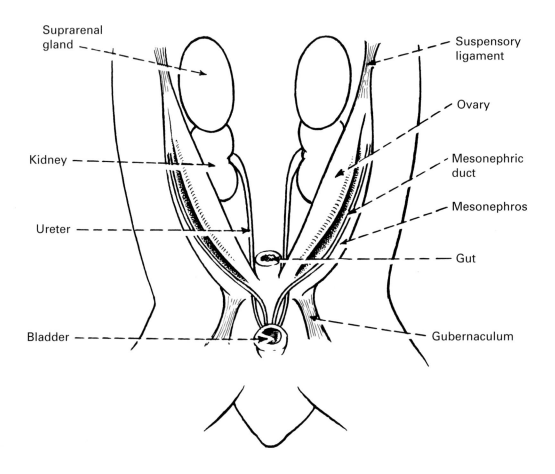

Another ligament, or gubernaculum, develops at the posterior or caudal end of the ovary. At first attached to the genital ridge, it later becomes attached to the developing uterus and becomes the ovarian ligament.

DEVELOPMENT OF UTERUS AND FALLOPIAN TUBES

When the embryo reaches a size of 10 mm at 35–36 days, a longitudinal groove appears on the dorsal aspect of the coelomic cavity, lateral to the Wolffian (mesonephric) ridge.

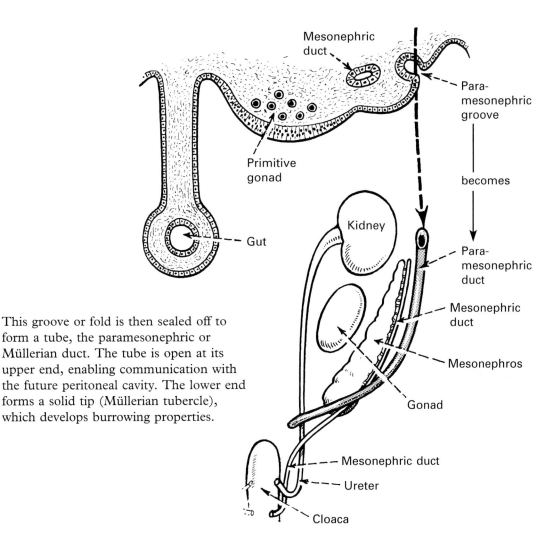

This groove or fold is then sealed off to form a tube, the paramesonephric or Müllerian duct. The tube is open at its upper end, enabling communication with the future peritoneal cavity. The lower end forms a solid tip (Müllerian tubercle), which develops burrowing properties.

DEVELOPMENT OF UTERUS AND FALLOPIAN TUBES

The Müllerian ducts from either side grow in a caudal direction, extraperitoneally. They also bend medially and anteriorly and ultimately fuse in front of the hind gut. The mesonephric duct becomes involved in the walls of the paramesonephric ducts.

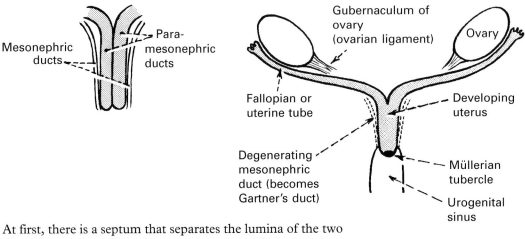

At first, there is a septum that separates the lumina of the two ducts. Later the septum disappears and a single cavity is formed, the uterus. The upper parts of both the ducts remain separate and form the fallopian tubes.

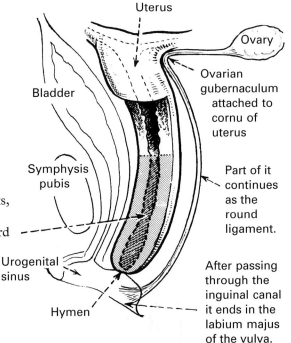

While this is happening, the ovary is also affected. Its gubernaculum is ultimately attached to the Müllerian duct at the cornu of the developing uterus. This pulls the ovary medially such that its long axis becomes horizontal.

The lower end of the fused Müllerian ducts, beyond the uterine lumen, remains solid, proliferates and forms a solid cord. This cord will canalise to form the vagina, which opens into the urogenital sinus.

At the point of entry into the urogenital sinus, a part of the Müllerian tubercle persists and forms the hymen.

DEVELOPMENT OF EXTERNAL GENITALIA

At an early stage, the hind gut and the various urogenital ducts open into a common cloaca.

A septum (urorectal) grows down between the allantois and the hind gut during the 5th week.

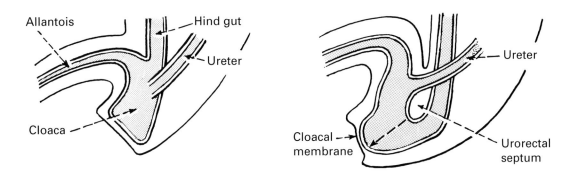

Eventually, this septum fuses with the cloacal membrane, dividing the cloaca into two compartments – the rectum dorsally and the urogenital sinus ventrally. At the same time, the developing uterus grows down and makes contact with the urogenital sinus.

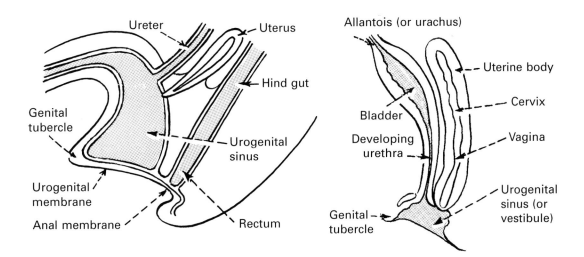

At the end of the 7th week, the urogenital membrane breaks down and the urogenital sinus opens on to the surface.

The developing uterus and vagina push downwards and cause an elongation and narrowing of the upper part of the urogenital sinus. This will form the urethra.

DEVELOPMENT OF EXTERNAL GENITALIA

Meanwhile, on the surface of the embryo, around the urogenital sinus, five swellings appear. At the cephalic end, a midline swelling grows, the genital tubercle, which will become the clitoris. Posterior to the genital tubercle and on either side of the urogenital membrane a fold is formed – urethral folds. Lateral to each of these another swelling appears – the genital or labial swelling. These swellings approach each other at their posterior ends, fuse and form the posterior commissure. The remaining swellings become the labia minora.

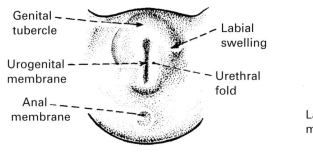

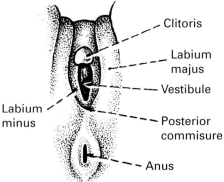

Certain small, but clinically important, glands are formed in and around the urogenital sinus.

In the embryo, the epithelial buds arise from the urethra and also from the epithelium of the urogenital sinus. In the male, these two sets of buds grow together and give rise to the glands of the prostate. They remain separate in the female, with the urethral buds forming the urethral glands and the urogenital buds giving rise to the paraurethral glands of Skene. The ducts of the latter open into the vestibule, on either side of the urethra.

Two other small glands arise by budding from the epithelium of the posterior part of the vestibule, one on either side of the vaginal opening. These are the greater vestibular or Bartholin's glands. Similar smaller glands also arise in the anterior portion of the vestibule.

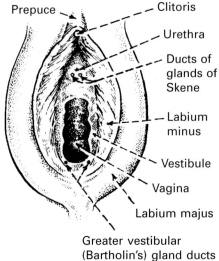

DEVELOPMENT OF MALE EXTERNAL GENITALIA

As in the female, a mesodermal mass, the urorectal septum, grows downwards and separates the urogenital sinus from the rectum and anus. The urogenital portion of the cloacal membrane disintegrates and an open gutter is formed through which the urine drains. This gutter is continuous anteriorly with the primitive urethral groove on the phallus.

The ectoderm on the under surface of the phallus disappears, exposing the underlying endodermal plate.

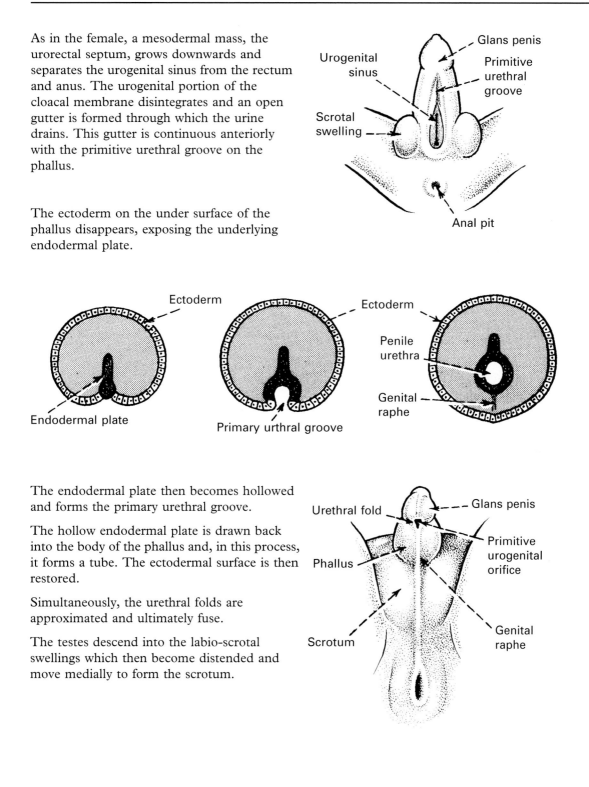

The endodermal plate then becomes hollowed and forms the primary urethral groove.

The hollow endodermal plate is drawn back into the body of the phallus and, in this process, it forms a tube. The ectodermal surface is then restored.

Simultaneously, the urethral folds are approximated and ultimately fuse.

The testes descend into the labio-scrotal swellings which then become distended and move medially to form the scrotum.

CHAPTER 2

ANATOMY OF THE REPRODUCTIVE TRACT

The Perineum   12
The Vulva   13
  Mons Pubis and Labia Majora   13
  Clitoris and Labia Minora   13
Bartholin's Gland   15
  Histology of Bartholin's Gland   15
Muscles of the Perineum   16
  Ischiocavernosus   16
  Bulbospongiosus   16
  Superficial Transverse Perineal
    Muscle   16
  External Anal Sphincter   16
The Urogenital Diaphragm   17
  The Urogenital Diaphragm
    (Triangular Ligament)   17
Ischiorectal Fossa   18
  Boundaries   18
Muscles of the Pelvis   19
Pelvic Diaphragm   20
  Functions of the Pelvic Diaphragm   20
Pelvic Fascia   21
  The Pelvic Fascia   21
The Vagina   22
  Histology   24
  Vaginal Secretion   24
  The Vaginal Epithelium   24
Uterus   25
  Corpus and Cervix   26
  Corpus (Uterine Body)   26
  Cervix   26
  Isthmus Uteri   26

Cavity of the Corpus   27
Cervix   27
Relationship of Uterus
  and Ureter   28
Ligaments of the Uterus   29
Histology   31
Fallopian Tube   32
Broad Ligament   33
  Blood Vessels   33
  Vestigial Structures   33
Ovary   34
  Histology   35
Changes in the Genital Tract
  with Age   38
  The Vulva   38
  The Vagina   38
  The Ovary   38
  The Uterus   38
Blood Supply of the Pelvis   39
  Supply to Uterus, Vagina
    and Bladder   39
  Collateral Blood Supply   41
  Abdominal Aorta   41
  External Iliac Artery   41
  The Femoral Artery   41
Lymphatic Drainage of the
  Genital Tract   42
Nerves of the Pelvis   43
Autonomic Nerve Supply of the
  Pelvis   44

THE PERINEUM

THE *PERINEUM* (Gk. 'around the natal area')

The *anatomical* or true perineum is the diamond-shaped outlet of the pelvis and the soft tissues that cover it.

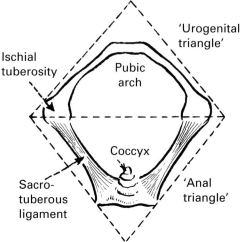

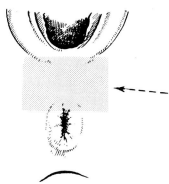

The *gynaecological* perineum is the area between the posterior commissure and the anus. This is the area referred to in gynaecology and obstetrics as 'the perineum'.

The anterior or urogenital triangle of the true perineum is covered by the external genitalia and other structures and is called the vulva. (L. *vulva* or *volva*: a covering.)

The *VULVA* consists of the following:

Mons pubis
Clitoris
Urethral orifice
Vestibule
Labia majora
Labia minora
Vaginal orifice
Hymen

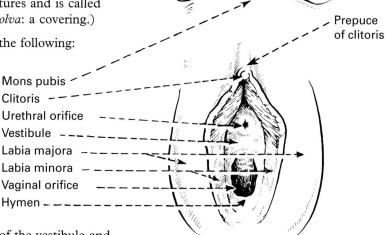

Subcutaneous: the bulb of the vestibule and the greater vestibular (Bartholin's) glands.

THE VULVA

MONS PUBIS AND LABIA MAJORA

The mons pubis is a pad of fatty tissue overlying the symphysis pubis and covered by skin and pubic hair. The labia are folds of skin and fat which pass from the mons back to the perineum. The lateral labial surfaces are pigmented and hairy, and the inner surfaces smooth and contain many sebaceous, sweat and apocrine glands.

The substance of the labia consists of vascular fatty tissue with many lymphatics, and also vestigial remnants of the dartos muscle. (The labium is the homologue of the scrotum.)

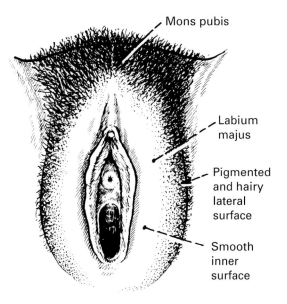

Mons pubis

Labium majus

Pigmented and hairy lateral surface

Smooth inner surface

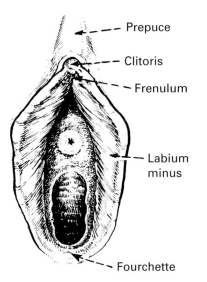

Prepuce

Clitoris

Frenulum

Labium minus

Fourchette

CLITORIS AND LABIA MINORA

The clitoris is the vestigial homologue of the penis and is formed the same way from two corpora cavernosa and a glans of spongy erectile tissue which has a copious blood supply from the clitoral artery. The clitoris is highly innervated.

The labia minora are two cutaneous folds enclosing the urethral and vaginal orifices. Anteriorly, each divides to form a hood or prepuce, and a frenulum for the clitoris. Posteriorly, they unite in a frenulum or fourchette, which is obliterated by the delivery of a baby. The labia minora contain no fat but many sebaceous glands.

THE VULVA

The **VESTIBULE** is the area between the labia minora. It is perforated by the urethral and vaginal orifices and the ducts of Bartholin's and Skene's glands. The fossa navicularis between the vagina and the fourchette is, like the fourchette, obliterated by childbirth. The lesser vestibular glands are mucosal glands discharging on to the surface of the vestibule.

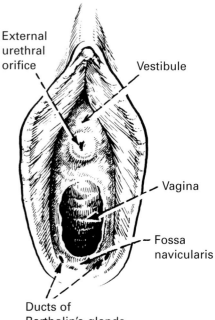

External urethral orifice

Vestibule

Vagina

Fossa navicularis

Ducts of Bartholin's glands

The **EXTERNAL URETHRAL ORIFICE** is, in the healthy state, a small protuberance with a vertical cleft. The tiny orifices of the paraurethral (Skene's) ducts lie just inside or outside the meatus. The paraurethral glands are homologues of the prostate and form a system of tubular glands, surrounding most of the urethra.

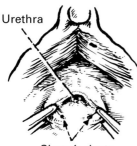

Urethra

Skene's ducts

The **VAGINAL ORIFICE** is a midline aperture incompletely closed by the **HYMEN**. The hymen is a thin septum of tissue lined by squamous epithelium with a small hole (sometimes several) for the passage of menstrual blood. It is stretched or torn by coitus and more or less obliterated by childbirth. A few tags of skin called carunculae myrtiformes are left.

Normal virgin hymen

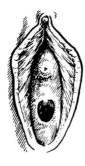

Hymen after coitus (or after using tampon)

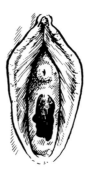

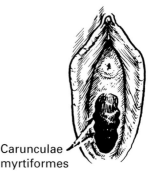

Carunculae myrtiformes

BARTHOLIN'S GLAND

The **BULB of the VESTIBULE** consists of two masses of erectile tissue on either side of the vagina, lying beneath the skin and bulbospongiosus muscle, but superficial to the perineal membrane. They are connected anteriorly by a narrow transverse strip and are the homologue of the bulb of the penis.

BARTHOLIN's (Greater vestibular) glands are the homologues of the bulbourethral (Cowper's) glands in the male but lie superficial instead of deep to the perineal membrane. Each gland is partly covered by the erectile tissue of the bulb and drains by a duct about 2 cm long which opens into the vaginal orifice lateral to the hymen.

Bartholin's gland is not palpable in the healthy state.

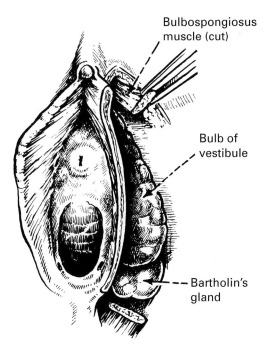

Bulbospongiosus muscle (cut)

Bulb of vestibule

Bartholin's gland

The erectile tissue of the bulb becomes tumescent during sexual excitement and the glands secrete a mucoid discharge, which acts as a lubricant.

HISTOLOGY OF BARTHOLIN'S GLAND

The gland is formed of racemose glands lined with columnar or cuboid epithelium. The duct demonstrates the very intimate embryological connection between genital and urinary tracts by being lined with transitional epithelium.

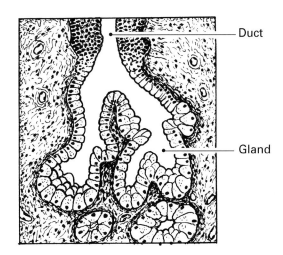

Duct

Gland

MUSCLES OF THE PERINEUM

ISCHIOCAVERNOSUS

This muscle compresses the root of the clitoris during sexual excitement, to produce erection by venous congestion.

BULBOSPONGIOSUS

This muscle conceals the vestibular bulb and Bartholin's glands. Its function is to diminish the vaginal orifice during coitus.

SUPERFICIAL TRANSVERSE PERINEAL MUSCLE

A small muscle that helps to fix the perineal body.

EXTERNAL ANAL SPHINCTER

Normally in a state of contraction to keep the anus closed. It also helps to fix the perineal body.

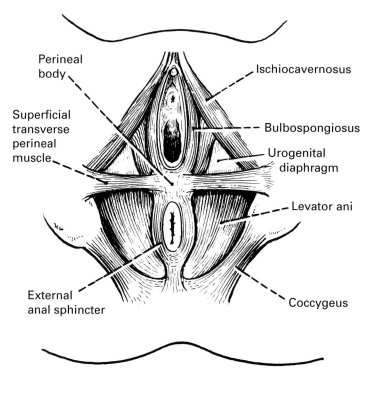

The *Perineal body* is a fibromuscular node between the anus and vagina with attachments to eight muscles:

    One Sphincter ani
    One Bulbospongiosus
    Two Transversi perinei superficiales
    Two Transversi perinei profundi (deep: not shown here)
    Two Levatores ani

The whole mass is what gynaecologists mean when they talk about 'the perineum'. If it is damaged during childbirth and not properly repaired and healed, it will not function properly and the efficiency of the whole pelvic diaphragm may suffer, leading to urinary or faecal incontinence.

THE UROGENITAL DIAPHRAGM

THE UROGENITAL DIAPHRAGM (Triangular Ligament)

This area of the perineum is more developed and surgically more important in the male. It consists of two sheets of fascia with a layer of muscle in between. It covers the pubic arch and is pierced by the urethra and, in the female, by the vagina.

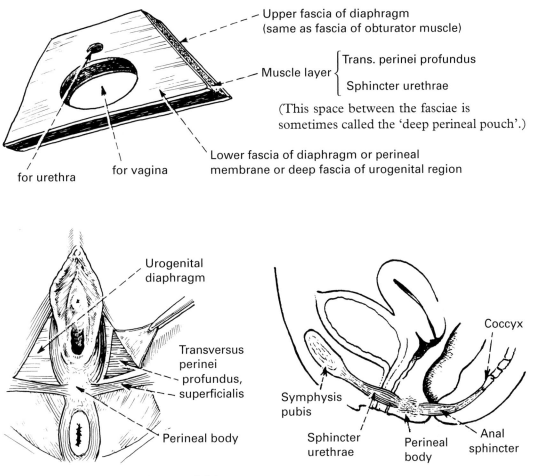

Upper fascia of diaphragm
(same as fascia of obturator muscle)

Muscle layer ⎰ Trans. perinei profundus
⎱ Sphincter urethrae

(This space between the fasciae is sometimes called the 'deep perineal pouch'.)

Lower fascia of diaphragm or perineal membrane or deep fascia of urogenital region

for urethra   for vagina

Urogenital diaphragm

Transversus perinei profundus, superficialis

Perineal body

Coccyx

Symphysis pubis

Sphincter urethrae   Perineal body   Anal sphincter

All the perineal muscles lie superficial to the perineal membrane, except the transversus perinei profundus, which helps to fix the perineal body.

(See page 16 on the function of the sphincter.)

The 'sphincter urethrae' is the system of musculature that assists the bladder muscle in closing the urethra. It is made up of the transversus perinei, the bulbospongiosus, and the levator ani; the anchoring bony points are the lower border of the symphysis pubis and the coccyx.

ISCHIORECTAL FOSSA

A wedge-shaped space between the ischial tuberosity and the anus, filled with fat and crossed by vessels and nerves.

BOUNDARIES

Laterally, the obturator fascia and ischial tuberosity.

Posteriorly, the sacrotuberous ligament.

Anteriorly, the urogenital diaphragm.

Medially, the sphincter ani and levator (anal) fascia.

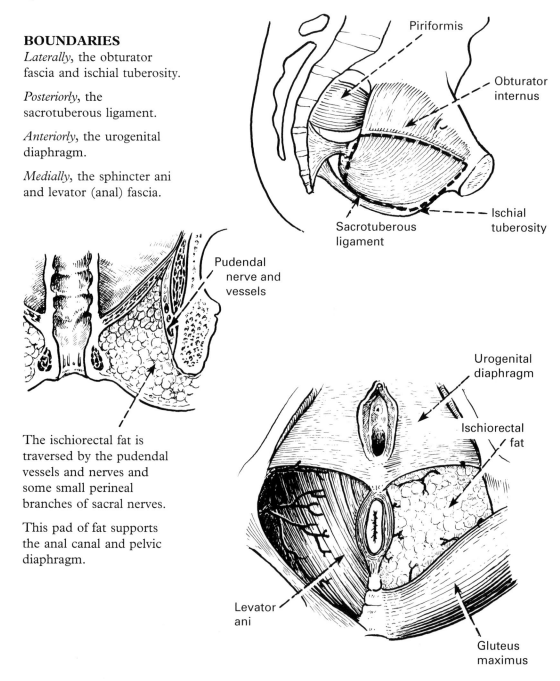

The ischiorectal fat is traversed by the pudendal vessels and nerves and some small perineal branches of sacral nerves.

This pad of fat supports the anal canal and pelvic diaphragm.

MUSCLES OF THE PELVIS

Levator ani ⎫
Coccygeus ⎬ Pelvic diaphragm

Obturator internus

Piriformis

The *Levator ani* arises from the back of the pubis, the obturator fascia (by a 'tendinous arch' or 'white line'), and the ischial spine.

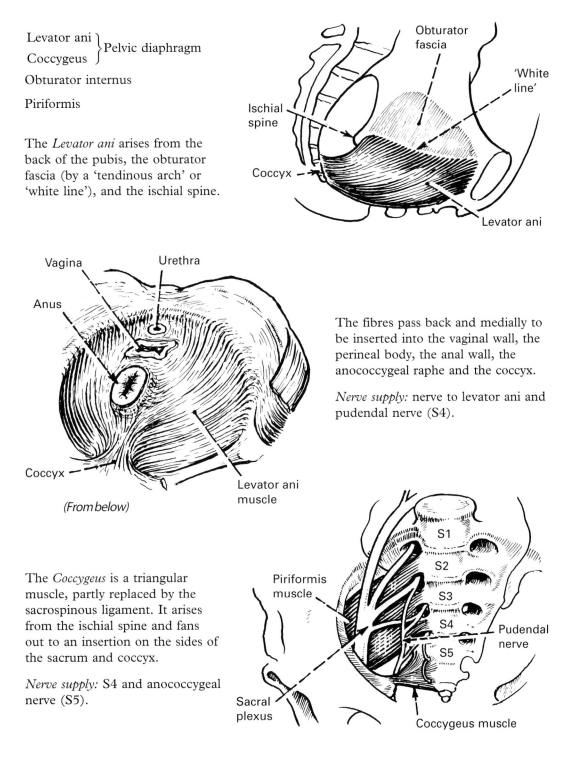

(From below)

The fibres pass back and medially to be inserted into the vaginal wall, the perineal body, the anal wall, the anococcygeal raphe and the coccyx.

Nerve supply: nerve to levator ani and pudendal nerve (S4).

The *Coccygeus* is a triangular muscle, partly replaced by the sacrospinous ligament. It arises from the ischial spine and fans out to an insertion on the sides of the sacrum and coccyx.

Nerve supply: S4 and anococcygeal nerve (S5).

PELVIC DIAPHRAGM

The *Obturator internus* arises from the anterolateral wall of the pelvis (and obturator membrane) and passes backwards through the lesser sciatic foramen to be inserted into the trochanter of the femur (L5, S1 and S2).

The *Piriformis* arises from the front of the sacrum and passes through the greater sciatic foramen to be inserted into the trochanter of the femur (S1 and 2).

These muscles are primarily lateral rotators of the hip and postural muscles.

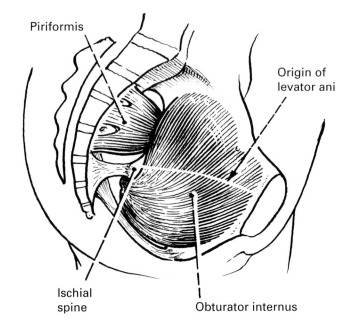

Piriformis

Origin of levator ani

Ischial spine

Obturator internus

FUNCTIONS OF THE PELVIC DIAPHRAGM
Apart from helping to fix the perineal body and assist the vaginal and anal sphincters, the main function of the pelvic diaphragm is to support the pelvic viscera.

The muscles used to be named as follows:

$$\left.\begin{array}{l} \text{pubococcygeus} \\ \text{iliococcygeus} \end{array}\right\} = \text{levator ani}$$

$$\text{ischiococcygeus} = \text{coccygeus}$$

In the lower animals, their function is to move the tail (the coccyx). In man, they have to meet the requirements of the erect position and resist the strain imposed by any increase in intra-abdominal pressure such as when laughing, coughing, straining at stool, etc. In addition, a complete relaxation of the muscles should be possible during parturition so that the vaginal foramen may enlarge almost to the size of the bony pelvic outlet.

PELVIC FASCIA

THE PELVIC FASCIA

Parietal Layer

The aponeuroses and fascial sheaths of the pelvic muscles (the 'wallpaper' of the pelvis).

Visceral Layer

The fascial sheaths of the organs and the fatty tissue filling the space between them (the 'stuffing' of the pelvis).

In certain areas, this stuffing is condensed and strengthened by plain muscle fibres and elastic tissue to form the ligaments of the uterus (pp. 28–31).

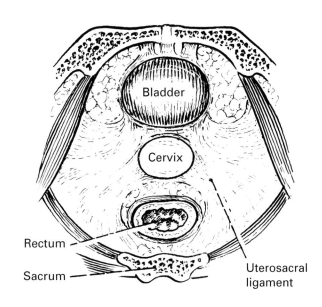

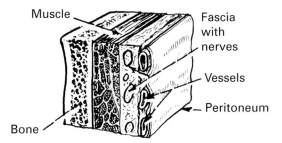

Relations of the Fascia

The nerve trunks, which leave the pelvis, are 'outside' the fascia. The vessels are 'inside' and lie between the fascia and peritoneum.

These fascial prolongations on structures leaving the pelvis form points at which pus may track from a pelvic abscess to a point in the buttock or groin or above the inguinal ligament, as demonstrated in this image.

(The greater sciatic notch is not shown.)

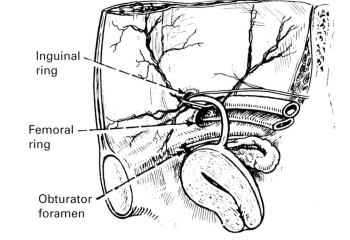

THE VAGINA

The vagina is a tubular structure extending from the vulva to the uterus.

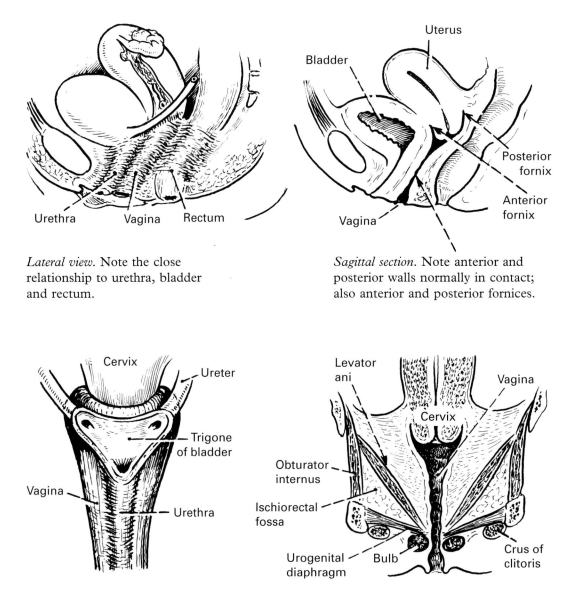

Lateral view. Note the close relationship to urethra, bladder and rectum.

Sagittal section. Note anterior and posterior walls normally in contact; also anterior and posterior fornices.

Anterior view shows the very intimate relationship with the bladder base and ureters.

Coronal section shows the relationship of vagina and pelvic floor.

THE VAGINA

In the nulliparous adult, the vagina is H-shaped in section and marked by longitudinal furrows – the columns of the vagina – and numerous transverse ridges or rugae. This configuration permits great distension during childbirth and is much less marked in parous women.

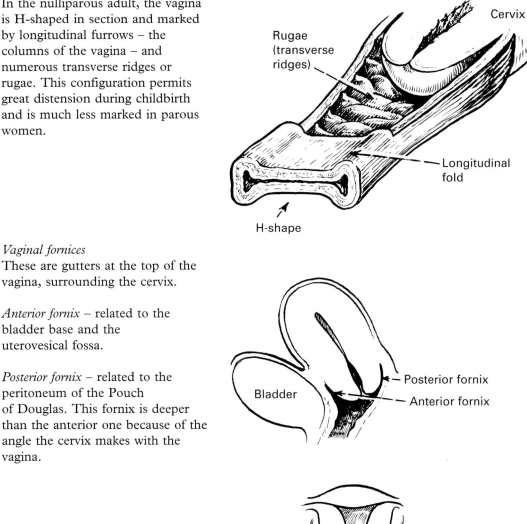

Vaginal fornices
These are gutters at the top of the vagina, surrounding the cervix.

Anterior fornix – related to the bladder base and the uterovesical fossa.

Posterior fornix – related to the peritoneum of the Pouch of Douglas. This fornix is deeper than the anterior one because of the angle the cervix makes with the vagina.

Lateral fornices – related to the ureters and the uterine vessels.

THE VAGINA

HISTOLOGY
Its length is about 9 cm along the posterior wall and 7.5 cm along the anterior. The width gradually increases from below upwards.

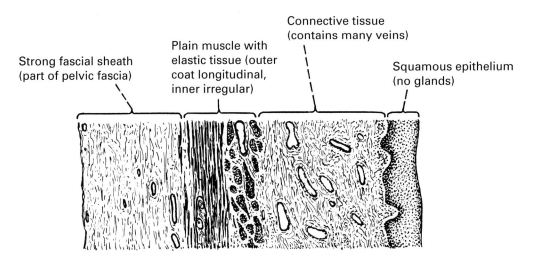

Strong fascial sheath (part of pelvic fascia)

Plain muscle with elastic tissue (outer coat longitudinal, inner irregular)

Connective tissue (contains many veins)

Squamous epithelium (no glands)

The vagina pierces the urogenital diaphragm and is encircled at its lower end by the voluntary bulbospongiosus, which has some sphincteric action, although the levator ani muscle is more effective.

VAGINAL SECRETION
This is composed of alkaline cervical secretion, desquamated epithelial cells and bacteria. The epithelium is rich in glycogen which is converted by Doderlein's bacillus into lactic acid. The vaginal pH is about 4.5 and provides a fairly effective barrier against infection.

THE VAGINAL EPITHELIUM
This is composed of several layers of squamous cells with no keratinisation. It develops papillae, which dip into the fibrous corium. It is much thinner in the child, and the rugae are absent. This appearance recurs in old age. Cyclic changes are discussed on page 53.

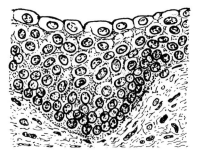

UTERUS

The uterus is a hollow viscus composed of smooth muscle, whose sole function is gestation.

It lies between the rectum and the bladder and is continuous with the vagina.

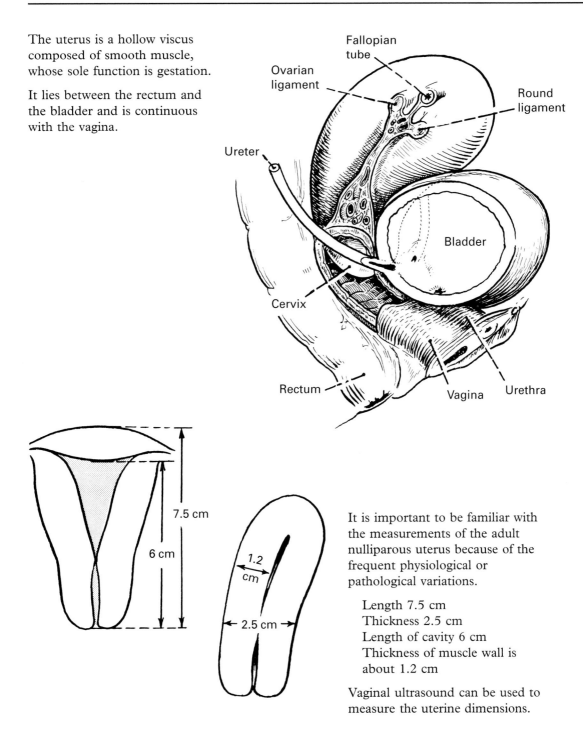

It is important to be familiar with the measurements of the adult nulliparous uterus because of the frequent physiological or pathological variations.

Length 7.5 cm
Thickness 2.5 cm
Length of cavity 6 cm
Thickness of muscle wall is about 1.2 cm

Vaginal ultrasound can be used to measure the uterine dimensions.

UTERUS

CORPUS AND CERVIX

The upper two-thirds of the uterus are called the corpus or body, and the lower third is the cervix or neck. They are quite distinct in function, and therefore in structure as well, although the transition from muscle to fibrous tissue is gradual.

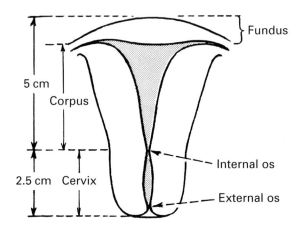

CORPUS (UTERINE BODY)

Its function is to provide a mucous membrane (endometrium) suitable for implantation, and thereafter to contain the growing fetus until it is mature. It is composed mainly of smooth muscle.

CERVIX

Its function is to provide an alkaline secretion favourable to sperm penetration, and once the uterus is gravid, to act as a sphincter. It is composed mainly of fibro-elastic tissue.

ISTHMUS UTERI

This name is sometimes given to the upper few millimetres of the cervical canal below the internal os, an area to which the specific function of developing into the lower segment has been ascribed. The epithelium is intermediate between corpus and cervix; but if it were not for the importance of the lower segment in the theory of the physiology of pregnancy, it is unlikely that anatomists would have provided either an identity or a name for the isthmus uteri.

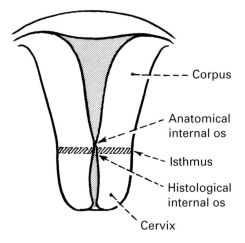

UTERUS

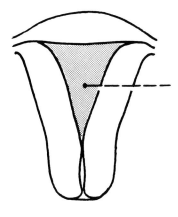

CAVITY OF THE CORPUS

The anterior and posterior walls are almost in contact, but in coronal plane the cavity is triangular.

The muscle wall at each cornu is pierced by the very narrow interstitial portion of the fallopian tube.

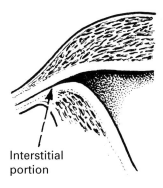

Interstitial portion

CERVIX

The external os is small before parturition and is sometimes called the os tincae (mouth of a small fish). After the birth of a child, it becomes a transverse slit – 'the parous os'.

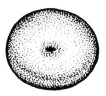

Nulliparous os

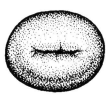

Parous os

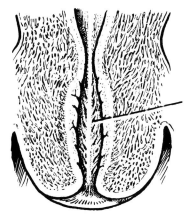

The cervical canal is fusiform and marked by curious folds called the 'arbor vitae'.

The cervix is divided into supra- and infravaginal portion by the attachments of the vagina.

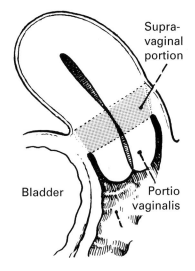

Supra-vaginal portion

Bladder

Portio vaginalis

UTERUS

RELATIONSHIP OF UTERUS AND URETER

The ureter is directly related to the uterine artery and the vaginal vault but is not in direct contact with the uterus.

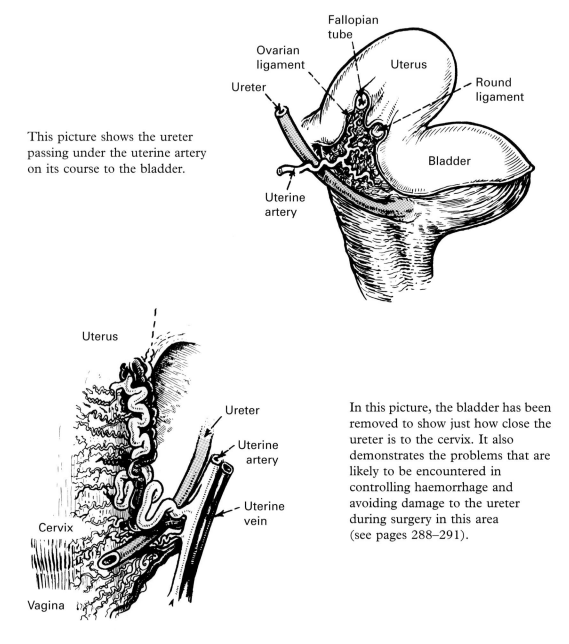

This picture shows the ureter passing under the uterine artery on its course to the bladder.

In this picture, the bladder has been removed to show just how close the ureter is to the cervix. It also demonstrates the problems that are likely to be encountered in controlling haemorrhage and avoiding damage to the ureter during surgery in this area (see pages 288–291).

UTERUS

LIGAMENTS OF THE UTERUS

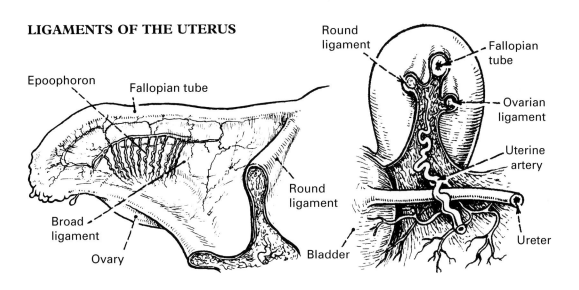

The *broad ligament* is a fold of peritoneum passing from the uterus to the side wall of the pelvis. It contains the fallopian tube, the round and ovarian ligaments, the mesonephric remnants, the ovario-uterine anastomosis and, in its base, the ureter.

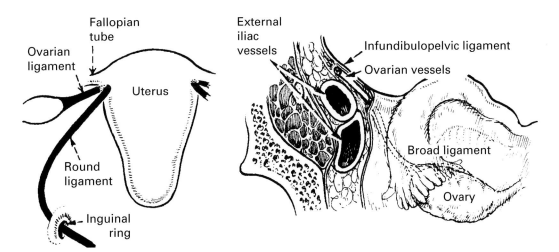

The ovarian and round ligaments are the vestigial gubernaculum. The round ligament ends in the inguinal canal and its fibres disperse in the labium majus.

The part of the broad ligament between the infundibulum and pelvic wall is called the infundibulopelvic ligament and contains the ovarian vessels and nerves. Note the proximity of external iliac vessels.

UTERUS

LIGAMENTS OF THE UTERUS—(cont'd)

The main supports of the uterus are the fibromuscular condensations of tissue in the pelvic fascia (page 21).

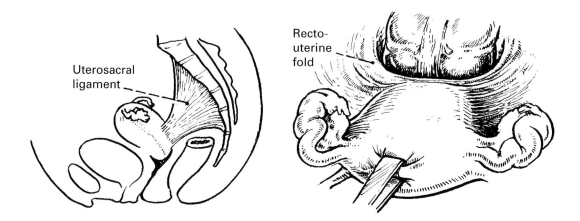

The *uterosacral ligaments* pass from the back of the uterus to the front of the sacrum and are easily identified by the covering recto-uterine fold of peritoneum. These ligaments maintain the anteverted position of the uterus, and they are accompanied by uterine vessels and nerves.

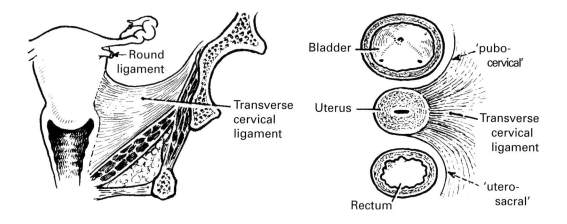

The *transverse cervical ligaments* (Mackenrodt's, cardinal ligaments) pass from the uterus and vagina to a wide insertion in the lateral pelvic wall. They lie below the broad ligament and contain vessels and nerves. The uterosacral ligament may be regarded as the posterior edge of the transverse cervical; its anterior edge is sometimes called the pubocervical, but this is not well defined.

UTERUS

HISTOLOGY

The uterus has an incomplete peritoneal coat, which is very adherent. The anterior bare area is to allow movement of the bladder. There is a complete fascial sheath continuous with the vagina, and the body is made of smooth muscle interspersed with fibro-elastic tissue. There is a reversion of the ratio of muscle to connective tissue as the cervix is approached, and the cervix is nearly all fibrous.

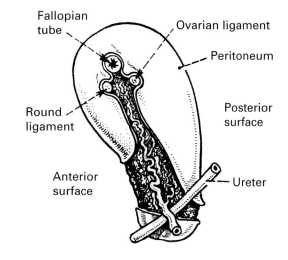

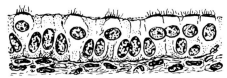

Endometrium (low power)

The epithelium of the cavity is called the endometrium and consists of a single layer of cuboid or columnar ciliated cells on a cellular stroma. The stroma is deeply pierced by invaginations of the epithelium called uterine glands, which secrete a small amount of mucus to maintain moistness.

For cyclical changes in the endometrium see pages 49–51.

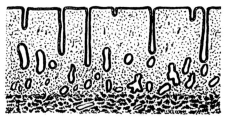

Uterine gland (high power)

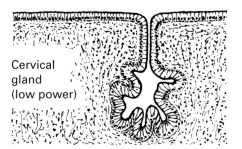

Cervical gland (low power)

The cervix is lined by a single layer of high columnar ciliated epithelium, which covers the folds of the arbor vitae (pp. 29–30) and lines the cervical glands. The glands secrete an alkaline mucus, which is favourable to the activity of spermatozoa.

FALLOPIAN TUBE

The tube extends from the cornu of the uterus into the peritoneal cavity and is about 10 cm long. The two tubes are twice the width of the pelvis, and they do more than just provide a passage for the ovum into the uterus. They must be sufficiently mobile to assist the ovum onwards by peristalsis; and sufficiently long to allow the ovum time for maturation after it has been fertilised in the ampulla and before it is ready for implantation in the uterus. The tube and ovary together are called the adnexa ('viscera adnexa' – organs next to) of the uterus.

Interstitial part

1 cm long and very narrow (less than 1 mm).

Isthmus

2 cm long, straight and cord-like. 1 mm diameter.

Ampulla

5 cm long, thin walled and convoluted.

Infundibulum

2 cm long. The terminal expansion, with fimbrial processes which help to attract the ovum.

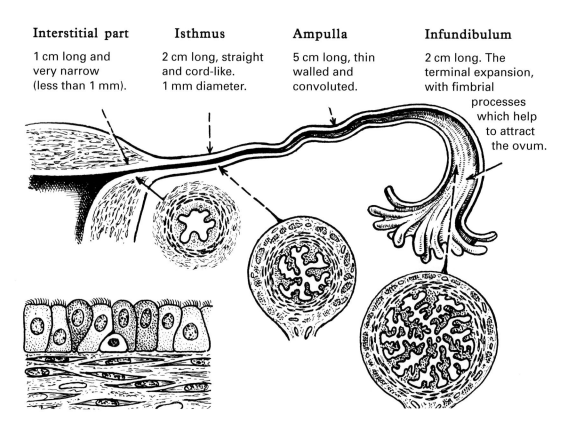

The tube has a lining of ciliated cells interspersed with non-ciliated secretory cells ('peg' cells). There is little or no submucosa. The epithelium is arranged in a complex pattern of plications, which becomes more marked as the outer end is approached.

BROAD LIGAMENT

BLOOD VESSELS

There is an anastomosis between the uterine and ovarian arteries, and the fallopian tube is supplied by vessels in an arcade pattern (cf. bowel).

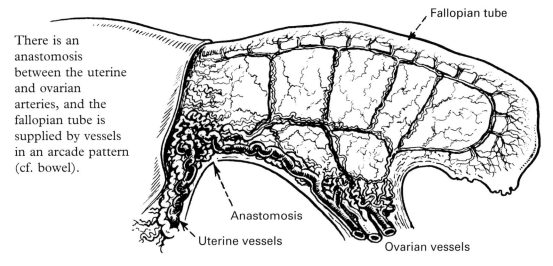

VESTIGIAL STRUCTURES

The epoöphoron and the paroöphoron are remnants of the mesonephros, and the duct (Gartner's duct) is the vestige of the mesonephric duct, which passes into the uterine muscle about the level of the internal os and continues downwards in the vaginal wall.

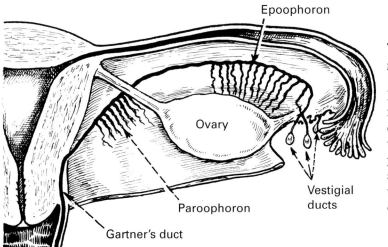

These structures may give rise to cysts (hydatids of Morgagni, Kobelt's tubules, fimbrial cysts) whose embryonic derivation is uncertain. They are probably mesonephric and can be grouped together as 'vestigial cysts'.

OVARY

The ovary is about 3 cm long and 1.5 cm
wide, roughly the size and shape of a date.
It has its own mesentery, the mesovarium
from the posterior leaf of the broad
ligament, and is attached to the cornu of
the uterus by the ovarian ligament, which
is continuous with the round ligament, the
vestigial gubernaculum.

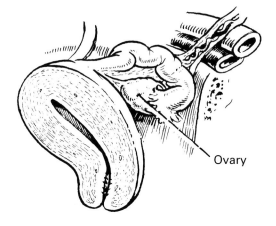

Ovary

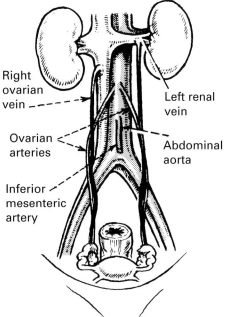

Right
ovarian
vein

Left renal
vein

Ovarian
arteries

Abdominal
aorta

Inferior
mesenteric
artery

The ovary is developmentally an abdominal
organ and its blood supply is from the
abdominal aorta. The ovarian vessels lie in
the infundibulopelvic ligaments.

Note: The left ovarian vein empties into the
left renal vein.

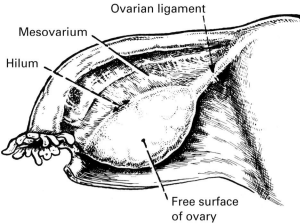

Ovarian ligament

Mesovarium

Hilum

Free surface
of ovary

The free surface of the ovary has no
peritoneal covering, only a surface
epithelium. The part attached to the
mesovarium through which all vessels
and nerves pass, is called the hilum.

OVARY

HISTOLOGY

Cross section shows the ovary to be roughly divided into a vascular medulla and a cortex.

The cortex is composed of a specialised ovarian stroma with a cuboidal surface epithelium which, like the tubal ostium, is intraperitoneal.

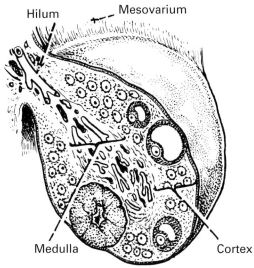

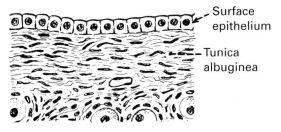

Note the condensed layer of stroma under the surface epithelium, called the tunica albuginea.

The hilum is characterised by the presence of paroöphoron tubules, which are of smooth muscle lined with ciliated epithelium; and by vestigial remnants of the sex cords called the rete ovarii, the analogue of the seminiferous tubules. These tissues are one reason for the extraordinary variety of ovarian tumours that can develop.

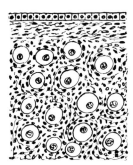

Cortex in an infant

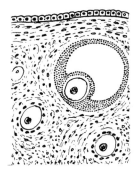

Cortex in an adult

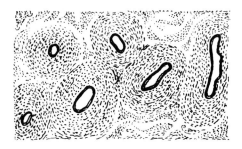

The hilum, showing cross section of paroophoron tubules.

OVARY

The **CORPUS LUTEUM** ('yellow body': the high lipid content required for steroid production gives the mature corpus luteum a yellow colour). During growth, the Graafian follicle gradually approaches the surface of the ovary and eventually extrudes the ovum through the stigma, into the waiting fimbriae of the tube. The follicle cells then quickly become luteinised by the retention of fluid to form the corpus luteum whose function is to secrete progesterone and prepare the endometrium for implantation of the fertilised ovum.

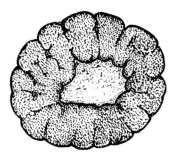

Corpus luteum (low power)

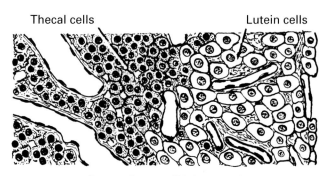

Thecal cells   Lutein cells

Corpus luteum (high power)

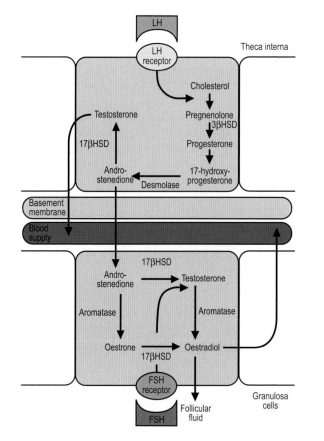

The growing corpus luteum is supplied with capillaries from the ovarian stromal vessels, and both theca and granulosa lutein cells secrete all the hormones. Under the influence of luteinising hormone (LH), theca cells metabolise cholesterol into androstenedione. The granulosa cells then metabolise the androstenedione produced by the theca cells into oestradiol under the control of follicle stimulating hormone (FSH). Thus, both cell types and both gonadotrophins are crucial to oestrogen synthesis.

OVARY

Corpus albicans

As the physiological cycle proceeds, degeneration gradually occurs, and eventually the corpus luteum is hyalinised – a corpus albicans – and is absorbed in about a year. Consequent scarring accounts for the irregular surface of the ovary in the more mature woman.

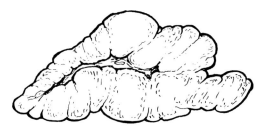

Follicular atresia

In utero, there are 7 million ovarian follicles. Atresia of the follicles commences *in utero*. At birth, the ovary contains a million follicles. There is continued loss of ovarian follicles with advancing age. Only about 400 can ever become mature follicles, but at each cycle and probably during childhood several follicles may start to develop and for a time produce hormones. This abortive attempt ends in atresia and the atretic follicle is absorbed; but the process may account for anovular cycles and for the oestrogens produced by young pre-pubertal girls whose breasts are beginning to develop. The rate of follicular loss appears constant until the age of 37 and thereafter the rate of loss accelerates until the menopause.

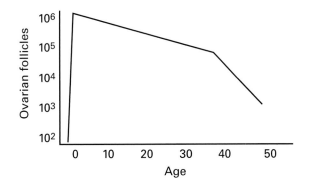

CHANGES IN THE GENITAL TRACT WITH AGE

Apart from normal growth, the appearances of the genital tract depend entirely on the supply of oestrogens.

THE VULVA

This is only a cleft in the perineum before puberty. Then the labia minora become more prominent and the fat of the mons and the labia majora is increased. Apart from the effects of coitus and parturition (p. 14) the most obvious sign of ageing is the gradual increase in size of the labia minora compared with the labia majora.

THE VAGINA

The rugae are absent before puberty and gradually (over several years) disappear after the menopause. In old women, the vagina is thin, atrophic and completely smooth.

THE OVARY

This is at its largest during the reproductive stage and shrinks thereafter. All the oocytes are gone by the time of the menopause, and the cortex consists of fibrous tissue.

THE UTERUS

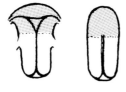

Infantile: the cervix is longer than the corpus, and there is no flexion.

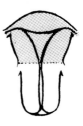

Pubertal: with the gradual increase in oestrogens, the corpus grows in relation to the cervix.

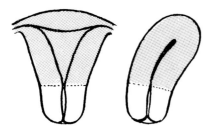

Adult: the corpus is now twice as long as the cervix and the normal degree of flexion has appeared.

After the menopause, the uterus gradually atrophies and in an old woman, the cavity may be less than 5 cm and the cervix simply an aperture in the senile vaginal vault.

BLOOD SUPPLY OF THE PELVIS

The common iliac artery bifurcates at the level of the sacrovertebral junction into external and internal iliac arteries. The internal iliac runs for about 4 cm and divides into an anterior and a posterior trunk, which are the main pelvic supply. The branches are subject to great variation.

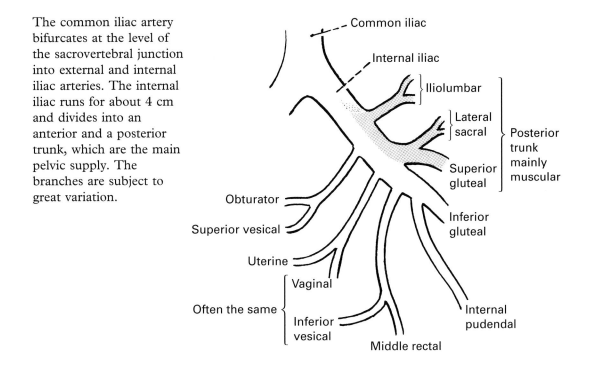

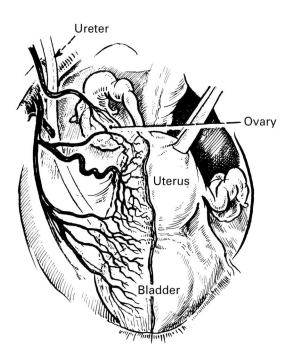

SUPPLY TO UTERUS, VAGINA AND BLADDER
This picture shows an arrangement often met with.

BLOOD SUPPLY OF THE PELVIS

The vessels of the uterus and vagina are much coiled to provide extra length during pregnancy. Note the nearness of the ureter.

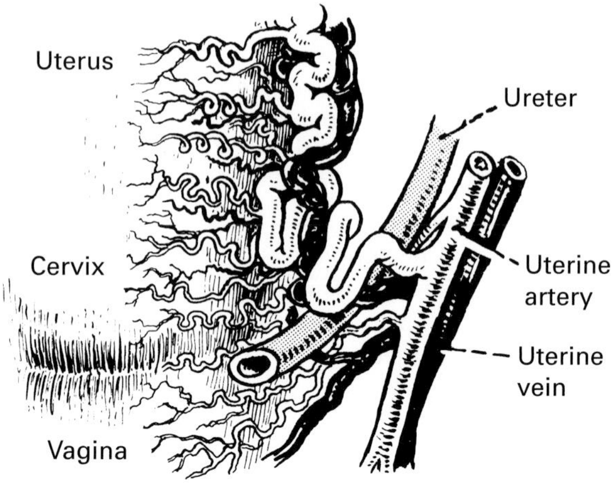

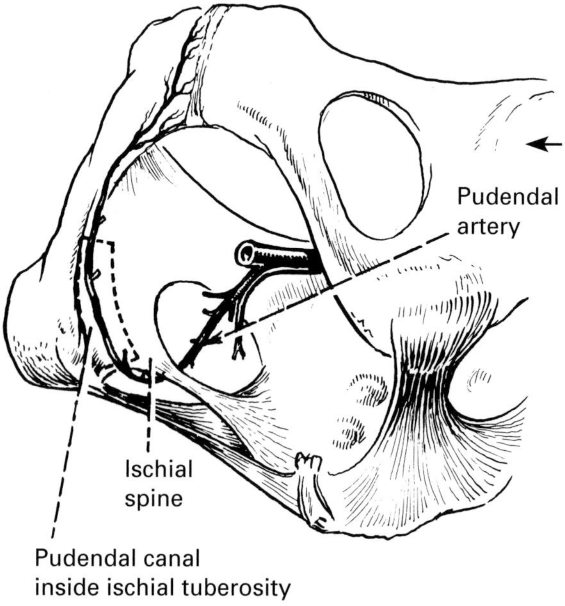

This picture shows the course of the pudendal artery passing behind the ischial spine and along the pudendal canal to the perineum.

In the ischiorectal fossa, the pudendal artery divides into inferior rectal and perineal branches.

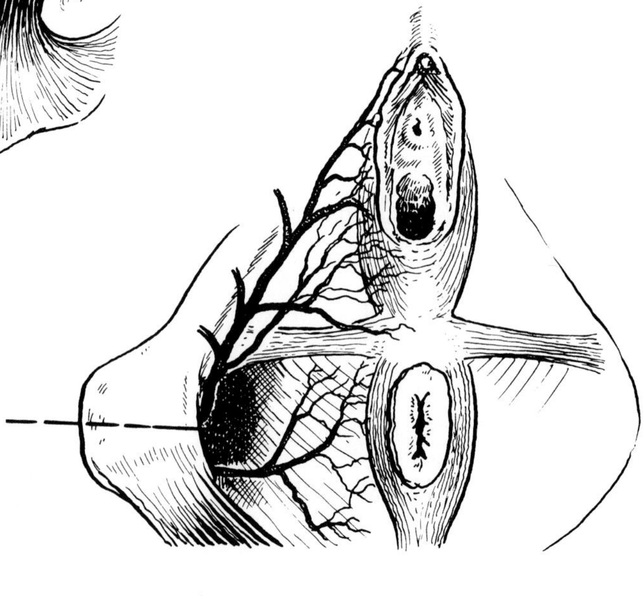

BLOOD SUPPLY OF THE PELVIS

COLLATERAL BLOOD SUPPLY

If the internal iliac artery has to be ligated, the collateral circulation should be adequate. It depends on anastomoses with the abdominal aorta, external iliac and femoral arteries.

ABDOMINAL AORTA

1. Ovarian artery → uterine artery.
2. Inferior mesenteric → superior rectal → inferior rectal (pudendal).
3. Median sacral → lateral sacral.

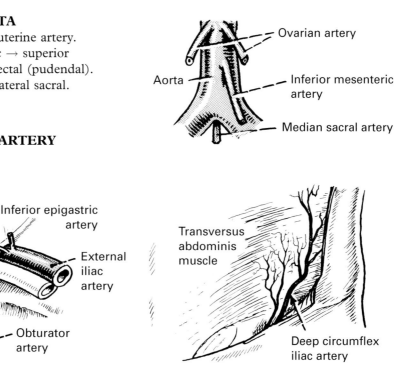

EXTERNAL ILIAC ARTERY

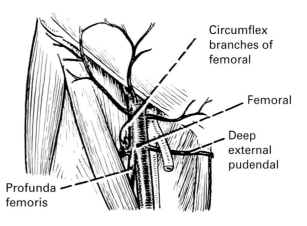

The inferior epigastric anastomoses with the obturator; the deep circumflex iliac with the iliolumbar and lumbar arteries.

THE FEMORAL ARTERY

The deep external pudendal anastomoses with the internal pudendal.

The superior and inferior gluteal arteries anastomose with the perforating and circumflex branches of the femoral and profunda femoris. (This is the 'cruciate' anastomosis.)

LYMPHATIC DRAINAGE OF THE GENITAL TRACT

The lymphatic plexuses accompany the blood vessels and drain into groups of glands, which are constant in position and are given names.

It will be seen that while the uterus is likely to drain into the external iliac group on the lateral wall of the pelvis, the vagina drains into the internal iliac group and the ovary drains directly into the aortic glands.

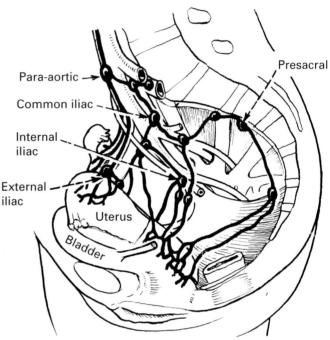

The superficial inguinal glands also receive lymph drainage from the vulva and the lower vagina. (But these structures may also drain via the pudendal vessel channels into the internal iliac group.)

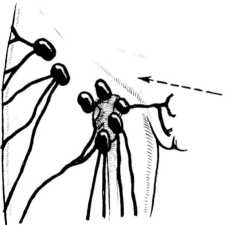

Because lymphatic plexuses and glands are a path of metastatic spread of cancer, treatment by either irradiation or surgery must involve an attack on the area of lymphatic drainage of the organs concerned. The lymphatic network is very widespread and the metastatic paths are not always the same; it is now recognised that the chance of cure is much reduced once the spread to the glands has occurred, whatever be the treatment given.

NERVES OF THE PELVIS

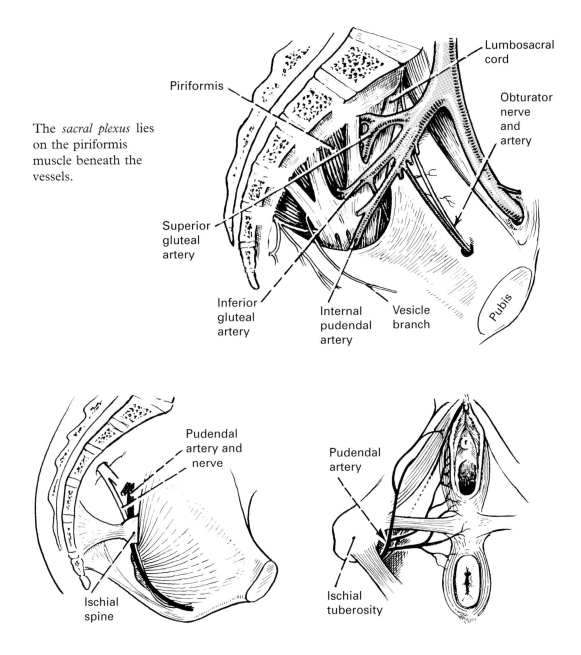

The *sacral plexus* lies on the piriformis muscle beneath the vessels.

Piriformis

Lumbosacral cord

Obturator nerve and artery

Superior gluteal artery

Inferior gluteal artery

Internal pudendal artery

Vesicle branch

Pubis

Pudendal artery and nerve

Ischial spine

Pudendal artery

Ischial tuberosity

The pudendal artery and nerve pass behind the ischial spine to gain the ischiorectal fossa.

The pudendal nerve crosses the ischiorectal fossa to supply the vulva and perineum.

AUTONOMIC NERVE SUPPLY OF THE PELVIS

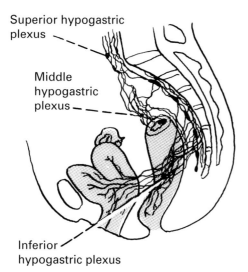

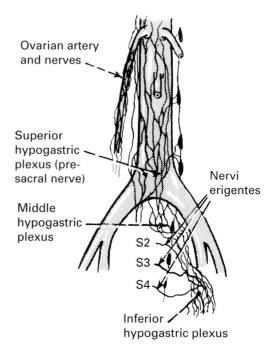

Sympathetic fibres enter via the lumbosacral chain and the mesenteric nerves. These are called the presacral nerves at the bifurcation of the aorta. They pass forward in the uterosacral ligaments to reach the viscera and are known there as the hypogastric plexus or plexus of Frankenhauser.

Parasympathetic nerves (nervi erigentes) join the hypogastric plexuses from sacral roots 2, 3 and 4.

There is an additional sympathetic supply by the nerves accompanying the ovarian vessels.

The function of the autonomic nerves is not understood. The cervix or vagina may be grasped by forceps in some patients with only minimal sensation, and a uterine sound or intrauterine contraceptive device in the uterine cavity may only cause a vague 'visceral' discomfort. However, there are cases where cervical stretch at a procedure or during passage of a clot causes vasovagal symptoms, and on occasion collapses.

CHAPTER 3

PHYSIOLOGY OF THE REPRODUCTIVE TRACT

Ovulation   46
   Female Reproductive Physiology   46
   Hypothalamus   49
   GnRH   50
   FSH   50
   LH   50
   Ovulation   50
Cyclical Ovarian Hormonal Changes   51
   Oestrogens   51
   Progesterone   51
   Endometrial Cycle   51
Action of Ovarian Hormones   52
   Oestrogen   52
   Progesterone   52
   Target Tissues   52
Effects of Ovarian Hormones   53
   Genital Tract   53
   Breast   53
   Hypothalamus   53
   Cardiovascular System   53
   Skeleton   53
   Psychological Characteristics   53
Puberty   54
The Menopause   55

OVULATION

FEMALE REPRODUCTIVE PHYSIOLOGY

During reproductive life, the cyclical development of ovarian follicles is the dominant process. The associated hormonal production has significant effects on the female genital tract, hypothalamus and pituitary.

In men, gamete production continues throughout life, whereas women develop their life supply of gametes during intrauterine life. See Chapter 1. The numbers decline even before birth, and there will be around 300,000 remaining at puberty.

The surface of the ovary is covered by a cuboidal 'germinal' epithelium. This layer is contiguous with the peritoneum. Underneath the epithelial layer is a thin layer of fibrous tissue, beneath which is the true cortex.

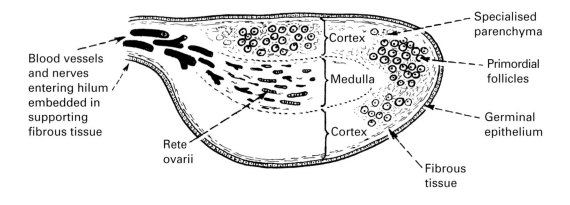

The cortex consists of a specialised stroma or parenchyma; the primordial follicles are embedded in this layer.

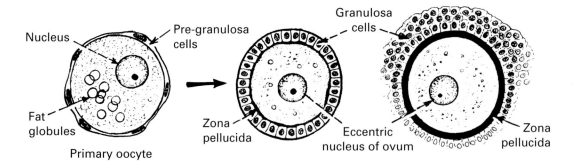

The primordial follicle consists of a primary oocyte surrounded by a single layer of flattened cells, the pre-granulosa, said to be derived from the cells of the sex cords.

The pre-granulosa cells become cuboidal and proliferate to form a shell several layers thick. At this stage, a hyaline membrane is formed immediately around the ovum – the zona pellucida.

OVULATION

The granulosa cells continue to proliferate until the follicle is approximately 200 μm in diameter. Fluid spaces now appear between the granulosa cells. They coalesce to form a cavity, the antrum, pushing the ovum to one side. The granulosa cells immediately surrounding the ovum are now known as the corona radiata, and the whole mass of cells in this situation is termed the cumulus oophorus.

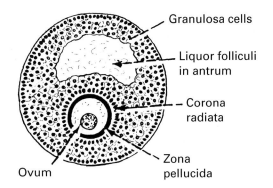

At the same time, the surrounding parenchymal cells arrange themselves concentrically around the follicle. The cells opposite the ovum become smaller and more epithelial in appearance. As the follicle increases in size, this epithelial change spreads to the parenchymal cells around the circumference of the follicle. This band of cells constitutes the theca interna. The cells are surrounded by sinusoidal capillaries, thus forming an endocrine gland-like structure. External to this band, the parenchymal cells are also arranged concentrically but retain their fusiform shape.

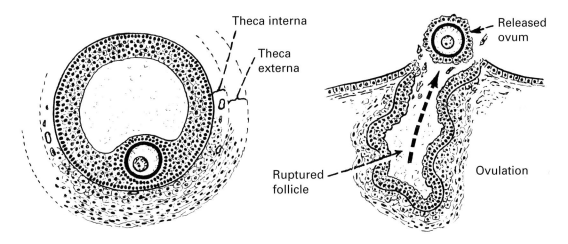

The follicle, which is called the Graafian follicle, continues to grow to a size of more than 1.0 cm. Approximately four to five follicles may attain this size and project on the surface of one ovary. One of these follicles ruptures on the surface, releasing the ovum surrounded by some of the granulosa cells. Ovulation is initiated by the gonadotrophin surge occurring in response to the long loop oestradiol positive feedback. Vascular changes occur in the follicle within minutes of the luteinising hormone (LH) surge, possibly due to release of histamine or other kinins. Proteolytic enzymes are released and collagen disintegrates. It is likely that insulin-like growth factors (IGFs) such as IGF-1 regulate granulosa differentiation. It is not known whether ovarian adrenergic nerve fibres or smooth muscle cells are involved. Prostaglandins may play a role.

OVULATION

From fetal life to the menopause, follicular growth is continuous. Oestrogen initiates the process. Three phases can be distinguished:

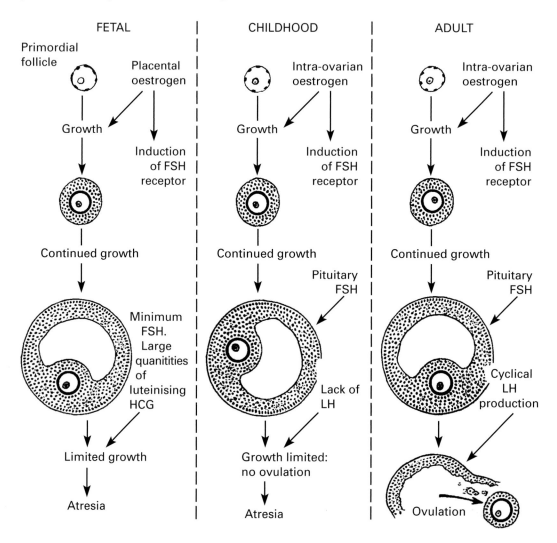

HCG = Human Chorionic Gonadotrophin.
FSH = Follicle Stimulating Hormone.
LH = Luteinising Hormone.

Normally only one follicle ovulates. Cohorts of follicles enter the growth phase in succession, and follicles of various sizes are usually found. The follicle destined to ovulate is among a cohort stimulated to grow by follicle stimulating hormone (FSH) secreted by the pituitary during the last few days of the cycle. Only about 400 of the original 2 million follicles will reach the ovulatory stage and there is continuous wastage of follicles from fetal life onwards.

OVULATION

Ovulation is the final event in a step-wise stimulatory mechanism starting in the hypothalamus, which contains gonadotrophin releasing cells. These produce a gonadotrophin releasing hormone (GnRH).

HYPOTHALAMUS

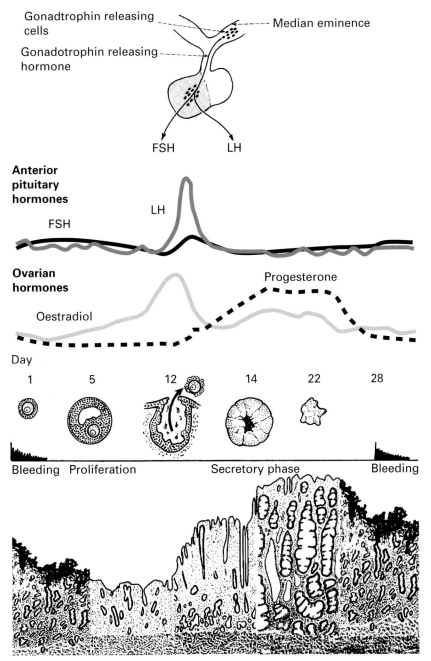

Endometrial cycle

OVULATION

GnRH

This substance begins to be secreted just before puberty in pulses every hour and continues in this fashion for the rest of life. There is only a single releasing hormone responsible for the production of both FSH and LH. The type of gonadotrophin secreted by the pituitary appears to be determined by other factors related to the phase of the menstrual cycle.

FSH

FSH stimulates follicular development and production of oestrogen. A peak of FSH is reached by the 6th day of the menstrual cycle. At this point, the rising oestrogen has a negative feedback effect, and the FSH curve languishes for a day or two; then, it resumes its upward trend to achieve a second peak at the time of ovulation on day 12.

Inhibin is produced by the corpus luteum and inhibits the production of FSH while it is active. As a result, follicular growth ceases. After the 22nd day, when the corpus luteum becomes inactive, FSH secretion and growth of follicles are resumed.

LH

Very low levels of LH are recorded in the early part of the cycle, but a sudden surge, coinciding with the second peak of FSH, induces ovulation and formation of the corpus luteum. Shortly thereafter, the level of LH returns to pre-ovulatory values.

OVULATION

FSH production is usually inhibited by rising oestradiol levels; however, a change occurs as the dominant follicle develops. Changes occur in the receptors on the follicular cells as the cycle progresses. Although the blood FSH is temporarily reduced after the 6th day, the larger follicles have accumulated sufficient FSH to maintain growth and oestrogen production. As the blood concentration of oestrogen continues to increase, it appears to reach a critical level at the 12th day, and in place of its usual negative feedback effect on the pituitary, it suddenly exerts a positive feedback effect with a consequent rise in FSH (the second peak) and secretion of LH.

Gonadotrophin Secretion (International Units per Litre)

	Menstruation		Follicular phase		Ovulation		Luteal phase	
	Mean	Range	Mean	Range	Mean	Range	Mean	Range
FSH	10	3–13	8	3–15	20	4–32	5	2–0
LH	8	3–12	8	6–14	65	43–88	8	2–13

CYCLICAL OVARIAN HORMONAL CHANGES

OESTROGENS
The plasma values of the three main oestrogens, oestradiol, oestrone and oestriol, are almost parallel throughout the cycle. The levels are low during menstruation and very gradually increase. Significant changes are noted around the 7th–8th day of the cycle, the levels rising to a maximum around the 12th day – ovulation peak. A fall occurs 24 h later, followed by a further increase a week later – the maximum phase of corpus luteum activity.

PROGESTERONE
Progesterone is almost absent from the plasma in the early stages of the menstrual cycle. At the time of ovulation, there is a steep rise, and a maximum value is achieved around the 20th–22nd day. Thereafter, a steep fall occurs.

ENDOMETRIAL CYCLE

Early Proliferative Phase
The endometrium shows proliferation of its stroma and glands, the latter elongating. The cells lining the glands are cuboidal, with definite limiting membranes, and the stromal cells are thin and spindly.

Late Proliferative Phase
The glands are very large and dilated – late proliferative phase. The blood vessels are also more prominent, and capillaries are dilated.

These proliferative changes are due to the influence of oestrogen secreted by the ovary at this time.

Secretory Phase
Following ovulation, the corpus luteum produces large quantities of progesterone, which induce secretory changes in the glands and swelling of the stromal cells. There is a rich blood supply, and the capillaries become sinusoidal.

Menstruation
Towards the end of the 28-day cycle, the stroma becomes even more vascular and oedematous, small haemorrhages and thrombi appear, and the endometrium ultimately breaks down due to withdrawal of the hormonal support. Vessel necrosis is preceded by intense vasospasm, possibly stimulated by prostaglandin F2-α.

The superficial layers of endometrium, together with blood and leucocytes, are shed and discharged – menstruation. Within a day or two, the raw surface is healed over by epithelium proliferating from the basal portions of glands.

ACTION OF OVARIAN HORMONES

OESTROGEN

Oestrogens have multiple effects including stimulation of growth and development of secondary sex features in the female.

PROGESTERONE

This hormone prepares the endometrium for implantation of the fertilised ovum and has no homologue in the male. In a clinical sense, it has an antioestrogen action.

TARGET TISSUES

Hypothalamus
Breasts
Genital tract
}

Tissues of these structures are particularly sensitive to oestrogen stimulation. The cytoplasm of their cells contains a specific oestrogen receptor molecule that has an affinity for oestrogen 100,000 times greater than the carrier protein, which retains the hormone in the bloodstream. Oestrogen also acts at the cell membrane, regulating ligand-gated ion channels.

Progesterone receptors appear in the cytoplasm only after the cell has been primed by oestrogen.

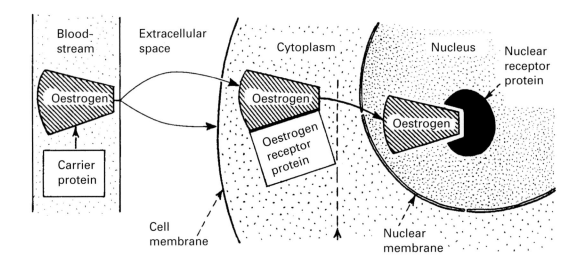

Transfer of the oestrogen molecule to the cell nucleus occurs more readily during the FSH phase of the cycle than during the LH phase, when progesterone levels are the highest. The number of oestrogen receptors is reduced after the menopause, but they never disappear.

The steroids, being lipids, are transported by quite separate lipophilic proteins, and the tissues stimulated by the steroids have their receptors in the cell cytoplasm, instead of on the cell surface as in the preceding steps of the ovulatory process.

EFFECTS OF OVARIAN HORMONES

GENITAL TRACT

Oestrogen stimulates growth and vascularisation, while progesterone increases endometrial gland secretion. In the cervix, secretion is considerably increased by oestrogen (to produce a favourable medium for spermatozoa), while progesterone reduces this. In the vagina, oestrogen causes cornification of cells and enlargement of nuclei, with increased deposits of glycogen.

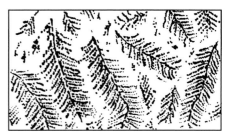

'Ferning' pattern in vaginal smear due to oestrogen stimulation.

BREAST

Oestrogen stimulates growth of the stroma, duct system and pigmentation, while cyclical progesterone stimulates growth of gland alveoli. Secondary sexual characteristics are controlled by oestrogen.

HYPOTHALAMUS

The hypothalamic–pituitary axis mediates the effects of ovarian hormones and controls the menstrual cycle through FSH and LH.

CARDIOVASCULAR SYSTEM

Oestrogen and progesterone have a number of different effects on the vascular tree, including effects on endothelial function, lipid profile and clotting factors.

SKELETON

Oestrogen is an antiresorptive agent that helps to retain calcium in the bones; at puberty, it causes the growth spurt and then the closure of long bone epiphyses.

PSYCHOLOGICAL CHARACTERISTICS

Mood may fluctuate with the menstrual cycle. Some women experience adverse psychological and physical symptoms premenstrually, termed premenstrual syndrome (PMS) or premenstrual tension (PMT).

PUBERTY

Puberty is the period of rapid growth when the child develops the physical characteristics of the adult. In addition to growth in stature, enlargement and changes in the function of reproductive organs occur. The mechanisms are poorly understood, but the main feature is an awakening of centres in the hypothalamus, with an increase in the pulsatile release of GnRH, leading to secretion of gonadotrophins. The reason for the absence of pulsatile GnRH secretion in infancy is not known.

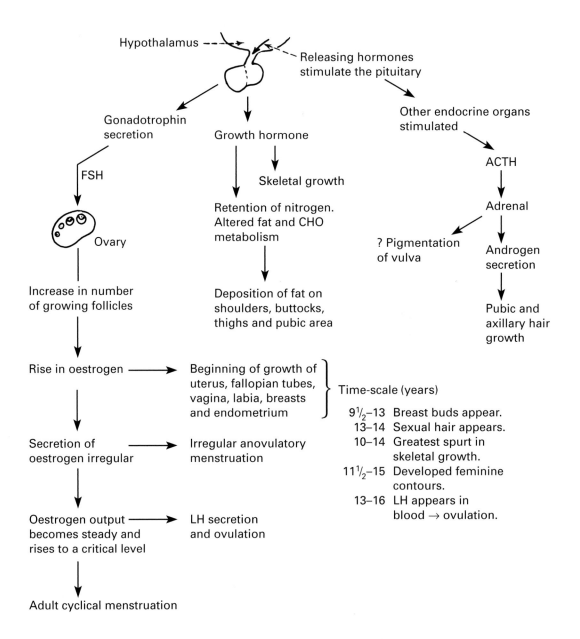

Hypothalamus

Releasing hormones stimulate the pituitary

Gonadotrophin secretion

Growth hormone

Other endocrine organs stimulated

ACTH

FSH

Skeletal growth

Ovary

Retention of nitrogen. Altered fat and CHO metabolism

Adrenal

? Pigmentation of vulva

Androgen secretion

Increase in number of growing follicles

Deposition of fat on shoulders, buttocks, thighs and pubic area

Pubic and axillary hair growth

Rise in oestrogen ⟶ Beginning of growth of uterus, fallopian tubes, vagina, labia, breasts and endometrium

Time-scale (years)

Secretion of oestrogen irregular ⟶ Irregular anovulatory menstruation

9½–13 Breast buds appear.
13–14 Sexual hair appears.
10–14 Greatest spurt in skeletal growth.
11½–15 Developed feminine contours.
13–16 LH appears in blood → ovulation.

Oestrogen output becomes steady and rises to a critical level ⟶ LH secretion and ovulation

Adult cyclical menstruation

THE MENOPAUSE

Menopause is the name given to the stage in life when the woman gradually loses her cyclical ovarian activity. In many ways, it is a reversal of the changes occurring at puberty. It usually takes place between the ages of 47 and 52 and is termed premature if it occurs before 45.

Menstruation rarely ceases abruptly but tends to become somewhat irregular and less frequent over a year or a little longer. The cessation does not appear to be due to a complete disappearance of ovarian follicles. Primordial follicles have been found in the ovaries of postmenopausal women. It would appear that there has to be a critical number of actively growing follicles before the menstrual cycle can operate.

For details of the pathophysiology and clinical features etc. of the menopause, see Chapter 18.

CHAPTER 4

DISORDERS OF SEX DEVELOPMENT

Maturation of Germ Cells: Meiosis	58
Genetic Abnormalities	59
Clinical Syndromes	*59*
Investigations of Genetic Defects	*59*
Laboratory Studies	*59*
Turner's Syndrome (Sex Chromosome Deletion: X)	*60*
Klinefelter's Syndrome (Sex Chromosome	
Acquisition: X)	*61*
Congenital Abnormalities	62
Complete Androgen Insensitivity (CAIS)	*62*
Congenital Adrenal Hyperplasia (CAH)	*63*
Abnormalities of Ovary and Tube	64
Abnormalities of the Ovary	*64*
Abnormalities of the Fallopian Tube	*64*
Abnormalities of the Uterus	65
Absent or Rudimentary Uterus	*65*
Double Uterus (Bicornuate Uterus)	*65*
Uterus Didelphys	*65*
Bicornuate Uterus or Uterus Bicornis	*65*
Uterus with Accessory Horn	*65*
Arcuate Uterus	*66*
Septated Uterus	*66*
Uterus Unicornis	*66*
Abnormalities of the Vagina	67
Abnormalities of the Vulva	68
Ectopia Vesicae	*68*
Congenital Abnormalities of Cloacal Origin	*68*
Genital Abnormalities	*68*

MATURATION OF GERM CELLS: MEIOSIS

Cells in the adult contain 46 chromosomes, two of which are sex chromosomes, XX in the female and XY in the male. These are known as diploid cells.

Before fertilisation of the ovum can occur, the chromosomes must be reduced from 46 to 23 in both ovum and sperm. Each gamete will contain one sex chromosome and is known as a haploid cell.

The process of meiosis begins with a rearrangement of the genetic material within the nuclei of the germ cells of both male and female. The reduction from diploid to haploid occurs during fetal life in the female, but in the male it is delayed until puberty.

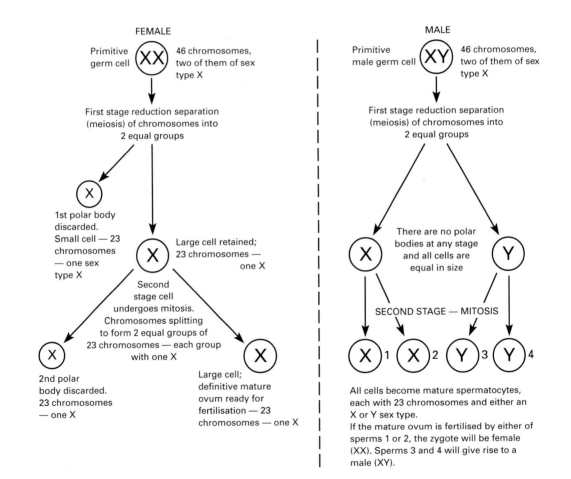

FEMALE

Primitive germ cell (XX) — 46 chromosomes, two of them of sex type X

First stage reduction separation (meiosis) of chromosomes into 2 equal groups

1st polar body discarded. Small cell — 23 chromosomes — one sex type X

Large cell retained; 23 chromosomes — one X

Second stage cell undergoes mitosis. Chromosomes splitting to form 2 equal groups of 23 chromosomes — each group with one X

2nd polar body discarded. 23 chromosomes — one X

Large cell; definitive mature ovum ready for fertilisation — 23 chromosomes — one X

MALE

Primitive male germ cell (XY) — 46 chromosomes, two of them of sex type X

First stage reduction separation (meiosis) of chromosomes into 2 equal groups

There are no polar bodies at any stage and all cells are equal in size

SECOND STAGE — MITOSIS

X 1 X 2 Y 3 Y 4

All cells become mature spermatocytes, each with 23 chromosomes and either an X or Y sex type.
If the mature ovum is fertilised by either of sperms 1 or 2, the zygote will be female (XX). Sperms 3 and 4 will give rise to a male (XY).

GENETIC ABNORMALITIES

CLINICAL SYNDROMES

The X chromosome favours development of female characteristics but full development is only possible if there are two such chromosomes. Any alteration in this number leads to abnormalities.

Development of the testis is entirely dependent on the presence of a Y chromosome. The testis, in addition to forming testosterone, which aids the development of male characteristics, produces a Müllerian inhibitory factor. Both male and female fetuses initially have both Müllerian and Wolffian systems.

In the absence of a testis, the whole Müllerian tract will develop, but curiously this does not depend on the presence of ovaries. These interrelationships result in a number of clinical syndromes with variations in individual cases.

INVESTIGATIONS OF GENETIC DEFECTS

In all cases, it is important to obtain a family history as complete as possible. Siblings and relatives of patients may give a history of amenorrhoea and infertility.

LABORATORY STUDIES

Chromosome Analysis

Cells are cultured, usually lymphocytes from a blood sample but other cells can also be used. The standard technique terminates the mitotic process at metaphase using a mitotic inhibitor such as colchicine. The resulting chromosomes are separated, counted, arranged in their groups and studied. Some chromosomal abnormalities are not visible with routine analysis. Fluorescence in-situ hybridisation (FISH) is a more rapid technique used to identify specific DNA sequences.

GENETIC ABNORMALITIES

TURNER'S SYNDROME (Sex Chromosome Deletion: X)

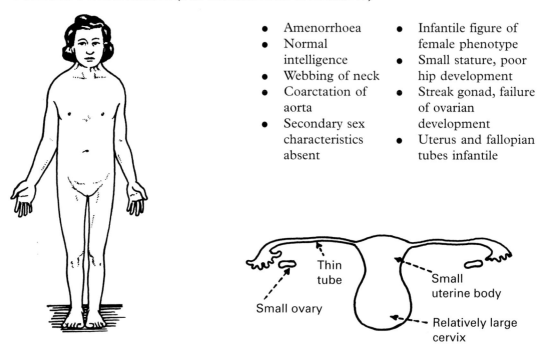

- Amenorrhoea
- Normal intelligence
- Webbing of neck
- Coarctation of aorta
- Secondary sex characteristics absent

- Infantile figure of female phenotype
- Small stature, poor hip development
- Streak gonad, failure of ovarian development
- Uterus and fallopian tubes infantile

Thin tube

Small ovary

Small uterine body

Relatively large cervix

The commonest chromosomal pattern is 45XO. Not all features of the condition are always present. In patients who are mildly affected, there may be a partial deletion of the X chromosome (Xx) or mosaicism (XO/XX). In such cases, normal ovaries can develop and menstruation can occur.

In males some of the somatic stigmata of Turner's may appear. This may be due to partial deletion of the Y chromosome – Xy, or to mosaicism – XO/XY.

Treatment
This diagnosis should be considered early in girls with short stature as hormone replacement therapy is required to encourage secondary sexual characteristics and skeletal development. For young women, the combined pill is often a socially acceptable maintenance therapy that results in a 'menstrual cycle'.

GENETIC ABNORMALITIES

KLINEFELTER'S SYNDROME (Sex Chromosome Acquisition: X)
There is a Y chromosome with an increase in the
number of X chromosomes. The commonest
abnormality is 47XXY. The phenotype is male. The
clinical features vary but the majority have
hypogonadism and infertility. Facial hair is scanty and
pubic hair has a female distribution. Gynaecomastia
can also be present. Mild developmental problems and
learning difficulties can occur but the vast majority of
individuals have normal intelligence. There is an
association between mental impairment and the
number of X chromosomes.

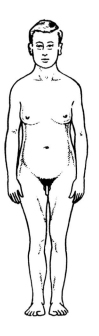

**SUPER-FEMALE (Sex Chromosome Acquisition: X, Sometimes at Both Stages
of Meiosis)**
This is a term sometimes used when the patient possesses extra X chromosomes but no Y
chromosome. The pattern may be XXX, XXXX or even XXXXX. Physically these
individuals are normal females, but the important point is that there is usually some mental
impairment and the degree of this increases with each extra X chromosome. Diagnosis is
made by chromosomal analysis.

CONGENITAL ABNORMALITIES

COMPLETE ANDROGEN INSENSITIVITY (CAIS)

This condition was previously known as testicular feminisation and may be mistaken for a sex chromosome abnormality. The chromosomal pattern is 46XY; however, there is insensitivity of the androgen receptor to respond to androgenic stimulation. As a Y chromosome is present, the testes form normally, producing anti-Müllerian hormone (AMH) and testosterone. AMH causes the regression of the Müllerian ducts (see Chapter 1), and the uterus, fallopian tubes and upper part of vagina therefore do not form. As the tissues are insensitive to androgens, the lower genital tract fails to virilise and a short vagina is formed. The patient is phenotypically female. Usually the diagnosis is made in early adult life when the patient complains of amenorrhoea.

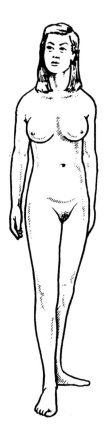

- Female phenotype.
- Normal or large breasts with small nipples.
- Absent or scanty pubic hair and axillary hair.
- Female external genitalia with blind vagina.
- Absent or rudimentary internal genitalia.
- Undescended testes anywhere along course of normal descent (20% become malignant in 4th decade).
- Testes secrete oestrogens and androgens. Probably Leydig cells produce feminising hormones.

Patients with CAIS usually inherit it from their mother in an X-linked pattern, but new mutations are also common.

Most carriers are unaffected, but some may show scanty pubic and axillary hair and have delayed menarche.

Until full growth is achieved, no therapy should be attempted. After puberty and fusion of epiphyses, the gonads should be removed surgically. This is a precautionary measure in view of the increased incidence of tumours in such gonads. Following this treatment, the patient is liable to have menopausal symptoms and should be given oestrogen replacement therapy for symptom control and for skeletal and cardiovascular prophylaxis until age 50 years at least. As the uterus is absent, progesterone is not required.

All of these foregoing syndromes, whether genetic or not, can pose social, psychological and sexual problems. The patient may have to make a great deal of mental adjustment and in such cases sensitive counselling will be required. Karyotyping and referral for genetic counselling should be considered.

Partial androgen insensitivity can also occur. A variety of clinical features occur, but ambiguous genitalia is a common presentation.

CONGENITAL ABNORMALITIES

CONGENITAL ADRENAL HYPERPLASIA (CAH)

This is an abnormality of cortisol production that can affect both male and female infants. The commonest enzyme deficiency is of 21-hydroxylase. The adrenals also produce mineralocorticoids and steroid hormones, and deficiencies of one pathway lead to excess production in other pathways. The severity of the enzyme deficiency can vary and will lead to different clinical conditions.

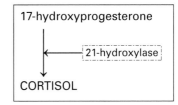

Adrenal dysfunction is due to congenital deficiency of the enzyme 21-hydroxylase. It should be detected and treated at birth.

- Deficiency of 21-hydroxylase leads to low cortisol secretion.
- Low cortisol leads to high ACTH secretion.
- High ACTH secretion leads to adrenal hypertrophy.
- As the pathway to cortisol is blocked, the alternative pathway to androgen formation is taken.
- The fetus and neonate show signs of virilisation.
- If aldosterone production is affected, the salt losing effects can be potentially life threatening if the condition is not detected promptly.

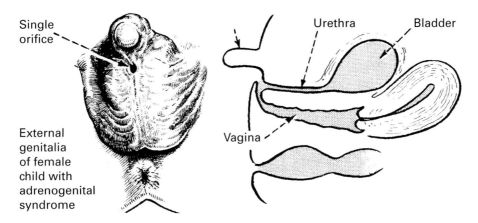

Single orifice

External genitalia of female child with adrenogenital syndrome

Urethra   Bladder

Vagina

Treatment

In female infants with virilised genitalia, chromosome analysis will reveal a 46 XX karyotype. Addisonian crisis may develop at any time and may be fatal. The diagnosis must be recognised as soon as possible and corticosteroid replacement therapy given immediately. This will reverse the changes in the endocrine organs, reducing the ACTH level and ultimately the adrenal hypertrophy. Further virilisation will be prevented but surgery may be required for female infants with virilised genitalia.

The abnormal genitalia should alert the attendant at the birth and help should be sought from a paediatrician. Milder forms of CAH can present later in childhood and adolescence with precocious puberty or oligoamenorrhoea.

CAH is an autosomal recessive condition and prenatal diagnosis is possible. Maternal treatment with corticosteroid can potentially reduce the intrauterine virilisation, although this remains experimental.

ABNORMALITIES OF OVARY AND TUBE

Congenital abnormalities arise from the following:-

- Incomplete development of the Müllerian ducts.
- Imperfect development of the gonad.
- Imperfect development of the cloacal region.
- Sex chromosome abnormalities.

Because of the close relationship between the genital and urinary tracts, renal tract imaging should always be carried out when a genital abnormality is found.

ABNORMALITIES OF THE OVARY

Absence of one ovary may occur in an otherwise normal woman. Before operating on one ovary, always look at the other.

With ovarian dysgenesis, the ovaries appear as 'streaks'. In place of the ovary there is a strip of whitish connective tissue continuous with the ovarian ligament. It may contain vestiges of a rete, and occasional cells which may be of germ cell type, but no follicles. These 'streak' ovaries are sometimes the seat of tumour growth, such as gonadoblastoma and dysgerminoma, and should always be removed.

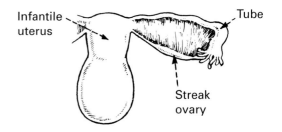

ABNORMALITIES OF THE FALLOPIAN TUBE

Absence is rare. The tube may be imperfectly developed.

This illustration shows a condition in which the proximal half of the left tube has failed to develop. The right adnexa are normal. All of these conditions are rare, but their importance lies in their association with infertility.

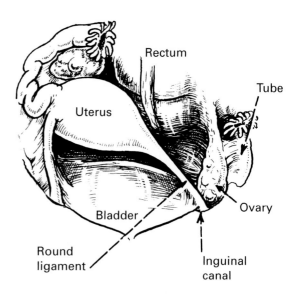

ABNORMALITIES OF THE UTERUS

ABSENT OR RUDIMENTARY UTERUS

The uterus consists of two nodules connected by a membrane ('ribbon' uterus). The other structures are normal. If a cavity exists in a nodule, cryptomenorrhoea (concealed bleeding) and dysmenorrhoea may arise and retrograde flow may lead to pelvic endometriosis.

This can be associated with atresia of the vagina (Mayer–Rokitansky syndrome).

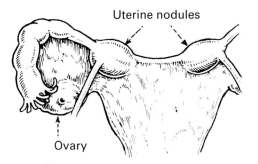

DOUBLE UTERUS (BICORNUATE UTERUS)

One or other variant of this condition is the commonest abnormality of the genital tract. It is due to failure of fusion of the Müllerian ducts, or failure of one to develop. There are a number of terms that describe the abnormality.

UTERUS DIDELPHYS

Double uterus and cervix, usually with double vagina.

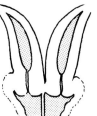

Two uterine corpora with two cervices. Both cervices need to be sampled at cervical screening. There are occasional reports of discrepancies with vaginal assessment during labour due to unrecognised double cervices.

BICORNUATE UTERUS OR UTERUS BICORNIS

Note the ligament, which may pass from rectum to bladder.
There is a cleft present at the fundus.

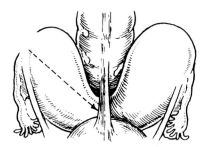

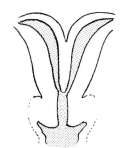

UTERUS WITH ACCESSORY HORN

The accessory horn has no cervix. If it menstruates, cryptomenorrhoea will follow. Spermatozoa can reach the horn by crossing the peritoneal cavity, and pregnancy can occur within a rudimentary horn.

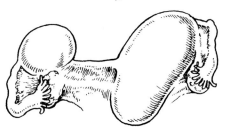

ABNORMALITIES OF THE UTERUS

ARCUATE UTERUS
The cavity has an indentation at the fundus.

This is probably the mildest form of uterine abnormality.

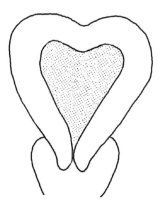

SEPTATED UTERUS
The uterus appears normal externally, but the cavity has a septum.

UTERUS UNICORNIS
One Müllerian duct has failed to develop.

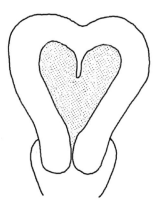

All of these abnormalities may be associated with obstetric implications. These include increased rates of infertility, miscarriage, preterm delivery and malpresentation. This, however, depends on the extent of the abnormality, and many women will have uncomplicated pregnancies.

ABNORMALITIES OF THE VAGINA

Gynatresia (occlusion of the genital canal) may be due to complete absence of the vagina, or incomplete development. When this is associated with absence of the uterus, it is known as Mayer–Rokitansky syndrome.

Septae can also occur. These are usually transverse septum producing the same effect as an imperforate hymen; sometimes, they may also be a vertical septum producing a double vagina. This often occurs in association with a double uterus.

When a transverse septum is identified, it may represent an imperforate hymen. This often presents with a thin bluish membrane because of a haematocolpos. If the tissue is thicker, it could represent a more extensive vaginal atresia. Where a uterus is present, dysmenorrhoea and cryptomenorrhoea will occur.

a. Absence of the whole genital tract except for the lower one third of the vagina. Coitus is possible but there is no possibility of pregnancy.

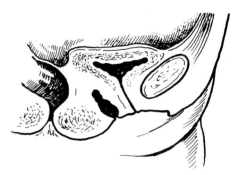

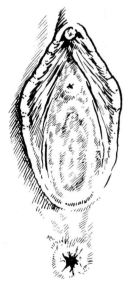

b. Complete absence of vagina. There is a slight depression over the hymen. Normal coitus is not possible.

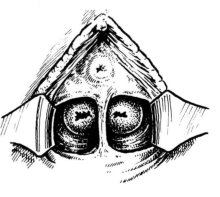

c. Vertical septum, double vagina and cervices.

Normal pregnancy and delivery are possible. Vaginal abnormalities can occur alone, but are usually associated with other abnormalities of the genital and renal tract. Imaging using ultrasound and/or MRI should be performed. Laparoscopic inspection of the pelvis may be required.

ABNORMALITIES OF THE VULVA

- Absence of the vulva or duplication of the vulva is exceedingly rare.
- There is a wide variation in the size of normal labia.

ECTOPIA VESICAE

Is an extreme defect seen in the newborn, but one which is susceptible to surgical treatment. There is failure of development of the symphysis pubis, mons, lower abdominal wall and anterior wall of the bladder. The tissues exposed are the posterior wall of the bladder, the ureteric orifices and the floor of the urethra.

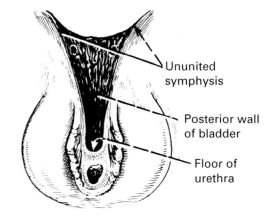

Ununited symphysis

Posterior wall of bladder

Floor of urethra

CONGENITAL ABNORMALITIES OF CLOACAL ORIGIN

These are due to failure of the cloacal septum to divide the cloaca perfectly into hindgut and urogenital sinus. The less serious degrees may persist unnoticed in adults as some form of ectopic anus.

Patients with these abnormalities can defecate through the vestibule or vagina, apparently without suffering from incontinence.

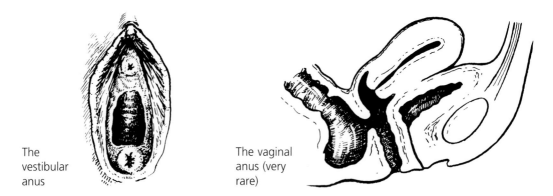

The vestibular anus

The vaginal anus (very rare)

In all of these vulval abnormalities, infection is a problem – of the urinary tract in ectopia vesicae, and of the genital tract in the other two.

GENITAL ABNORMALITIES

The results of these conditions as they relate to gynaecological practice have already been mentioned in the section dealing with amenorrhoea.

CHAPTER 5

HISTORY AND EXAMINATION

Taking the History	70
Parity and Obstetric History	*70*
Contraceptive and Fertility Requirements	*70*
Smear History	*71*
Menstrual History	*71*
Useful Definitions	*71*
Pelvic Pain	72
Other Gynaecological Symptons	74
Premenstrual Symptoms	*74*
Vaginal Discharge	*74*
Vaginal Prolapse	*74*
Urinary Symptoms	*74*
Gynaecological Examination	*74*
Abdominal Examination	75
Examination of the Vulva	78
Bimanual Pelvic Examination	79
Speculum Examination	80
Examination of the Breasts	82
Laparoscopy	83
Technique	*83*
Complications	*85*
Indications	*85*

TAKING THE HISTORY

The key to any consultation is taking an accurate and complete history. This is relevant in all medical disciplines and particularly in gynaecology. Do not assume that the referral letter contains all the relevant information. It is important to ask what the main problem is – it may be hidden away among a list of relatively unimportant or misleading complaints.

Women may find discussing gynaecological symptoms difficult and require

Privacy	Time	Sympathy
The consultation should be held in a room with adequate facilities and privacy. Permission should be sought for any students who are present	The patient should be allowed to tell her own story before any attempt is made to elicit specific symptoms	The doctor's manner must be one of interest and understanding

Gynaecological history follows the standard principles of medical history taking but there are a number of other issues that are relevant to gynaecology.

Standard history taking	Additional features relevant to gynaecology
Age Presenting complaint Past medical history Medication history Allergies Social history Family history Systemic enquiry	Parity Obstetric history Contraception and fertility requirements Smear history Menstrual history – this will often be part of the presenting complaint

PARITY AND OBSTETRIC HISTORY

The first number refers to the number of pregnancies beyond 24 weeks. This cut off largely relates to the gestation of potential viability although any liveborn infant before 24 weeks would also be counted among this number. The second number refers to pregnancies of less than 24 weeks. In practical terms, the easiest way to ask about this is to ask if the woman has any children and then ask if she has had any other pregnancies. Pregnancies in this category are likely to be miscarriages, terminations or ectopic pregnancies. It is important to be sensitive about the terminology when discussing pregnancy loss. The term 'abortion' is out dated and should not be used when discussing miscarriage.

Details of the mode of delivery of any children are always important in gynaecology, but other factors such as perineal trauma and postnatal infection are also relevant.

CONTRACEPTIVE AND FERTILITY REQUIREMENTS

This information will be relevant to many gynaecological issues as potential treatments may affect fertility, and many contraceptive treatments will have a useful effect; for example, the combined oral contraceptive pill and menstrual loss and dysmenorrhoea. Infertility may also be the presenting complaint.

TAKING THE HISTORY

SMEAR HISTORY

Women should be asked when their last cervical smear was performed and if the result was normal. Any abnormal smears and colposcopy history should be noted. Within the UK, routine smears are generally performed by primary care, but cervical cytology may be required for symptomatic women.

MENSTRUAL HISTORY

At the very minimum, the last menstrual period (LMP) should be recorded. For premenopausal women, the length of a menstrual period and frequency of period should be recorded. This is conveniently expressed as a numerical fraction. Thus, 5/28 means the cycle lasts for 5 days and occurs every 28 days. Make sure that you obtain the number of days from the start of one period to the start of the next. Irregular cycle may produce fractions such as 5–10/21–35.

USEFUL DEFINITIONS

Menarche – first menstrual period.

Menopause – date of final menstrual period. This can only be defined with certainty after a year has elapsed since the final menstrual period. It is also useful to ask about menopausal symptoms and hormone replacement therapy (HRT) use. The classic menopausal symptom is vasomotor flushes, but a myriad of other symptoms can also be experienced (see Chapter 18 The Menopause).

Perimenopause – the years of transition where irregular cycles occur. For most women, this lasts for 4 years before the final menstrual period occurs.

Menorrhagia – heavy periods. This is one of the commonest reasons that women are referred to gynaecology. You should ask for how long and how often bleeding occurs. The passage of clots and flooding through sanitary protection are signs that the menstrual flow is excessive. It can also be useful to ask about frequency of changing sanitary protection and whether 'double' protection is required, that is, having to wear a sanitary towel and tampon at the same time.

Abnormal Bleeding

Postcoital bleeding – bleeding occurring after intercourse.
Intermenstrual bleeding – bleeding between periods.
Postmenopausal bleeding – bleeding more than one year since LMP.

Irregular Bleeding

Primary amenorrhoea – failure to menstruate by age 16.
Secondary amenorrhoea – no menstruation for 6 months after periods are established.
Oligoamenorrhoea – infrequent, erratic periods.

Remember that anovulatory cycles occur at the extremes of menstrual life. It is therefore physiological to have erratic infrequent periods in the first few years after menarche and in the perimenopause.

PELVIC PAIN

This may or may not be related to the menstrual cycle. Premenstrual pain may represent endometriosis. *Dysmenorrhoea* refers to painful menses, usually of a crampy nature. This is usually central low abdominal cramp but can be referred to the thighs and lower back.

Primary dysmenorrhoea – periods have been painful since established menstruation has occurred.

Secondary dysmenorrhoea – periods have become painful. This is thought to be more likely to be associated with pelvic pathology.

Mittelshmertz – mid-cycle pain related to ovulation.

There are a number of other organ systems that can be responsible for pelvic pain. The most likely sources within the pelvis are the gastrointestinal and urinary tracts. It is important to ask about these systems when assessing for a source of pain. For example, acute right iliac fossa pain could represent an ovarian cyst accident or appendicitis among other diagnoses. Classically, appendicitis will also present with anorexia.

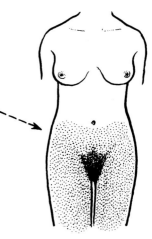

Areas of referred pain during menstruation

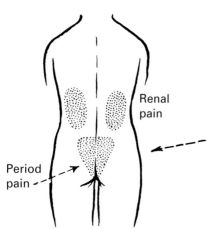

Renal pain

Period pain

The nature and pattern of pain will also be useful. Bladder pain is central and low, but renal pain will radiate to the loins.

PELVIC PAIN

The severity of pain can be judged to some extent by the patient's behaviour. Pain that causes a woman to take time off work or wakes her from sleep is likely to be caused by an underlying pathology. Pain that causes nausea and vomiting is important. Associated symptoms such as fainting, shoulder tip or pain with defecation imply potential intra-abdominal blood loss, and ectopic pregnancy should be strongly considered.

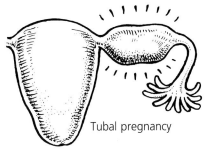
Tubal pregnancy

Dyspareunia – Pain or exacerbation of underlying pain during sexual intercourse is an important symptom. *Deep dyspareunia* implies pathology of the upper genital tract. Patient will describe the pain as 'deep inside' during intercourse. Superficial dyspareunia is more likely to represent a vaginal cause. Superficial causes of dyspareunia include causes such as local infections, that is, Candida or scarring from episiotomy or vaginal tears during childbirth. *Vaginismus* is also a common cause of dyspareunia, where the vaginal muscles tense during attempted penetration. It can affect tampon insertion and smear taking and can usually be demonstrated with vaginal examination. It may be present in women with entirely healthy vaginal tissues, but understandably women who experience dyspareunia for any reason can tense up because of anticipation of pain so the presence of vaginismus does not exclude pelvic pathology. A careful one finger vaginal examination to identify if there are any specific areas of tenderness can be useful if the patient will not tolerate a speculum or two-finger bimanual.

OTHER GYNAECOLGICAL SYMPTOMS

PREMENSTRUAL SYMPTOMS

Many women experience premenstrual mood disturbance. A range of other physical symptoms occur, including breast tenderness, bloating and headaches. Ideally, women should keep a diary of these symptoms to explore the relationship to their menstrual cycle.

VAGINAL DISCHARGE

Women who complain of a vaginal discharge should be asked about the colour, odour and any associated vaginal irritation or systemic upset. It can also be useful to determine any relationship to the menstrual cycle as the discharge may be physiological in nature.

VAGINAL PROLAPSE

Women with prolapse present with a sensation of something coming down within the vagina. They may also experience backache and a dragging sensation.

URINARY SYMPTOMS

Women are frequently referred to gynaecology with the complaint of urinary incontinence. This may or may not be associated with vaginal prolapse. Other urinary symptoms should be considered.

Urinary incontinence can be 'stress' incontinence, where the woman leaks when she coughs or exercises or it can be urge incontinence where the woman complains of a sudden sensation of urinary urgency and is incontinent before she makes it to the toilet. The latter symptom is often associated with urinary frequency and nocturia. In practice, many women complain of a mixed pattern of symptoms.

GYNAECOLOGICAL EXAMINATION

General Principles

The majority of women have varying degrees of anxiety about vaginal examination. Examination is usually more informative in a relaxed patient and a number of simple measures can be used to make the patient feel at ease.

Women should be given an appropriate area to change in privacy. A sheet should be provided to allow the woman to cover herself. A chaperone should be present for any intimate examination. This should apply for both male and female practitioners. The chaperone provides two purposes, firstly as a source of support and distraction for the patient but also to provide evidence that no improper behaviour has taken place. Formal consent should be given for any intimate examination by a student including under anaesthesia.

An explanation of the purpose of the examination should be given to the woman and permission sought to perform the examination. Simple terms should be used to explain the likely sensations experienced. The examination should be thorough but gentle. The patient should feel confident that you will stop the examination if she wishes.

ABDOMINAL EXAMINATION

This must never be omitted, whatever be the patient's complaint. Many gynaecological tumours form large swellings, which leave the pelvis altogether, and an undisclosed pregnancy may be present. Always examine the upper abdomen. Be certain that the bladder is empty. Ask the patient to tell you if you are hurting her.

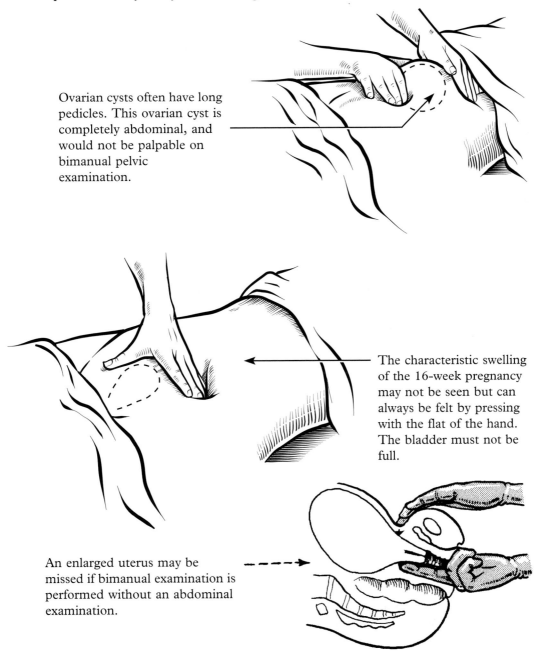

Ovarian cysts often have long pedicles. This ovarian cyst is completely abdominal, and would not be palpable on bimanual pelvic examination.

The characteristic swelling of the 16-week pregnancy may not be seen but can always be felt by pressing with the flat of the hand. The bladder must not be full.

An enlarged uterus may be missed if bimanual examination is performed without an abdominal examination.

ABDOMINAL EXAMINATION

All the classical techniques of inspection, palpation, percussion and auscultation are advised, but the most important is gentle palpation with the flat of the hand to detect solid or semi-solid tumours.

The examiner must bear in mind the various intra-abdominal structures which may give rise to swellings.

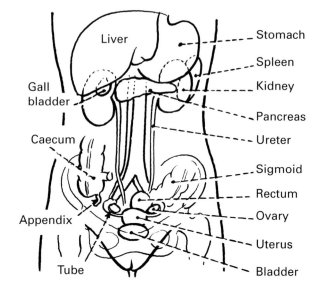

Liver — Stomach
— Spleen
Gall bladder — Kidney
— Pancreas
Caecum — Ureter
— Sigmoid
— Rectum
Appendix — Ovary
— Uterus
Tube — Bladder

The hypochondria should be examined to exclude liver and spleen enlargement or gallbladder tenderness, before palpating the lower abdomen.

An attempt to palpate the kidneys should be made. Tenderness may be elicited in the loin, suggesting urinary tract infection.

ABDOMINAL EXAMINATION

Inspection may show the characteristic shape of a large ovarian cyst. The outline is rounded and uniform, the skin is stretched and a fluid thrill may be elicited.

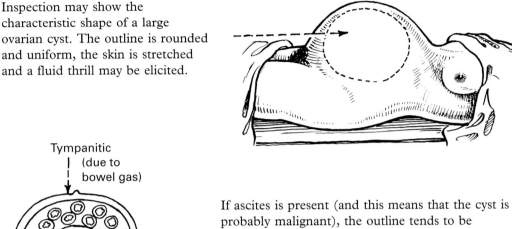

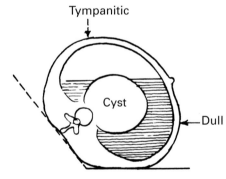

If ascites is present (and this means that the cyst is probably malignant), the outline tends to be cylindrical, with some flattening at the top. The umbilicus is everted, and the percussion note is dull in the flanks but tympanitic above because of the upward floating of the intestines.

If the patient is turned on her side, and the percussion is repeated after about 30 s, the dull and tympanitic areas are reversed – 'shifting dullness'.

Unfortunately, obesity is an increasing problem, and abdominal examination can be particularly challenging. With an 'abdominal apron' of fat, the symphysis pubis may be mistaken for a hard lower abdominal mass on palpation. Investigation techniques can also be technically difficult. Abdominal ultrasound is significantly limited by abdominal fat, but transvaginal scanning will be useful.

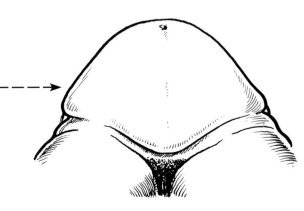

EXAMINATION OF THE VULVA

The dorsal position is most convenient for patient and doctor although examination in a lateral position is useful to assess vaginal prolapse. During palpation, visual inspection of the labia, clitoris, anus and surrounding skin should be performed. Raised or ulcerated areas should raise the question of vulval malignancy. There are specific skin conditions that affect the vulva, including lichen sclerosus, which often presents with itchy white patches and labial fusion. Common benign lesions include sebaceous cysts. Excoriation suggests an underlying irritation.

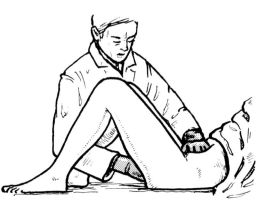

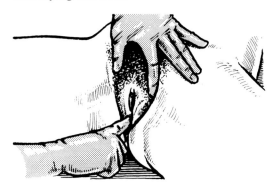

1. A single finger presses on the perineum, avoiding the sensitive vestibule, and accustoming the patient to the examiner's touch.

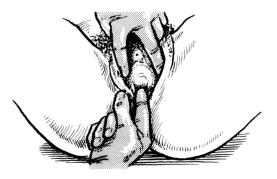

2. Urethral meatus and vestibule are exposed. Pressure from the finger will squeeze any pus from the peri-urethral glands.

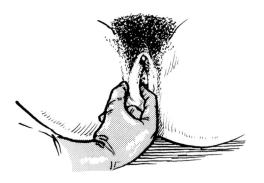

3. Bartholin's gland is palpated (on both sides). It is difficult to feel the normal gland.

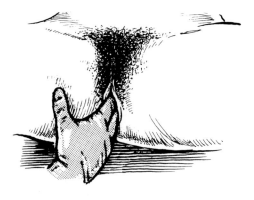

4. If there is room, a second finger is inserted and the perineal floor is palpated by stretching.

BIMANUAL PELVIC EXAMINATION

This technique needs practice. The external hand is the more important and supplies more information. It is customary to use two fingers in the vagina, but an adequate outpatient examination may be made with only one finger. Very little information is gained if the patient finds the examination painful. In a virgin or a child, vaginal examination should not be performed, unless there are exceptional circumstances, and examination under anaesthesia should be considered.

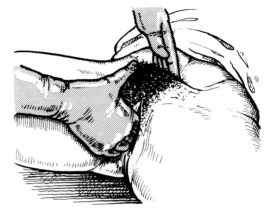

Pelvic models are available, with interchangeable uterine and adnexal components to simulate normal and pathological conditions, for practice examination.

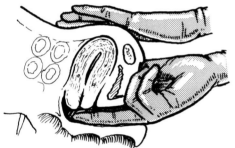

1. The vagina and cervix are palpated and any hardness or irregularity noted.

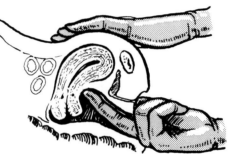

2. The whole uterus is identified, and size, shape, position, mobility and tenderness are noted.

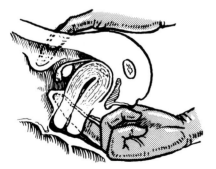

3. The lateral pelvis is palpated and any swelling noted. Normal adnexa are difficult to feel, unless the ovary contains a corpus luteum.

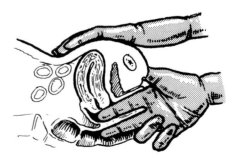

4. Sometimes rectovaginal examination is helpful, particularly if the rectovaginal septum is to be examined, for example, in assessment of extent of malignant disease.

SPECULUM EXAMINATION

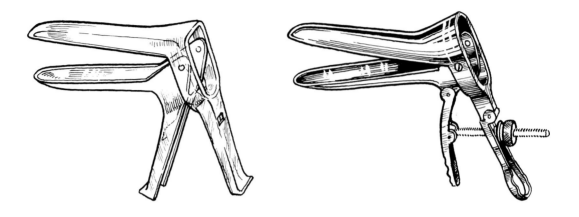

The bi-valve speculum is the most useful (Cusco's pattern is shown here). It is made of either steel or Perspex (disposable) and is designed to open after insertion so that the cervix and vagina can be visualised. Versions with a screw or ratchet are available to hold the device open so that cytological smear or bacteriological swab can be taken as required.

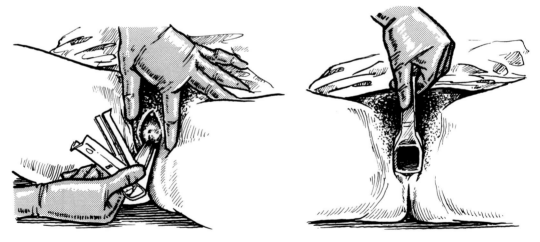

1. The speculum is applied to the vulva at an angle of 45° from the vertical. This allows the easiest insertion.

2. When fully inserted, it is gently opened out and held in position with the cervix between the blades. A good light is needed for inspection. Care is required when removing the speculum to ensure that the blades have not caught the cervix or vagina and that the blades have not been held open by the ratchet or screw.

SPECULUM EXAMINATION

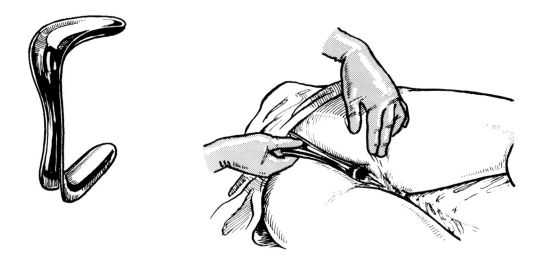

SIMS' SPECULUM (the duckbill speculum) is designed to hold back the posterior vaginal wall so that air enters the vagina because of negative intra-abdominal pressure, and the anterior wall and cervix are exposed.

In this picture, the patient is in Sims' position (semi-prone) which is useful if the anterior wall is to be studied (e.g. if fistula is suspected).

EXAMINATION OF THE BREASTS

A gynaecological examination provides a suitable opportunity for examining the breasts. Signs of pregnancy or lactation may be observed or a lump may be palpated. The breast is a much commoner site of cancer than the genital tract.

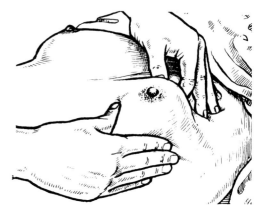

The examination should be made with the patient seated and also lying on her back. The breast is gently but thoroughly palpated with the fingers, and the axilla is also palpated.

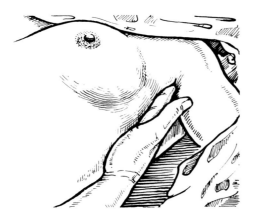

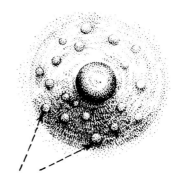

Montgomery's tubercles, seen in early pregnancy.

Routine X-ray mammography is offered by the NHS every 3 years between 50 and 65 years of age. In women with a first degree relative diagnosed with breast cancer before 50 years, mammography may be appropriate and referral to a breast cancer family history clinic is ideal.

LAPAROSCOPY

Inspection of the pelvic organs through an endoscope passed through the abdominal wall. This is a common procedure, frequently performed in day surgery units, but it does carry a small risk of visceral injury which must be taken into account.

TECHNIQUE

The patient is anaesthetised, the bladder emptied and a bimanual examination should be performed to assess for pelvic masses and to assess the direction of the uterus. A forceps is fixed to the anterior lip of the cervix and the uterus is cannulated. This allows the uterus to be moved about once the endoscope is passed, and dye can be injected through the cannula to test the patency of the tubes.

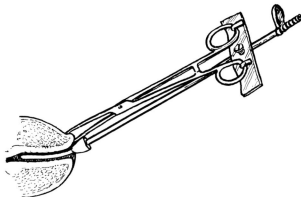

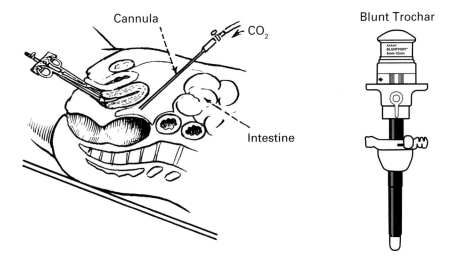

Laparoscopy can be performed by various techniques. A cut down technique can be used to open the rectus sheath and underlying peritoneum just below the umbilicus. A blunt trocar is then inserted, and the abdominal cavity is filled with CO_2 gas to allow visualisation of pelvic organs. The patient is tilted head down to encourage the intestines to fall away from the pelvis. Alternatively, a Veress needle can be used to fill the abdominal cavity, and a sharp trocar is inserted through the rectus sheath. There are also devices that allow insertion of a trocar with direct visualisation.

LAPAROSCOPY

Many instruments for laparoscopy are now disposable and incorporate retractable safety features to help avoid perforation of viscera. Any secondary ports should be inserted under direct vision, and care taken to avoid vessels within the anterior abdominal wall, for example, inferior epigastric artery.

The laparoscope is passed through the initial port and the inspection made of the abdomen and pelvis. The uterus should be manipulated to allow visualisation of the adnexa and Pouch of Douglas. A camera attached to the eyepiece of the laparoscope permits assistants and observers to share the surgeon's view on a video screen and permits video recording of the findings or procedure.

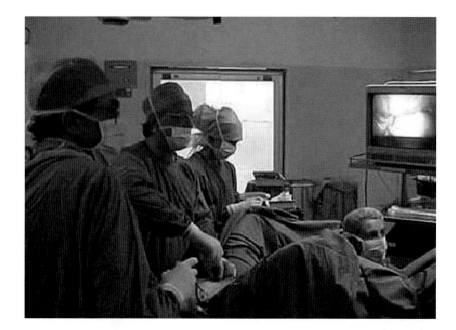

Additional ports are needed to insert surgical instruments. For diagnostic laparoscopy, this is usually simply a manipulation of the tissues to allow adequate inspection. For operative laparoscopy, a range of standard surgical instruments, such as forceps, scissors and suture holders, are available. There are also a number of instruments designed to apply diathermy and other modalities. Many procedures are now performed entirely by laparoscopy or assisted by laparoscopy.

LAPAROSCOPY

COMPLICATIONS

1. Perforation of a viscus, especially bowel. Patients who are overweight or have had previous abdominal surgery are more at risk of this complication. There is no primary entry technique that will remove the risk of perforation; however, adequate pressures of CO_2 should be used for secondary port entry to raise the abdominal wall away from visceral structures. Good laparoscopic technique keeps any operating instruments in clear view away from viscera.

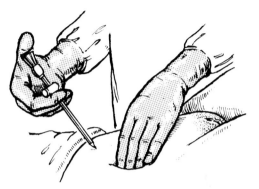

2. Haemorrhage from damage to vessels, or from a trocar puncture.
3. Infection is very rare and nearly always the result of unnoticed bowel damage. Complications are more frequent with operative laparoscopy than with diagnostic laparoscopy.

INDICATIONS

1. Diagnostic. Such conditions as salpingitis, early tubal pregnancy and ovarian pathology can be identified or excluded. Laparoscopy is useful in the investigation of complaints of pelvic pain.
2. Infertility investigation. Besides inspection, the patency of fallopian tubes can be demonstrated by observing the passage of dye injected through the cervix (hydrotubation).
3. Sterilisation. See page 353–355.
4. Other applications of laparoscopy include the following:
   Division of adhesions
   Oophorectomy
   Ovarian cystectomy
   Salpingectomy and salpingostomy
   Laparoscopic hysterectomy
   Colposuspension
   Vaginal vault suspension for vault prolapse.

CHAPTER 6

ABNORMALITIES OF MENSTRUATION

Normal and Physiological Changes
in the Menstrual Cycle 88
Amenorrhoea *88*
Menarche *88*
Physiological Amenorrhoea 89
Pregnancy *89*
Lactation *89*
Menopause *89*
Causes of Amenorrhoea *89*
Uterine and Lower Genital Tract
Disorders 90
Imperforate Hymen or Transverse
Vaginal Septum *90*
Asherman's Syndrome *91*
Müllerian Agenesis *91*
Congenital Androgen
Insensitivity *91*
Ovarian Disorders 92
Gonadal Dysgenesis *92*
Premature Ovarian Failure *93*
Resistant Ovary Syndrome *93*
Polycystic Ovarian Syndrome *94*
Pituitary Disorders 97
Hyperprolactinaemia *97*
Hypothalamic Disorders 101
Diagnosis *101*
Causes *101*
Investigation of Amenorrhoea 102
Investigation *102*
Hirsutism 105
Aetiology *105*
Physiology of Testosterone *105*
Virilisation 106
Clinical Features *106*
Investigation *106*
Management of Hirsutism 107
Local Treatment *107*
Drug Treatment *108*
Menstrual Disorder 109
Dysfunctional Uterine
Bleeding 110
Clinical Features *110*

Estimation of Blood Loss *110*
Investigation of the
Endometrium 111
Outpatient Procedures *111*
Investigations of Endometrium 112
Methods of Endometrial Biopsy *112*
Dilatation and Curettage *112*
Investigations of Endometrium -
Complications 113
Management of Heavy Menstrual
Bleeding 114
Medical Management *114*
Surgical Management *115*
Endometrial Ablation Techniques *115*
Dysmenorrhoea 120
Nature of the Pain *120*
Aetiology *120*
Clinical Features of Primary
Dysmenorrhoea *121*
Management *121*
Drug Treatment *121*
Adenomyosis 122
Pathology *122*
Microscopic Appearances *122*
Endometriosis 123
Pathology *123*
Secondary Pathology *124*
Histology *125*
Clinical Findings *126*
Symptomatology *126*
Physical Examination *126*
Laparoscopy *126*
Imaging Techniques *127*
Differential Diagnosis *127*
Histogenesis *127*
Treatment *127*
Premenstrual Syndrome 129
Clinical Features *129*
Investigations *129*
Treatment *130*
Management Options for Severe PMS *130*

NORMAL AND PHYSIOLOGICAL CHANGES IN THE MENSTRUAL CYCLE

Normal menstrual cycles have a length of 21–35 days (mean 28 days). A normal period lasts for 3–7 days. Menstrual blood loss of 30–50 ml/month is normal. Menstrual blood loss is considered as excessive when it is greater than 80 ml/month. It is, however, rarely measured in clinical trials, and heavy menstrual loss should be defined clinically.

AMENORRHOEA

Amenorrhoea is the absence of menstruation for 6 months in a woman who had previously menstruated normally (sometimes called 2° amenorrhoea)

or

amenorrhoea is the term given when a girl has failed to menstruate by the age of 16 (sometimes called 1° amenorrhoea).

In practice, the distinction between 1° and 2° amenorrhoea is not generally helpful in making a diagnosis. A similar process of investigation should be carried out whether or not the patient had previously menstruated. Amenorrhoea occurs in a number of physiological conditions, and these should be borne in mind when initiating investigation.

MENARCHE

Menarche is the onset of menstruation at puberty. The median age at which menarche occurs (13 y) is relatively late in the events occurring around puberty. For most young women, the growth spurt and secondary sexual characteristics, such as breast development (thelarche) and the growth of pubic and axillary hair, usually precede the onset of menstruation by about 2 years.

Absent or late puberty may present with amenorrhoea. If a girl over the age of 14 presents with amenorrhoea, investigations should depend on whether or not other signs of puberty are present.

PHYSIOLOGICAL AMENORRHOEA

PREGNANCY

During pregnancy, the levels of oestrogen and progesterone remain high, thus ensuring the integrity of the endometrium, and causing amenorrhoea. Initially, the corpus luteum is the source of oestrogen and progesterone. Later in pregnancy, the production of oestrogen and progesterone is taken over by the placenta. Pregnancy should be considered in the differential diagnosis of all women who present with amenorrhoea.

LACTATION

Soon after delivery, prolactin is secreted in large quantities by the anterior pituitary. There is partial suppression of luteinising hormone (LH) production so that ovarian follicles may grow, but ovulation does not occur, and amenorrhoea is the result. If the mother does not breast feed, menstruation will return in 2–3 months, but if she does breast feed, the period of amenorrhoea will be prolonged.

MENOPAUSE

The menopause is the cessation of menstruation (mean age 51 y) due to exhaustion of the supply of ovarian follicles. Oestrogen production therefore falls. This fall in oestrogen production is accompanied by a rise in follicle stimulating hormone (FSH) levels, which continues for a considerable time. In a proportion of women, menstruation ceases abruptly, but in many, the menstrual cycles alter. Frequently, they become shorter initially, but later they lengthen and tend to be irregular, before ceasing entirely. This phase is known as the menopause transition, and the final period is recognised only in retrospect, after 1 year of amenorrhoea. See Chapter 18.

CAUSES OF AMENORRHOEA

Amenorrhoea may be classified in a number of ways. One of the most helpful classifications is shown below:

1. Uterine or lower genital tract causes
2. Ovarian causes
3. Pituitary causes
4. Hypothalamic causes.

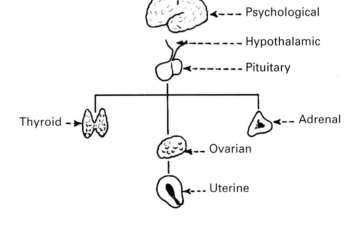

UTERINE AND LOWER GENITAL TRACT DISORDERS

IMPERFORATE HYMEN OR TRANSVERSE VAGINAL SEPTUM

This condition usually presents with primary amenorrhoea. There is no visible bleeding although the usual cyclical symptoms are present. In that there is no flow of blood, the term amenorrhoea can be used, but the cause is an obstruction by a vaginal septum or an imperforate hymen rather than a functional abnormality.

Three degrees are recognised.

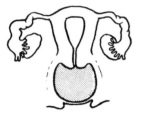

Haematocolpos. Only the vagina is distended by altered blood.

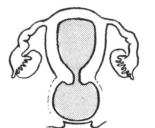

Haematometra. The uterus is also distended.

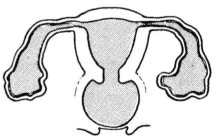

Haematosalpinx. In long-standing cases the tubes are also involved.

Clinical Features

The patient is usually a girl of 17 or so, complaining of primary amenorrhoea and pelvic pain of increasing severity. In long-standing cases, the pressure of the distended vagina may cause urinary retention. Pregnancy must be excluded.

Examination

A pelvic mass is palpated and may even be visible. The vaginal membrane or hymen is bulging.

Treatment

Incision and drainage. Very large amounts of inspissated blood may be released, and if the septum is particularly thick, a vaginal reconstruction procedure may subsequently be required.

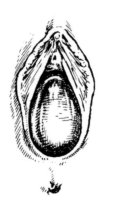

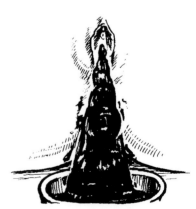

UTERINE AND LOWER GENITAL TRACT DISORDERS

ASHERMAN'S SYNDROME

In Asherman's syndrome, the uterine cavity is obliterated by adhesions. The condition is usually caused by uterine surgery: most commonly curettage, for example during termination of pregnancy. In developing countries, infections such as tuberculosis and schistosomiasis are commoner causes of Asherman's syndrome.

The adhesions should be broken down hysteroscopically. High dose oestrogens are used to stimulate endometrial proliferation following the procedure. Some authorities advocate the use of a Foley catheter placed in the uterus for a short time after adhesiolysis to prevent recurrence. Pregnancy rates following treatment are in the order of 80%. Such pregnancies may be complicated by abnormal placentation, for example by placenta accreta.

MÜLLERIAN AGENESIS

See Chapter 1

The Müllerian ducts fuse by the 10th week of gestation to form the fallopian tubes, uterus and upper portion of the vagina. Agenesis or lack of development of the Müllerian ducts (the Mayer–Rokitansky–Kuster–Hauser syndrome) leads to absence of these structures. Absence or hypoplasia of the vagina is a constant feature, but the uterine abnormalities vary. Provided there is a cavity lined by endometrium, menstruation can be normal.

The diagnosis of Müllerian agenesis is made in women with primary amenorrhoea and an absent vagina, but normal female chromosomes. Ovarian function is normal.

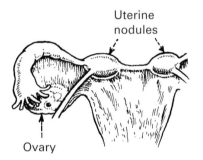

Uterine nodules

Ovary

CONGENITAL ANDROGEN INSENSITIVITY

Previously known as testicular feminisation syndrome, congenital androgen insensitivity is the third commonest cause of primary amenorrhoea. The individual is phenotypically female although the uterus is absent. The karyotype is 46XY (see p. 62).

OVARIAN DISORDERS

Ovarian disorders

1. Gonadal dysgenesis
2. Premature ovarian failure
3. Resistant ovary syndrome
4. Disorders of ovulation such as polycystic ovarian syndrome
5. Hormone-producing tumours, such as granulosa cell tumours (oestrogen-producing) or Leydig cell tumours (androgen-producing).

GONADAL DYSGENESIS

Women with gonadal dysgenesis have abnormal ovarian development, leading to absent or streak ovaries. The number of germ cells that migrate to the ovary during intrauterine life is reduced. These woman present with primary or secondary amenorrhoea, and have persistently elevated gonadotrophins on testing.

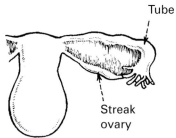

In women under 30 years of age at the time of presentation, a karyotype should be performed. Turner's syndrome (p. 60) is the classic form of gonadal dysgenesis, but other karyotypes, including 46XX are also found. If a Y chromosome is present, consideration should be given to gonadectomy because of the risk of neoplasia.

OVARIAN DISORDERS

PREMATURE OVARIAN FAILURE

In this condition, ovarian follicles are depleted from the ovary before the normal age of the menopause, and a premature menopause ensues. In addition to amenorrhoea, the patient may complain of menopausal symptoms such as hot flushes, loss of libido, etc. This condition is not uncommon: 1% of women will have ovarian failure by the age of 40. Premature ovarian failure is found in around 10% of women with amenorrhoea.

Cause

The majority of women with premature ovarian failure have no obvious cause for their condition. It is associated with chromosomal abnormalities such as Turner's syndrome (XO). It may occur in association with autoimmune disease, following infections such as mumps, or following chemotherapy or pelvic radiotherapy.

Diagnosis

The diagnosis is made by finding elevated serum FSH levels (>20 IU/L). As FSH levels are elevated physiologically mid-cycle, at least two FSH levels should be obtained at six weekly intervals. If a high FSH level is followed 2 weeks later by menstruation, the cause of the elevated FSH may be more likely to represent ovulation rather than menopause.

Treatment

Women with premature ovarian failure should be advised that they are likely to be infertile, although spontaneous pregnancies have been reported. Pregnancy can be achieved by IVF (*in vitro* fertilisation) with donor oocytes.

Oestrogen replacement should be considered to reduce the risk of osteoporosis and cardiovascular disease. A progestogen is also required to protect the endometrium from the stimulatory effects of oestrogen. This can be in the form of hormone replacement therapy, but, alternatively, the combined oral contraceptive pill would be a suitable option and may be more acceptable to young women.

RESISTANT OVARY SYNDROME

In this condition, the ovarian follicles fail to develop, despite high circulating levels of gonadotrophins. The clinical and biochemical features are that of premature ovarian failure. An ovarian biopsy will reveal ovarian follicles, and thus distinguish the condition from premature ovarian failure. In practice, this is not helpful; it may stimulate adhesion formation and the absence of follicles can be reliably determined only after the entire ovary has been examined. The treatment is the same as for premature ovarian failure.

OVARIAN DISORDERS

POLYCYSTIC OVARIAN SYNDROME

Polycystic ovarian syndrome (PCOS) is a functional derangement of the hypothalamo–pituitary ovarian axis associated with anovulation. The pathophysiology of PCOS remains poorly understood. Insulin resistance is a feature, and a genetic element to the disorder has been proposed. Women with PCOS are more at risk of developing Type II diabetes.

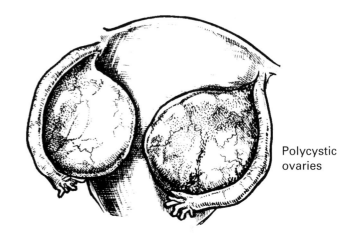

Polycystic ovaries

In women with PCOS, LH levels are relatively high and FSH levels are relatively low, leading to an elevated LH:FSH ratio. Oestradiol levels tend to be within the normal range. Production of androgens is stimulated by the elevated levels of LH; increased levels of testosterone, androstendione and DHA are secreted by the ovary. Some of these androgens are converted to oestrogen in peripheral tissues. In response to high androgen levels, sex hormone binding globulin (SHBG) is reduced by about 50%, leading to an increase in the proportion of unbound, active, androgens. Hence, androgenic side effects are common, despite only a modest rise or even normal levels of total serum testosterone levels.

Clinical Features

The clinical features of PCOS are variable. In the classic 'Stein Leventhal' syndrome, described in 1935, the presenting features are oligomenorrhoea, hirsutism and obesity. Other manifestations are common, however, and include menstrual disorders ranging from amenorrhoea to menorrhagia and signs of androgen excess, such as hirsutism, acne and infertility.

OVARIAN DISORDERS

POLYCYSTIC OVARIAN SYNDROME—(cont'd)

Diagnosis

No specific features of polycystic ovarian syndrome are diagnostic of the condition. According to the Rotterdam criteria, the diagnosis can be made if two out of three of the following criteria are present:

1. *Oligoamennorhoea*

2. *Ultrasound*
   Ultrasound will show multiple follicular cysts up to 6–8 mm diameter within the ovary. This is described as a necklace of pearls appearance. The volume of the ovarian subcortical stroma is increased. Such findings on ultrasound support rather than confirm a diagnosis of PCOS, as 25% of normal women will demonstrate these features on ultrasound.

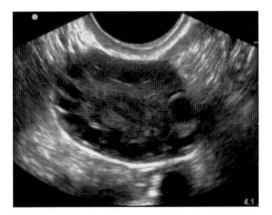

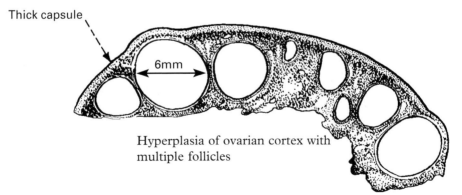

Thick capsule

6mm

Hyperplasia of ovarian cortex with multiple follicles

3. *Elevated free testosterone levels*
   A modest increase in total testosterone is accompanied by a decrease in SHBG resulting in an increase in free testosterone levels.

   An elevated LH:FSH ratio may occur but is no longer a diagnostic criteria.
   A physiological raised LH level occurs during the LH surge.

OVARIAN DISORDERS

POLYCYSTIC OVARIAN SYNDROME—(cont'd)

Long-term Effects of PCOS

1. Women with PCOS who are anovulatory are at increased risk of endometrial hyperplasia and subsequent endometrial cancer ($\times$3) because of the high oestrogen and low progesterone levels.
2. The hyperinsulinaemia associated with insulin resistance leads to an increased risk of diabetes mellitus.
3. Women with PCOS who are obese and insulin resistant have an increased risk of hypertension and cardiovascular disease.

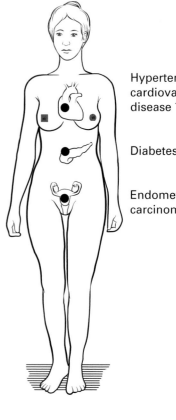

Hypertension/
cardiovascular
disease ↑

Diabetes ↑

Endometrial
carcinoma ↑

Treatment of PCOS

The treatment for PCOS is aimed at relieving symptoms and preventing adverse long-term effects. For women who are overweight, weight loss should be strongly supported as it reduces the clinical features of the condition and provides long-term health benefits.

1. *Infertility*

    Anovulatory women with infertility should be treated with clomiphene in the first instance. Women who fail to respond may require gonadotrophins $\pm$ gonadotrophin releasing hormone (GnRH) analogues.

2. *Amenorrhoea*

    Women with amenorrhoea may be treated with the combined oral contraceptive pill if contraception is required, or cyclical gestogens (e.g. medroxyprogesterone acetate 10 mg daily from day 15 to 25) if contraception is not required. The prevention of amenorrhea is important in PCOS to reduce the risk of endometrial carcinoma. The Mirena IUS is also useful to reduce the long-term risk of endometrial hyperplasia.

3. *Hirsutism*

    See p. 106.

PITUITARY DISORDERS

1. Hyperprolactinaemia
2. Pituitary adenoma
3. Craniopharyngioma
4. Other tumours such as meningioma
5. Pituitary necrosis (Sheehan's syndrome/ Simmond's disease).

Pituitary tumours are normally benign. However, as they grow in a confined space, they may cause symptoms by compressing surrounding tissue and structures. Functioning pituitary tumours may exert effects because of the hormones they release. The commonest of these are prolactin secreting pituitary tumours, accounting for 50% of all pituitary adenomas.

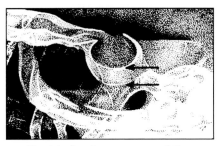

'Double floor' appearance of the pituitary fossa due to tumour

HYPERPROLACTINAEMIA
Prolactin is secreted from the anterior pituitary,
and the normal blood level is between 150 and 600 mU/L depending on the laboratory. During pregnancy, there is a 10-fold increase in serum prolactin levels. Non-physiological hyperprolactinaemia, which occurs when the woman is non-pregnant, can cause amenorrhoea or galactorrhoea (inappropriate lactation) or both. Hyperprolactinaemia is the principal cause of amenorrhoea in around 20% of women with this condition.

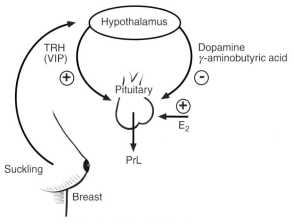

Control of prolactin release

PITUITARY DISORDERS

Aetiology

1. *Pituitary tumour*
   microadenoma <10 mm diameter
   macroadenoma >10 mm diameter

2. *Hypothyroidism*
   Thyroid function tests should be
   performed on all women with
   hyperprolactinaemia. In primary
   hypothyroidism, TRH is increased.
   As TRH stimulates pituitary
   prolactin production,
   hyperprolactinaemia results.
   Treatment with L-thyroxine should
   restore prolactin levels to normal.

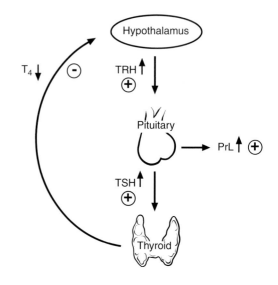

3. *Drugs*
   Drugs with dopamine agonistic activity
   cause hyperprolactinaemia by attenuating
   the inhibitory action of dopamine on
   pituitary prolactin production.

   Commonly used dopamine agonists
   Phenothiazines
   e.g. chlorpromazine
   thioridazine
   prochlorperazine
   Butyrophenones
   e.g. haloperidol
   Benzamides
   e.g. metoclopramide
   Cimetidine
   Methyldopa

   Other drugs which may cause hyperprolactinaemia
   Tricyclic antidepressants
   Monoamine oxidase inhibitors
   Opiates*
   Cocaine*
   *especially during chronic abuse

4. *Idiopathic*

PITUITARY DISORDERS

Diagnosis of Hyperprolactinaemia

The diagnosis of hyperprolactinaemia can be made on a single serum measurement. In the presence of oligo- or amenorrhoea, a serum prolactin of 800 mU/L or greater is likely to be of pathological significance. In the absence of an obvious alternative cause, radiological examination such as computerised tomography (CT) scanning or magnetic resonance imaging (MRI) should be performed to exclude a pituitary tumour.

Mechanism of Amenorrhoea

Raised prolactin

↓

Disturbance of normal hypothalamic GnRH release

↓

LH pulsatility suppressed

↓

Anovulation/amenorrhoea

PITUITARY DISORDERS

Treatment

Medication

Dopamine is the prolactin release inhibiting factor produced by the hypothalamus, and medical treatment for hyperprolactinaemia is based around dopaminergic stimulation.

1. *Bromocriptine*
   This is a semi-synthetic ergot alkaloid. Side effects include nausea and giddiness with fainting (syncope). Side effects may be minimised by commencing with a small dose and increasing gradually.

2. *Quinagolide*
   Quinagolide, a dopamine agonist, is given daily and may be tolerated better than bromocriptine.

3. *Cabergoline*
   Cabergoline is a dopamine agonist with a long half-life. It is administered weekly.

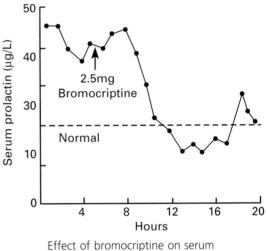

Effect of bromocriptine on serum prolactin. Duration 12–16 h.

Surgery

Transnasal

Trans-sphenoidal surgery can be used to resect both micro- and macroadenomas. Symptoms of hypopituitarism, particularly diabetes insipidus, may be a long-term consequence of surgery. The results of treatment vary greatly between centres. Knowledge of local data can be used to determine whether surgery or medical treatment is most appropriate for each patient.

HYPOTHALAMIC DISORDERS

Intermittent release of GnRH (gonadatrophin releasing hormone) stimulates production of FSH and LH by the anterior pituitary. Increased concentration of endogenous dopamine and opioids can affect the release of GnRH. This can be provoked by a number of conditions, detailed below.

Disorders of the hypothalamus result in hypogonoadotrophic hypogonadism, and hence amenorrhoea.

DIAGNOSIS

The diagnosis is made by exclusion. These patients have low gonadotrophins, normal prolactin levels, a normal pituitary gland on radiological evaluation, and they fail to bleed in response to progesterones.

CAUSES

1. *Anorexia nervosa*

    This is an eating disorder characterised by low body weight. It is much more common in women than in men and usually starts in the mid-teen years. The patient's weight is more than 15% below normal for her age and height.

    In moderate to severe disease, it is important to treat the psychological cause of the condition and this is best done by referral to a psychiatrist. Treatment with hormone replacement therapy will relieve symptoms of oestrogen deprivation and initiate the resumption of menstrual periods.

2. *Exercise*

    Female athletes are commonly amenorrhoeic, and the mechanism is one of suppression of GnRH production. This condition is related to the much reduced body fat (although not necessarily body weight), stress and to exercise itself. Again, oestrogen replacement (with added cyclical gestogens) should be considered.

3. *Kallmann's syndrome*

    This is a rare condition of congenital hypogonadotrophic hypogonadism in association with anosmia. Secondary sexual characteristics are absent. Ovulation can be induced with gonadotrophins.

INVESTIGATION OF AMENORRHOEA

In most cases, the failure to menstruate is due to some abnormality in the control mechanism involving the hypothalamic–pituitary pathway. A careful history and physical examination is essential and may provide pointers to likely abnormalities.

The history should include the following:
    change in weight
    presence of galactorrhoea
    presence of hirsutes (excess body or facial hair)
    presence of stress
    questions about excessive exercise.

A full physical examination should be performed. This should include the following:
    assessment of patient's body mass index (BMI) (weight in kg^2/height in m)
    presence of galactorrhoea
    presence of hirsutes
    blood pressure
    urinalysis
    assessment of secondary sexual characteristics
    assessment of external genitalia
    pelvic examination to assess internal genitalia.

In women who are *virgo intacta*, a pelvic examination should not be performed. If necessary, information about the presence of a uterus can be gained from ultrasound or MRI. However, inspection of external genitalia can still be performed and may reveal a condition such as cliteromegaly.

INVESTIGATION
The simplified scheme of investigation shown will identify which compartment is responsible for the amenorrhoea. In practice, estimation of serum prolactin and thyroid stimulating hormone (TSH) is performed concurrently with a progesterone challenge test.

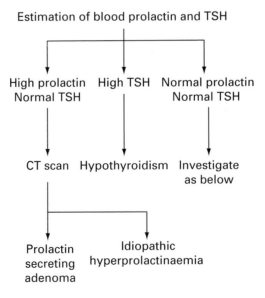

INVESTIGATION OF AMENORRHOEA

The progesterone challenge test involves giving a progesterone, for example, medroxyprogesterone acetate 10 mg daily for 5 days. It is essential to exclude pregnancy first. If the woman bleeds after progesterone is withdrawn, this indicates firstly that a uterus is present, and secondly that there is some circulating oestrogen. If the progesterone challenge test is negative, it is appropriate to give oestrogen and progesterone, (e.g. 1.25 mg of conjugated oestrogens for 21 days, with the addition of a progesterone for the last 5 days). Failure to bleed in response to this treatment confirms a uterine problem.

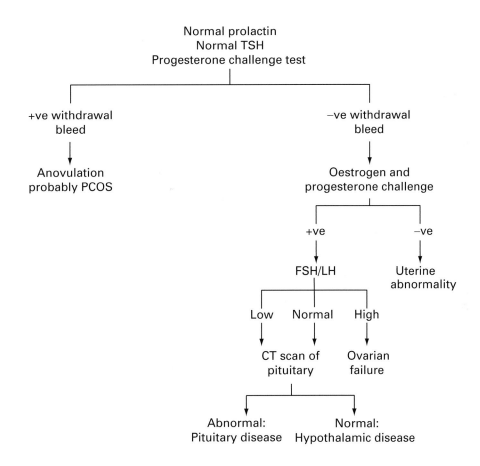

INVESTIGATION OF AMENORRHOEA

If the results of these tests are inconclusive, it suggests that the cause lies between the pituitary and ovaries, and further laboratory exploration must be undertaken.

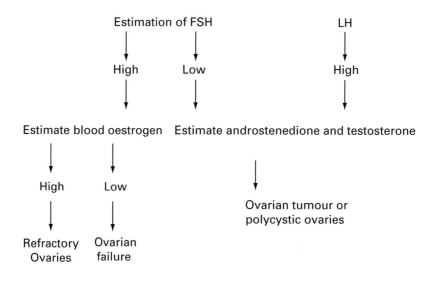

HIRSUTISM

Hirsutism in the female means an excessive production of hair with a tendency to male distribution. 'Excessive' is defined as beyond social acceptability or causing embarrassment to the patient.

Normal pattern hair is of two types:
  (i) fine downy, vellus hair which is non-pigmented.
  (ii) coarser pigmented terminal hair as in the axilla and pubis.

About one-third of women have some visible pigmented hair on the upper lip, and 5% have it on the chin and sides of the face.

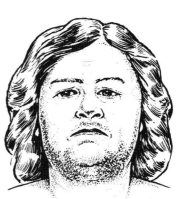

AETIOLOGY
1. Rise in secretion of free androgens.
2. Reduction in SHBG.
3. Increased end organ sensitivity to androgens.

SHBG level falls when testosterone production increases, and probably also in the case of drug-induced hirsutism. Oestrogen increases the levels of SHBG and lowers the amount of free androgen.

PHYSIOLOGY OF TESTOSTERONE
The three principal androgens are dihydrotestosterone, testosterone and androstenedione; the last mentioned is the least potent but is converted to dihydrotestosterone in the follicle cells.

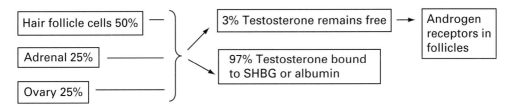

Causes:

1. *Idiopathic hirsutism*
   By far the commonest, it has no apparent androgen increase, and is probably due to increased local testosterone production at the target organ.

2. *Polycystic ovary disease*
   There is usually a higher level of free active testosterone because of reduced SHBG. See page 95.

3. *Androgen-producing tumours*
   These may arise in the ovary or adrenal glands. They should be considered if serum testosterone is greater than 5 nmol/L or if the history is of sudden onset.

4. *Congenital adrenal hyperplasia*
   This is an adrenal disease, caused by an enzyme defect (commonly 21-hydroxylase deficiency) resulting in elevated androgens.
   17-hydroxyprogesterone is elevated.

5. *Drugs such as:*
   phenytoin
   diazoxide
   minoxidil
   androgen-containing compounds

VIRILISATION

Masculinisation and virilisation are terms for extreme androgen effects.

CLINICAL FEATURES
The symptoms and signs include the following:
    male pattern balding
    cliteromegaly
    deepening of the voice
    increased muscle mass
    male body habitus.

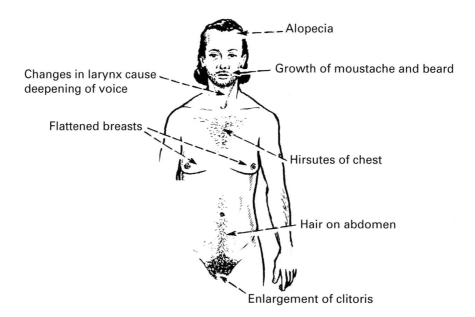

These symptoms are more likely to represent an androgen secreting tumour, but mild symptoms such as male pattern balding can occur with PCOS.

INVESTIGATION
    serum testosterone
    serum dehydroepiandrosterone sulphate (DHAS)
    (elevated in adrenal disease)
    17-hydroxyprogesterone (17-OHP)
    (elevated in congenital adrenal hyperplasia)
    24 h urinary free cortisol if Cushing's syndrome is suspected.

If the testosterone levels are significantly elevated, an androgen secreting tumour of the ovary or adrenal gland is likely. Ultrasound, CT scanning and perhaps even laparoscopy may be required to make the diagnosis.

MANAGEMENT OF HIRSUTISM

If the woman is untroubled by her symptoms, no treatment is needed. Women who are overweight should be advised to lose weight.

LOCAL TREATMENT

Ferriman Galwey Charts
These charts provide a semi-objective scoring system for hirsutism. If they are completed at each patient visit, the change in symptoms may be assessed.

Shaving
This method has to be repeated frequently.

Electrolysis
Decomposition of the hair follicle by the passage of an electric current. Low galvanic current is used through a fine electrode. The hair is electrolysed after about 10 s and plucked out painlessly.

Diathermy
The follicle is coagulated instantly and the hair pulled out.

Electrical destruction of individual hairs is permanent, but prolonged treatment is tedious and expensive and may cause scarring.

Depilatory Creams
These are alkaline solutions, which dissolve the hairs and allow them to be wiped away. They will injure the skin if left on too long.

Depilatory Waxes
The wax is melted and spread on to the skin. When it sets, it is pulled off, plucking the hairs with it. This is painful and leaves the skin tender and reddened.

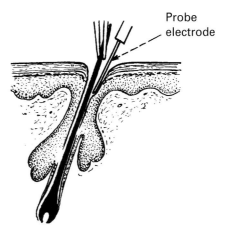

Probe electrode

MANAGEMENT OF HIRSUTISM

DRUG TREATMENT

1. *Combined oral contraceptive pill (COCP)*
   These drugs act firstly by suppressing LH production and thereby attenuating ovarian androgen synthesis. Secondly, the oestrogens stimulate SHBG production by the liver. The effect of the progestogen component can vary as some such as norethisterone and levonorgestrel have an androgenic derivation. Some of the available preparations contain antiandrogenic progestogens, these include Cyproterone Acetate and Drospirenone.

2. *Antiandrogens*
   As mentioned above, cyproterone is a progesterone, which inhibits LH production. It also binds to the androgen receptor and therefore acts as an antiandrogen. It can either be administered as with ethinyloestradiol (the contraceptive pill 'Dianette') or daily from days 5–14, with ethinyloestradiol on days 5–25 (the 'reverse sequential' regimen).

   Other antiandrogens include flutamide, a non-steroidal, and finasteride, a 5α reductase inhibitor. Finasteride inhibits the conversion of testosterone to dihydrotestosterone.

3. *Insulin sensitising agents*
   Metformin will improve insulin sensitivity and reduces free androgens in women with PCOS.

4. *Dexamethasone*
   Dexamethasone inhibits adrenal androgen production, and is useful in hirsutism caused by adrenal disease.

5. *GnRH analogues with addback hormone replacement therapy (HRT)*
   This treatment is expensive, but has been shown to be effective in clinical trials.

6. Eflornithine cream locally slows hair growth by inhibiting the enzyme orthinine decarboxylase.

NB. With all of the above, it may be 3 months or more before an improvement in symptoms can be expected, and the patient should be counselled regarding this.

MENSTRUAL DISORDER

Heavy menstrual bleeding is one of the commonest reasons why women in the Western world consult a gynaecologist. The vast majority of these women have benign or no pathology; however, the illustration demonstrates that for a minority of women there will be a malignant pathology.

Clearly, the age of the patient has a major influence on the likely cause of bleeding, for example, endometrial carcinoma is uncommon in premenopausal women and, similarly, endometriosis is uncommon in postmenopausal women.

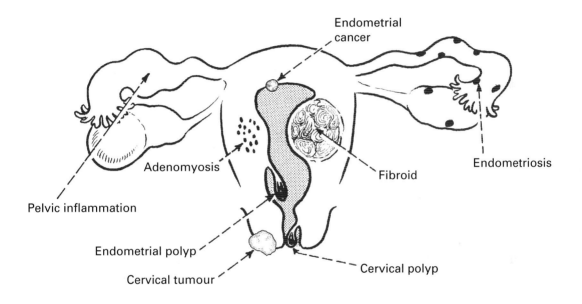

Careful history taking is crucial in the assessment of menstrual disorder. Women with heavy regular bleeding and no additional symptoms of concern such as intermenstrual or postcoital bleeding are most likely to have dysfunctional uterine bleeding. Benign pathologies such as fibroids are a common cause of heavy menstrual bleeding. See Chapter 11.

DYSFUNCTIONAL UTERINE BLEEDING

Dysfunctional uterine bleeding is one of the commonest causes of excessive menstrual bleeding in women of reproductive age.

Dysfunctional uterine bleeding is the term applied to cases of excessive bleeding where no organic lesion can be found. Presumably the cause lies in an abnormal function of the ovarian and endometrial control mechanisms associated with the menstrual cycle.

Where appropriate investigation may be required. This will depend on the age of the patient and any additional symptoms.

Pelvic ultrasound (ideally transvaginal) should be performed. Hysteroscopy and endometrial biopsy may be required, depending on scan findings, age of the woman, and presenting symptoms.

CLINICAL FEATURES

The patient will complain of heavy and/or irregular bleeding. *Normal menstrual cycles* have a length of 21–35 days (mean 28 days). A normal period lasts for 3–7 days. Menstrual blood loss of 30–50 ml/month is normal. Menstrual blood loss is considered as excessive when it is greater than 80 ml/month. It is however rarely measured during clinical trials, and heavy menstrual loss should be defined clinically.

ESTIMATION OF BLOOD LOSS

1. *Subjective methods*

   The subjective estimation of menstrual blood loss is often difficult. What is normal to one woman may be regarded as abnormal by another. The simplest method of determining excessive menstrual loss is to ask the patient about the number of sanitary pads and/or tampons used daily. The use of pictures to indicate the amount of staining on each pad/tampon may improve accuracy. The passage of significant clots usually indicates excessive menstrual loss. The social effect of heavy menstrual loss can be considerable and symptoms such as flooding through sanitary protection are important.

2. *Objective methods*

   Haemoglobin measurements will indicate if the patient is anaemic. An estimation of serum ferritin may show a depletion in iron stores. Whilst the detection of anaemia has important clinical implications, many women with a good diet are able to maintain normal haemoglobin levels, despite excessive menstrual loss.

   The optimum method of assessing menstrual blood loss accurately is to ask the patient to collect her used pads and tampons over the course of one menstrual period. These can then be soaked in sodium hydroxide, and the optical density compared to a known standard. This technique is generally only used as a research tool, but reveals that many women who complain of menorrhagia have a menstrual loss within the normal range. A blood loss of 80 ml is thought to represent the upper limit of a 'normal' period. Studies have also shown that some women with a blood loss of greater than 80 ml do not perceive that they have heavy periods.

INVESTIGATION OF THE ENDOMETRIUM

Transabdominal scanning can be useful and should be used for women who have never been sexually active (*virgo intacta*). The bladder requires to be full so that overlying bowel is moved away to optimise the view of the pelvis. Even with a full bladder, views of the endometrium may be limited and particularly difficult to obtain in obese patients.

Transvaginal ultrasound scan This technique offers a close view of the uterus and adnexae.

Features noted during transvaginal scanning of the pelvis

Thickness and regularity of the endometrium; in postmenopausal women, the endometrial thickness (ET) is less than 3 mm in an AP diameter. A thickened endometrium may represent a polyp or endometrial hyperplasia; however, the normal endometrial thickness varies in premenopausal women during the menstrual cycle, and it may be physiological.

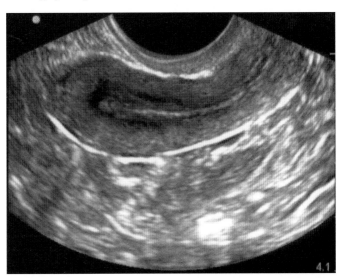

Presence of uterine fibroids The size and site of fibroids are important. Small fibroids of less than 3 cm are very common and usually do not change the treatment options.

Adnexal pathology can also be visualised in detail.

OUTPATIENT PROCEDURES

Hysteroscopy

Hysteroscopy is a technique used to visualise the endometrium under magnification. Abnormal areas of the endometrium can be seen, and a targeted biopsy taken. The procedure may be performed as an outpatient procedure if a sufficiently narrow hysteroscope and distension media are available. The distension media can be fluid: saline or dextrose or CO_2 gas.

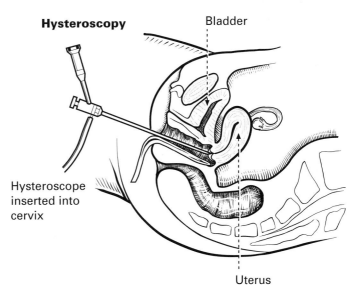

Hysteroscopy

Bladder

Hysteroscope inserted into cervix

Uterus

INVESTIGATION OF THE ENDOMETRIUM

The main purpose of endometrial biopsy is to assess for endometrial hyperplasia or identify endometrial carcinoma. The risk of endometrial cancer in premenopausal women is very low, but biopsy should be performed for women over 45 with menstrual disorder. In women under 45, the need for biopsy (possibly with hysteroscopy) should be guided by other factors including intermenstrual or irregular bleeding, and scan findings. See page 201 hyperplastic conditions of the uterus.

METHODS OF ENDOMETRIAL BIOPSY

Pipelle de Cornier
The Pipelle is inserted into the uterine cavity and the plunger withdrawn to produce a vacuum. A small sample of endometrium is thereby sucked into the tube and subsequently expelled into fixative.

Vabra Curettage
This method of obtaining material for histological examination can be done in the outpatient clinic. Adequate specimens can be obtained, but the procedure is painful.

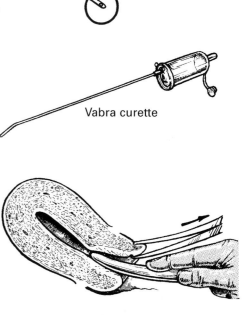

Vabra curette

DILATATION AND CURETTAGE
As a sole procedure, dilatation and curettage is now considered to be an outdated procedure; however, occasionally it may be required to provide a better sample of the endometrium. It is usually accompanied by hysteroscopic assessment of the cavity prior to sampling. It is often necessary to dilate the cervical canal in order to pass the curette. This procedure is normally performed under general anaesthesia as an inpatient.

Technique
The dilator must be held firmly in one hand and pressed into the canal against traction in the opposite direction exerted by the other hand. Resistance must be overcome slowly, and the dilator must not be passed farther than the length of the uterine cavity measured by the sound.

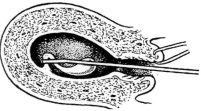

Curettage
Dilatation of the cervix is followed by curettage of the endometrium. The endometrium can then be examined histologically. Hysteroscopy and endometrial biopsy are largely diagnostic tools, but in the uncommon situation in which pathology such as an endometrial polyp is present, they may be therapeutic.

INVESTIGATIONS OF ENDOMETRIUM - COMPLICATIONS

1. *Trauma to cervix*
The volsellum forceps may tear the anterior lip of cervix if pulled on too forcibly.

The cervix splits at about 8mm dilatation

The next dilatation enlarges the false passage

2. *Perforation of the uterus or cervix*
This is not an uncommon occurrence and usually no ill-effects result. The usual site is the midline of the fundus, and it becomes evident when the curette passes farther than the length of the cavity as shown by the uterine sound. Immediate laparoscopy and/or laparotomy is required if there is any suspicion of damage to extrauterine viscera. This risk is higher during pregnancy as the uterus is softer.

3. *Uterine synechiae*
Over-vigorous curettage may remove all the endometrium from areas of anterior and posterior walls, permitting the myometrium to heal together forming adhesions – Asherman's syndrome. This is diagnosed and treated hysteroscopically.

MANAGEMENT OF HEAVY MENSTRUAL BLEEDING

MEDICAL MANAGEMENT
Tranexamic Acid
Administration: tranexamic acid 1 g qds during menstruation.

Mode of action: inhibits clot breakdown within endometrial vasculature.

Side effects are usually mild but can include nausea, vomiting and diarrhoea.

Up to 40% reduction in menstrual loss can be achieved.

Prostaglandin Synthetase Inhibitors
Administration: for example mefenamic acid, 500 mg tid during menstruation.

Mode of action: alters imbalance of vasodilator prostaglandin PGE2 and the vasoconstrictor prostaglandin PGF2a.

Side effects can include, diarrhoea, rashes, thrombocytopenia and haemolytic anaemia.

A 25% reduction in menstrual loss can be achieved.

Combined Contraceptive Pill
Administration: usual contraceptive regimen.

Mode of action: suppression of ovulation limits hormonal stimulation of the endometrium.

A reduction in menstrual loss can be seen in women both with and without menorrhagia.

Levonorgestrel Intrauterine System (LNG-IUS) Mirena
Administration: intrauterine system releasing 20 μg of levonorgestrel daily.

Mode of action: inhibits endometrial proliferation.

This device was originally designed as a contraceptive agent but is one of the most effective medical methods for reducing menstrual blood loss. One year after insertion, menstrual blood loss is reduced to 5% of the original amount. The main side effect of treatment is irregular bleeding in the first 3–6 months after insertion.

Progesterone
This is most useful for anovulatory bleeding.

Cyclical gestogens.

Administration: for example norethisterone 5 mg bd from days 5–26 of the menstrual cycle.

Mode of action: thought to provide progestogenic support to the endometrium when endogenous progesterone is lacking.

MANAGEMENT OF HEAVY MENSTRUAL BLEEDING

SURGICAL MANAGEMENT

Endometrial Ablation
Hysterectomy

Abdominal – total
　　　　　　　subtotal (conservation of cervix)
Vaginal – laparoscopically assisted vaginal hysterectomy
　　　　　total laparoscopic hysterectomy

ENDOMETRIAL ABLATION TECHNIQUES

These techniques use a variety of energy sources and can either be performed under hysteroscopic guidance or as a blind procedure. Endometrial ablation does not guarantee amenorrhoea, but symptoms are improved in most women. The major advantage of endometrial ablation over abdominal hysterectomy is the shorter inpatient stay and recovery associated with this operation. Complications of the procedure include excessive fluid absorption and uterine perforation with damage to intra-abdominal organs.

Endometrial ablation is only appropriate for women who have completed their family and effective contraception should be continued following the procedure.

Hysteroscopic Procedures
Trans-cervical resection of endometrium (TCRE)
Using an operating hysteroscope, the uterine cavity is distended with a glycine solution and either a wire loop diathermy instrument is used to cut strips of endometrium and underlying myometrium or a 'roller ball' electrode is used to coagulate the endometrium. These techniques are performed under direct vision.

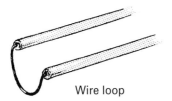

Wire loop　　　　　'Roller ball'

MANAGEMENT OF HEAVY MENSTRUAL BLEEDING

Second Generation Techniques
These techniques use a variety of thermal energies and are not performed under direct vision. They are relatively simple to perform; however, if the instrument is displaced, there is a risk of thermal injury to extrauterine structure, for example, bowel injury. The common techniques are microwave (MEA), a fluid filled balloon that is heated, Thermachoice and electrical energy, Novasure. There are a variety of safety mechanisms that these techniques employ; however, none of them is infallible, and recent advice has recommended that hysteroscopy should be performed prior to the procedure and that ultrasound should be used to confirm that the device is within the endometrial cavity during treatment.

An endometrial biopsy to exclude endometrial carcinoma is essential as part of any endometrial ablation procedure.

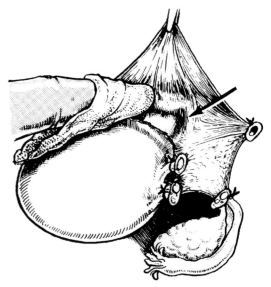

Total Hysterectomy (Removal of Uterus and Cervix)

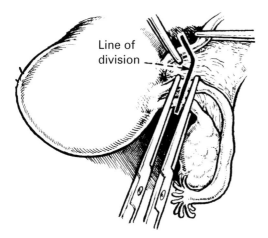

1. Division of adnexa. The ovarian ligament, fallopian tube and round ligament are clamped and divided.

2. Vesicouterine peritoneum is opened up and bladder is being dissected off cervix. (The 'lateral vesicouterine ligament' – marked by the arrow – conceals the ureter.)

MANAGEMENT OF HEAVY MENSTRUAL BLEEDING

Total Hysterectomy (Removal of Uterus and Cervix)—(cont'd)

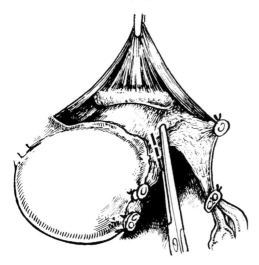

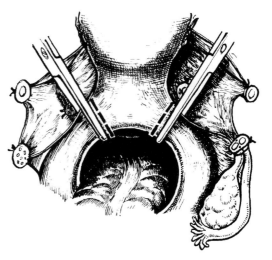

3. Parametrium containing the uterine arteries is clamped and divided.

4. The uterosacral ligaments are clamped and divided.

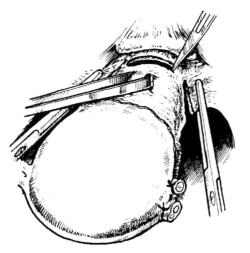

5. The top of the vagina is now clear of bladder and ureters and can be opened to allow excision of uterus and cervix.

MANAGEMENT OF HEAVY MENSTRUAL BLEEDING

Subtotal Hysterectomy

Subtotal hysterectomy involves removal of the body of the uterus only. The cervix is conserved. The operation is easier and safer than total hysterectomy, particularly if there are adhesions around the cervix (e.g. from previous caesarean section). The risk of ureteric damage is much less than with total hysterectomy. The major disadvantage of subtotal hysterectomy is that cervical smears continue to be required as there remains a risk of cervical cancer. There is a small risk of persistent light bleeding from the remnant of endocervix.

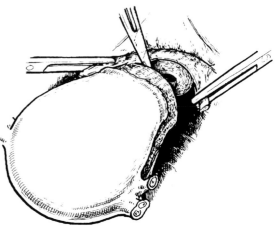

Bilateral Oophorectomy

Hysterectomy is often accompanied by bilateral oophorectomy. The pros and cons of this procedure are summarised below.

Advantages

    reduces risk of ovarian cancer
    effective treatment for premenstrual syndrome
    may improve efficacy of treatment if pelvic pain is included in symptoms.

Disadvantages

    leads to premature menopause and effects of oestrogen withdrawal, unless patient takes HRT.

MANAGEMENT OF HEAVY MENSTRUAL BLEEDING

Vaginal Hysterectomy

In vaginal hysterectomy, the uterus and cervix are removed via a vaginal approach. The operation is technically difficult in women without some degree of uterine prolapse. This approach avoids the need for an abdominal scar, and recovery is usually more rapid; however, the risk of major complications is slightly higher than with an abdominal procedure. There are a number of factors that may make an abdominal procedure the better option, for example, large fibroids, severe endometriosis.

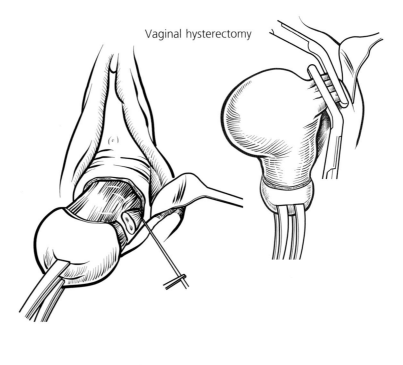

Vaginal hysterectomy

Laparoscopically Assisted Vaginal Hysterectomy (LAVH)
A laparoscopically assisted hysterectomy procedure allows the ovaries to be removed; this is difficult with a standard vaginal hysterectomy. The broad ligaments, including the ovarian vessels, the round ligaments, and the uterine arteries may be 'clamped and cut' by an endoscopic device which inserts multiple rows of stainless steel staples and divides the tissues. Alternatively, diathermy may be used to coagulate the tissues prior to division. The uterus is then removed vaginally and the vaginal vault closed per vaginam.

Total Laparoscopic Hysterectomy
The entire procedure is completed laparoscopically, and the uterus is removed per vaginam.

DYSMENORRHOEA

Dysmenorrhoea implies pain during menstruation, and most women experience some degree of pain at least on the first day of the period, when the loss is heaviest.

Cramp may occur premenstrually; if this is severe, it may be more likely to suggest underlying pathology, such as endometriosis.

The pain may be secondary to organic disease such as endometriosis or infection, but primary dysmenorrhoea, which is being discussed here, occurs in the presence of a normal genital tract.

NATURE OF THE PAIN
It is usually described as having two components: a continuous lower abdominal pain attributed to vascular congestion, which radiates through to the back and sometimes down the thighs, and an intermittent cramping pain.

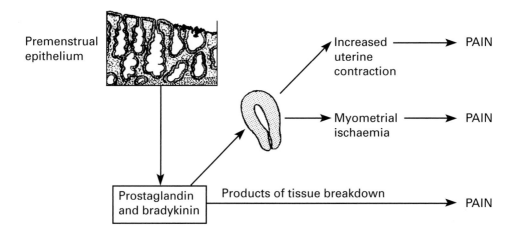

AETIOLOGY
There is increased myometrial activity during the periods in women with dysmenorrhoea and uterine blood flow is reduced, especially during intense contractions. It is thought that this hyperactivity is the result of excessive quantities of prostaglandins synthesised during the breakdown of the premenstrual endometrium.

DYSMENORRHOEA

CLINICAL FEATURES OF PRIMARY DYSMENORRHOEA
This condition is typically present from the time when ovulation is established, usually the late teens.

Prostaglandin (PG) synthetase inhibitors have been shown experimentally to abolish uterine contraction and ischaemia and the pain that accompanies them.

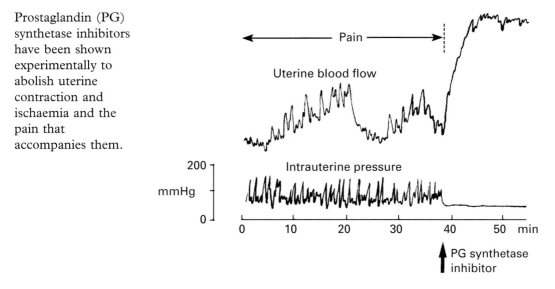

MANAGEMENT
In mild or moderate disease, treatment can be commenced after a full history and examination. In severe or unresponsive disease, investigation should be performed. A transvaginal scan and possibly laparoscopy should be considered.

DRUG TREATMENT
1. *The contraceptive pill.* Dysmenorrhoea is very unlikely in the absence of ovulation, probably because of the pseudo-atrophy of the endometrium. The disadvantages of this efficacious treatment are the well-known side effects and perhaps the prevention of pregnancy.
2. *Prostaglandin synthetase inhibitors* such as mefenamic acid inhibit prostaglandin production, reduce uterine contractions, and thereby alleviate dysmenorrhoea.
   In controlled studies, up to 90% of women report an improvement of symptoms with mefenamic acid.
3. *Levonorgestrel intrauterine system* MIRENA
   Progesterone is a smooth muscle relaxant and intrauterine administration will significantly reduce dysmenorrhoea.

ADENOMYOSIS

This is an infiltration of the myometrium by ectopic deposits of endometrium. It is usually only diagnosed once the uterus is examined histologically following hysterectomy. It can be visualised with ultrasound but MRI is better at differentiating adenomyosis from fibroids.

PATHOLOGY

The gross appearances are quite striking. The uterus is usually enlarged and this may be quite marked.

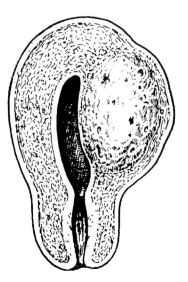

MICROSCOPIC APPEARANCES

The appearance of the endometrial deposits within the myometrium varies. In many cases, they consist of typical glands and stroma although the stroma may be more prominent than the glands. Cyclical changes may be observed, but this is not common. More often, the endometrium is of immature type, and if it does react, it usually shows only proliferative changes. Clinical features are pain and menstrual upset.

Endometrial deposits in the myometrium. Note the non-secretory gland epithelium. The surrounding myometrium undergoes moderate hyperplasia.

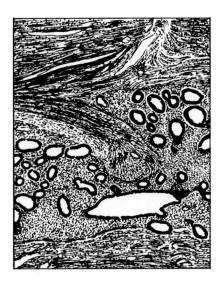

ENDOMETRIOSIS

Endometriosis is a condition where deposits of endometrium develop outside the uterine cavity. Its manifestations are very variable and often bear no relation to the extent of the disease.

PATHOLOGY

The gross appearance shows ectopic deposits, which can vary in number from a few in one locality to large numbers distributed over the pelvic organs and peritoneum.

The commonest sites of these deposits are the following:

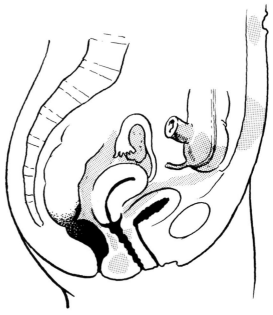

- Ovary
- Peritoneum of the rectovaginal cul-de-sac of the Pouch of Douglas
- Sigmoid colon
- Broad ligament
- Uterosacral ligaments.

Less common are the following sites:

- Cervix
- Round ligament
- Bladder
- Umbilicus
- Appendix
- Laparotomy scars.

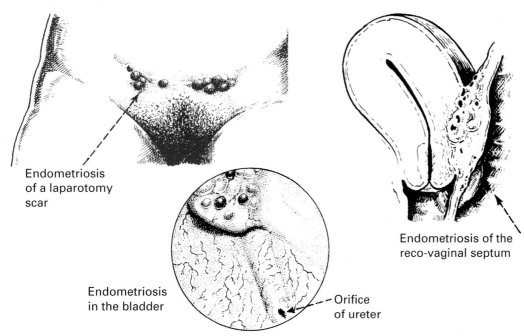

Endometriosis of a laparotomy scar

Endometriosis in the bladder

Orifice of ureter

Endometriosis of the reco-vaginal septum

ENDOMETRIOSIS

The commonest appearance of a typical lesion is that of a round protruding vesicle that shows a succession of colours from blue to black to brown. The variation in colour is due to haemorrhage with subsequent breakdown of the haemoglobin. Ultimately the area of haemorrhage heals by the formation of scar tissue. The result is a puckered area on the peritoneum. Commonly, however, the haemorrhage results in adhesion to surrounding structures. These adhesions are more apt to form between fixed structures such as the broad ligament, ovary, sigmoid colon, or the posterior surfaces of the vagina and cervix.

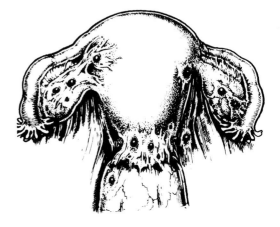

The ectopic deposits of endometrial tissue vary in size from pin-point to 5 mm or more. It is these larger deposits which tend to rupture leading to adhesions. These adhesions over the ovary can lead to the formation of quite large haemorrhagic cysts due to continued bleeding from deposits, the blood being unable to escape.

Investigation has shown that many lesions do not have a 'typical' appearance. The following is a list of other appearances which have been described.

- White, slightly raised opacities due to retroperitoneal deposits.
- Red flame-like or vascular swellings, more common in the broad ligament or uterosacral ligament.
- Small excrescences like the surface of normal endometrium.
- Adhesions under the ovary or between the ovary and the ovarian fossa peritoneum.
- Café-au-lait patches often in the Pouch of Douglas, broad ligament or peritoneal surface of the bladder.
- Peritoneal defects on uterosacral ligament or broad ligament.
- Areas of petechiae or hypervascularisation usually on the bladder and the broad ligament.

SECONDARY PATHOLOGY

This is due to the adhesions between the endometriotic deposits and adjacent organs. In long-standing cases, the pelvic cavity is obliterated by these adhesions. Retroversion of the uterus can occur as the adhesions form.

ENDOMETRIOSIS

HISTOLOGY

While the deposits consist of endometrial elements, rarely do they mirror the appearance of normal endometrium, especially in their architecture. In place of the compact orderly arrangement of glands and stroma, there are scattered patches of gland formations with some surrounding stroma. Sometimes gland formations predominate; occasionally only stromal cells can be seen.

Sometimes the deposits show evidence of cyclical activity, but the activity does not always coincide with what is happening in the uterine endometrium.

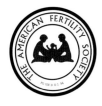

THE AMERICAN FERTILITY SOCIETY
REVISED CLASSIFICATION OF ENDOMETRIOSIS

Patient's name _____ Date _____

Stage I (Minimal)	– 1–5	Laparoscopy _____ Laparotomy _____ Photography _____
Stage II (Mild)	– 6–15	Recommended Treatment _____
Stage III (Moderate)	– 16–40	_____
Stage IV (Severe)	– >40	
Total _____		Prognosis _____

			<1 cm	1–3 cm	>3 cm
PERITONEUM	ENDOMETRIOSIS				
		Superficial	1	2	?
		Deep	2	4	6
OVARY	R	Superficial	1	2	4
		Deep	4	16	20
	L	Superficial	1	2	4
		Deep	4	16	20

		Partial	Complete
	POSTERIOR CUL DE SAC OBLITERATION	4	40

			<1/3 Enclosure	1/3 – 2/3 Enclosure	>2/3 Enclosure
OVARY	ADHESIONS				
	R	Filmy	1	2	4
		Dense	4	8	16
	L	Filmy	1	2	4
		Dense	4	8	16
TUBE	R	Filmy	1	2	4
		Dense	4^a	8^a	16
	L	Filmy	1	2	4
		Dense	4^a	8^a	16

[a]If the fimbriated end of the fallopian tube is completely enclosed, change the point assessment to 16

ENDOMETRIOSIS

CLINICAL FINDINGS

The incidence of endometriosis has been estimated at 3–7% of women, but the true incidence is unknown. Quite often, deposits are found incidentally in women who have no symptoms of endometriosis and are undergoing laparoscopy or laparotomy for some other condition. In addition, as indicated in the section on pathology, many peritoneal changes now known to be due to endometriosis were undiagnosed in the past.

The prevalence of endometriosis peaks between the ages of 30 and 45 years. As ectopic endometrium is stimulated by the same ovarian steroid hormones as the endometrium lining the uterine cavity, endometriosis is almost never found outside the reproductive years.

SYMPTOMATOLOGY

A. *Pain* affects more than 80% of women with endometriotic deposits. The pain tends to begin premenstrually, reaching a peak during menstruation and subsiding slowly.

The character of pain may vary as does its apparent origin. It may be generalised throughout the abdomen and pelvis like the pain of severe dysmenorrhoea. Alternatively, pain may be localised to a particular site within the pelvis. Deep dyspareunia affects around 40% of women with endometriosis.

B. *Menstrual disturbance* Menstrual disturbance affects around 20% of women with endometriosis. It may take the form of premenstrual 'spotting', menorrhagia or infrequent periods. Lesions in the wall of the bladder may result in 'menstrual haematuria'.

C. *Infertility* Endometriosis is found more commonly in women undergoing investigation for infertility than in the 'normal' population. It is not clear which condition arises first. Approximately 30% of patients with endometriosis complain of infertility. When endometriosis is extensive, and both fallopian tubes are occluded, the mechanism by which endometriosis prevents conception is obvious. However, milder forms of endometriosis are also associated with subfertility, and here the pathophysiology is less clear. The most likely mechanism appears to be that immunological factors within the peritoneal cavity inhibit normal gamete function, thus reducing fertilisation rates.

PHYSICAL EXAMINATION

Endometriosis cannot be diagnosed by physical examination alone. However, enlargement of the ovaries, fixed retroversion of the uterus, and tender nodules within the pelvis may each raise the suspicion of the disease. Endometriosis should always be considered when patients have symptoms referable to the pelvic cavity.

LAPAROSCOPY

Laparoscopic examination is the gold standard investigation for endometriosis. The lesions can be seen and their number and location estimated. Endometriosis of long standing may be very difficult to diagnose because of obliteration of the pelvic cavity by adhesions.

ENDOMETRIOSIS

IMAGING TECHNIQUES

Ultrasound, CT and MRI may suggest the presence of endometriosis (e.g. by the demonstration of a particular type of ovarian cyst) but are by themselves insufficiently reliable to make the diagnosis.

DIFFERENTIAL DIAGNOSIS

Owing to the mixture of symptoms and the variation in appearance of the pelvic structures, conditions such as pelvic inflammatory disease and tumours of the ovary and bowel must be considered and eliminated.

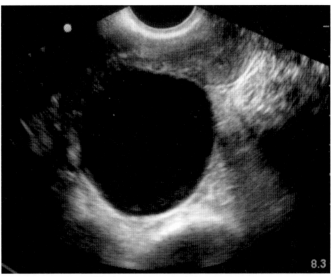

Endometrioma right ovary

HISTOGENESIS

There are three theories:

1. Retrograde spill of menstrual debris through the tubes. Retrograde menstruation takes place in most women, but it is unclear why some women should develop endometriosis while others are unaffected.
2. Metaplasia of embryonic cells. These are derived from the primitive coelom and may remain in and around the pelvis and differentiate into Müllerian duct tissue.
3. Emboli of endometrial tissue may travel by lymphatics or blood vessels and become established in various sites.

The first of these theories is the most favoured.

TREATMENT

Medical Treatment

Any treatment must be aimed at treating symptoms. As ovarian hormones are responsible for growth and activity in endometrium, many medical therapies are designed to reduce ovarian steroid production or oppose their action.

1. Progestogens
   Progestogens in a relatively high dose (e.g. medroxyprogesterone acetate 10 mg tid) induce decidualisation, and sometimes resorption of ectopic endometrium. Side effects include weight gain, bloating and irregular vaginal bleeding.

2. Combined contraceptive pill
   The combined oral contraceptive pill also induces decidualisation of ectopic endometrium. It may be given continuously for up to 3 months.

127

ENDOMETRIOSIS

3. Danazol

    Danazol is a steroid hormone closely related to testosterone, which inhibits pituitary
    gonadotrophins, and is antioestrogenic, antiprogestational, slightly androgenic, and
    anabolic. It is an effective treatment but is now outdated as irreversible androgenic effects
    such as hirsutism and deepening of the voice are common.

4. Gonadotrophic releasing hormone analogues (GnRH analogue)

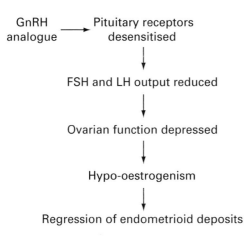

GnRH analogues are administered by
depot injection or nasal spray. Their mode
of action is shown above. These drugs are
generally effective in treating symptoms
caused by endometriosis; however,
menopausal side effects are common.
Add-back hormone replacement therapy
will usually prevent the vast majority of
vasomotor symptoms without stimulating
endometriosis. These preparations are
licensed for 6 months of use as there is
concern that long-term use will increase
the risk of osteoporosis and other effects of
oestrogen deprivation.

Conclusion

As with medical therapies for other conditions, the optimum treatment is dictated by the side
effect profile which is most acceptable to the patient. None of the drug treatments described
will prevent recurrence of endometriosis once therapy has been stopped, although there may
be a period of some months between stopping treatment and the re-emergence of symptoms.
No medical treatment has been shown to improve subsequent fertility.

Surgical Treatment

Where the woman has completed her family, radical surgery to remove both ovaries is likely to
provide a lasting cure for endometriosis as it removes the oestrogenic stimulus to endometrial
growth.

In many cases, the patient wishes relief from pain but also desires to retain the possibility of
future pregnancy. In these circumstances, only conservative surgery can be employed.

The intentions in conservative surgery are the following:

1. To ablate as many endometrial deposits in the pelvic cavity as possible.
2. To restructure the pelvic anatomy by destroying adhesions that interfere with ovarian
    and tubal function.
3. To destroy endometrial deposits in the ovaries.

PREMENSTRUAL SYNDROME

The premenstrual syndrome (PMS) includes a large group of symptoms, which appear regularly and predictably in the week before the onset of menstruation. The symptom pattern varies with the individual, but 95% of women are likely to acknowledge at least one of the symptoms listed below. Symptoms resolve completely by the end of menstruation. The severity can vary significantly and it has been classified as follows:

Mild – does not interfere with personal/social and professional life.

Moderate – interferes with personal/social and professional life, but the woman is still able to interact, although may be suboptimally.

Severe – unable to interact personally/socially/professionally – withdraws from social and professional activities.

Water retention	Pain	Autonomic reactions
Weight gain (up to 7lb) Painful breasts Abdominal distension Feeling of bloatedness	Headache Backache Tiredness Muscle stiffness	Dizziness/faintness Cold sweats Nausea/vomiting Hot flushes
Mood changes	Loss of concentration	Miscellaneous
Tension Irritability Depression Crying spells	Forgetfulness Clumsiness Difficulty in making decisions Poor sleeping	Feelings of suffocation Chest pains Heart pounding Numbness, tingling

CLINICAL FEATURES
Although the aetiology of PMS is unknown, it is clearly related to cyclical ovarian activity. Women who have no cyclical variation in sex steroids (e.g. postmenopausal women, pregnant or breastfeeding women, and women who have had bilateral oophorectomy) do not have PMS.

INVESTIGATIONS
There is no test that 'confirms' a diagnosis of PMS. It is helpful to ask the patient to complete a symptom diary on a daily basis over the course of several cycles in order to demonstrate that symptoms are related to the premenstrual phase.

In a few women, it may be helpful to institute treatment with a GnRH analogue for 3 months. This drug reliably suppresses ovarian activity. If symptoms are still present by the third month of treatment, they are unlikely to be related to PMS.

PREMENSTRUAL SYNDROME

TREATMENT
General advice to minimise stress, maintain a sensible diet and have regular exercise have been shown to have beneficial effects for women with PMS.

MANAGEMENT OPTIONS FOR SEVERE PMS
1. *Pyridoxine (vitamin B6)*
   This is based on disordered tryptophan metabolism in sufferers from endogenous depression. Pyridoxine corrects the reduced brain 5-hydroxytryptamine. High doses are associated with peripheral neuropathy and a maximum of 10 mg daily is recommended.

2. *Oil of evening primrose*
   Oil of evening primrose is widely prescribed for the treatment of PMS. It is available 'over the counter' and has few adverse effects. Its main benefit appears to be in the management of cyclical mastalgia.

3. *Progesterone*
   Progesterones are widely prescribed for the treatment of PMS. In the many placebo-controlled studies in which they have been evaluated, they have repeatedly been shown to be ineffective.

4. *The combined oral contraceptive pill (COCP)*
   The COCP abolishes cyclical hormone fluctuations; however, it has been shown to have been of limited benefit in the management of women with severe PMS. This may be due to the effect of the progestin component as newer progestogens may be beneficial. Preparations containing drospirenone, an antiandrogenic, antimineralocorticoid progestin appears to be effective in the treatment of PMS.

5. *Oestrogen*
   Oestrogen patches and implants are beneficial in the management of severe PMS. Doses of 100 μg patches were shown to be effective. Progestin is required and the Mirena IUS may be of benefit to minimise systemic side effects.

6. *Selective serotonin uptake inhibitors (SSRIs)*
   SSRIs such as fluoxetine have been shown to be significantly better than placebo for the treatment of PMS in controlled trials. As altered serotonergic function has been demonstrated in women with PMS, there is a clear rationale for their use.

7. *GnRH analogues*
   GnRH analogues are extremely effective in the treatment of PMS, and indeed may be useful in making the diagnosis (see above). Unfortunately, the menopausal side effects, associated bone loss, and expense mean these drugs are unsuitable as long-term treatment. Add-back HRT should be given at the same time as treatment with GnRH analogues for PMS.

8. *Bilateral salpingo-oophorectomy*
   Bilateral oophorectomy is extremely effective in the treatment of PMS. When combined with hysterectomy, oestrogen replacement can safely be given with no increase in symptoms. Clearly, hysterectomy and bilateral oophorectomy will rarely be indicated for the treatment of PMS alone. However, in women undergoing hysterectomy, the presence of significant PMS may be an indication for bilateral oophorectomy.

CHAPTER 7

GYNAECOLOGICAL INFECTIONS

Inflammation in the Lower
  Gynaecological Tract 132
  Defence Mechanisms 132
Vulval Inflammation 133
  Treatment 133
Vaginal Discharge and Infection 134
  Composition 134
  Source of Vaginal Discharge 134
  Clinical Features 134
Complaints of Vaginal
  Discharge 135
  Examination 135
  Leucorrhoea 135
Vaginal Discharge 136
  Candida Albicans 136
  Bacterial Vaginosis 137
  Trichomonas Vaginalis 137
Vaginitis 139
  Atrophic Vaginitis 139
  Vulvovaginitis in Children 139
  Foreign Bodies 139
  Other Causes of Vaginitis 139
Genital Herpes 140
  Clinical Findings 140
  Diagnosis 140
  Treatment 140
Genital Warts 141
  Clinical Findings 141
  Differential Diagnosis 141
  Histology 141
  Treatment 141
Bacterial Infections 142
  Chlamydia Trachomatis 142
Tropical Sexually Transmitted
  Infections 143
  Lymphogranuloma Venereum
    (LGV) 143

Granuloma Inguinale 143
Chancroid 143
Gonorrhoea 144
  Clinical Features 144
  Examination 144
  Treatment 144
  Sexual Partners 144
Syphilis 145
  Primary Syphilis 145
  Diagnosis of Syphilis 146
  Signs and Symptoms of
    Syphilis 147
  Toxic Shock Syndrome 147
Physiological Variation of the
  Cervix 148
  Cervical Ectopy 148
Pelvic Inflammatory Disease 149
  Acute PID 149
  Bacteriology 149
  Differential Diagnosis 149
  Management 149
  Chronic PID 150
Genital Tuberculosis 151
  Clinical Features 151
  Diagnosis 151
  Pathology 151
  Treatment 152
Human Immunodeficiency Virus 153
  Transmission 153
  Acquired Immune Deficiency
    Syndrome (AIDS) 153
  Intercurrent Infections Frequently
    Found in AIDS Patients 154
  Paediatric AIDS 154
  Treatment 154
  Antiretroviral Drugs are the
    Mainstay of Treatment 154

INFLAMMATION IN THE LOWER GYNAECOLOGICAL TRACT

Under normal conditions, the vulva, vagina and ectocervix are the habitat of various types of infective agents, but they are a threat only if normal defence mechanisms are altered.

DEFENCE MECHANISMS

1. *Vaginal acidity*

Glycogen is produced by vaginal epithelium influenced by oestrogens and is converted to lactic acid by Doderlein's bacillus (a type of *B. acidophilus*). This maintains the vaginal pH between 3 and 4 which inhibits most other organisms.

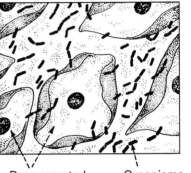

Normal vaginal flora

Desquamated cells

Organisms mostly lactobacilli

(Note absence of pus cells)

2. *Thick layer of vaginal squamous epithelium*

This is a considerable physical barrier to infection. Continual desquamation of the superficial kerato-hyalin layer and glycogen production, both dependent upon ovarian oestrogen action, combat bacteria. In children and postmenopausal patients, the epithelium lacks oestrogen stimulation and is thin and easily traumatised or infected.

3. *Closure of the introitus*

The vaginal canal is only a potential space kept closed by the surrounding muscles and provides another physical barrier. This, however, alters following sexual activity and pregnancy.

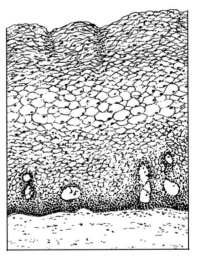

Functional vaginal epithelium: intermediate cells rich in glycogen

4. *Glandular secretions* from the cervix and Bartholin's glands maintain an outward fluid current helping to clear the canal of debris. In addition, cervical secretion contains immunoglobulins, especially IgA, and there are varying numbers of polymorphs, lymphocytes and macrophages.

VULVAL INFLAMMATION

Vulval inflammation is not uncommon but is usually an extension of infection from the vagina. A mild reaction may arise because of physical and anatomical conditions in the area, such as (a) moistness and (b) proximity of urethra and anus.

The area is not only naturally moist but also warm, particularly in obese patients. The folds of fat harbour moisture, and chafing occurs between them. The proliferation of bacteria is encouraged. Urinary incontinence and unsuspected glycosuria may add to this. It is important to test the urine for sugar in all patients.

Incidental factors may intensify any reaction resulting from these conditions, for example, the wearing of nylon underwear which is heat-retaining and non-absorptive. Chemical factors such as washing underclothes with detergents, and using toilet powders, perfumes and deodorants, which intensify the reaction, may be associated with this. The clinical result is irritation and itching leading to scratching. Continual itch-scratch-itch leads to maceration of the skin and may invite infection. Careful attention to personal hygiene is essential. Obese patients should be encouraged to lose weight and all the incidental factors mentioned above should be avoided.

Search for lice or scabies should be made where appropriate.

One of the complications of vulvar inflammation is *obstruction of the duct of Bartholin's gland.* Cystic dilatation and abscess formation are apt to follow. The condition occurs during a woman's sexual life. Any organism, staphylococcal, coliform or gonococcal, may be found.

The gland lies partly behind the bulb of the vestibule and is covered by skin and the bulbospongiosus muscle. The duct is 2 cm long and opens into the vaginal orifice lateral to the hymen.

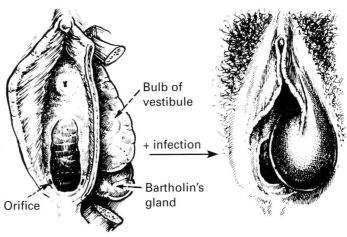

Bulb of vestibule

+ infection

Bartholin's gland

Orifice

TREATMENT
Marsupialisation (Gk. marsipos, a bag). The cyst or abscess is widely opened within the labium minus and drained, and its walls sutured to the skin leaving a large orifice, which it is hoped will form a new duct orifice and allow conservation of the gland. A ribbon-gauze pack is inserted for 48 h by some surgeons.

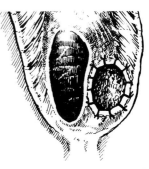

VAGINAL DISCHARGE AND INFECTION

A small amount of vaginal discharge is normal in adult life and may be excessive in the presence of cervical ectopy. Cervical ectopy is where the glandular epithelium from the endocervix is visible on the ectocervix.

COMPOSITION
The vaginal discharge is composed of tissue fluid, cell debris, carbohydrate, lactobacilli and lactic acid. The pH is about 4.5, a degree of acidity that inhibits the growth of organisms other than the lactobacilli.

SOURCE OF VAGINAL DISCHARGE

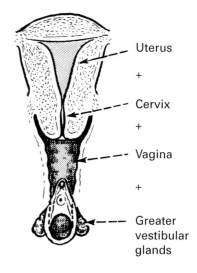

Vulva: Greater vestibular glands, glands of vulval skin.

Vagina: Mainly desquamated epithelial cells which liberate glycogen. The lactobacilli metabolise the glycogen to lactic acid. Vaginal transudate (secretion from tissues and capillaries of the mature vagina) is often described; vaginal epithelium is certainly not water resistant (like transitional epithelium). There are no mucosal glands.

Cervix: Alkaline mucous secretion which becomes copious and watery during ovulation.

Uterine glands also discharge into the vagina.

Uterus
+
Cervix
+
Vagina
+
Greater vestibular glands

CLINICAL FEATURES
Volume: The need to wear a pad or tampon continuously suggests excessive discharge.

Onset: Onset can be associated with the end of a pregnancy, the contraceptive pill, a course of antibiotic.

Colour: Normal discharge is white but stains yellow or pale brown on clothing or pads. A greenish-yellow colour suggests pyogenic infection, commonly accompanied by an unpleasant odour. Red or dark brown suggests blood.

Irritation: Any discharge can in time excoriate the vulva, but often *Candida* and *Trichomonas* cause itching.

COMPLAINTS OF VAGINAL DISCHARGE

Women will complain under the following conditions.

(a) There appears to be an excessive amount of staining on the clothing.
(b) They detect an offensive smell.
(c) They suffer local irritation.

There is often little correlation between symptoms and signs. Some women will complain of what is really normal; and gynaecologists regularly observe heavy and purulent discharge in women who deny any symptoms at all.

EXAMINATION

1. Vulva, perineum and thighs are inspected for signs of excoriation. The vestibular glands and urethral meatus are observed and palpated.
2. Vaginal walls and cervix are examined through a speculum. Normal vaginal epithelium is pink, the rugae are well marked and the epithelial surface of the cervix smooth and moist. Normal discharge is white and odourless.
3. A bimanual examination should always be made.
4. Specimens of discharge are taken for microscopy and culture. *Chlamydia* must be excluded. Cervical rather than vaginal swabs should be taken and a separate swab and appropriate medium are essential for *Chlamydia*. A urine sample can also be taken for *Chlamydia* DNA analysis.

LEUCORRHOEA

This means an excessive amount of normal discharge – a very subjective assessment. The patient will complain of constantly having to change her clothes but there will be no irritation and appearance will be normal. The smell will be the normal vulval odour (from the action of commensal bacteria on the secretions of the apocrine sex glands); microscopy will reveal normal appearances and culture will grow only lactobacilli.

The patient should be reassured and given an explanation of normal physiology. No local treatment is necessary.

VAGINAL DISCHARGE

CANDIDA ALBICANS

This is yeast and exists in two forms – slender branching hyphae or as a small globular spore which multiplies by budding.

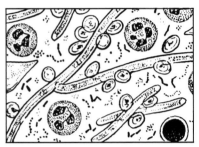

Mycelia and spores of *C. albicans*. Note the presence of leucocytes.

Source of Infection

This organism may exist as a normal commensal in the rectum and small numbers may be found in the vagina. Sexual transmission is also possible. Symptomatic infection is most likely to arise when there are predisposing conditions, examples of which are given below:

1. *Pregnancy.* The vagina provides a tropical microclimate and the high concentration of sex steroids in the blood maintains an increased glycogen formation in the vaginal epithelium and may alter the local pH.
2. *Immunosuppressive therapy.* This includes cytotoxic drugs and corticosteroids. There is also thought to be a natural degree of immunosuppression during pregnancy.
3. *Glycosuria.* This may be due to undiscovered diabetes, but again a mild degree of glycosuria may exist in a normal pregnancy because of the lowering of the renal threshold for sugar.
4. *Antibiotic therapy.* Systemic antibiotics destroy the normal bacteria, thus reducing the competition for nutrients, leaving the field clear for *C. albicans*.

Clinical Features

The patient is usually between 20 and 40, when oestrogen support of the epithelial glycogen content is at its highest. The complaint is of irritant discharge and dyspareunia. Examination reveals an inflamed and tender vagina and vulva with white plaques resembling curdled milk adhering to the vaginal wall and vulva. Removal of the plaque reveals a red inflamed area. Pre-pubertal or postmenopausal infection is less common.

Treatment

A single 500 mg clotrimazole pessary, with external application of 1% clotrimazole cream, offers convenient therapy. Routine treatment of partners is unlikely to reduce recurrence rates. In persistent or recurrent infection, confirmation of the diagnosis by culture and determination of sensitivity to treatment are important.

Oral antifungal medication can also be used.

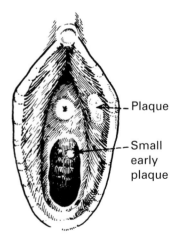

– Plaque

– Small early plaque

VAGINAL DISCHARGE

BACTERIAL VAGINOSIS

For a long time, a large number of cases of vaginitis were labelled non-specific because of disagreement regarding the infective agent. These cases were characterised by a non-irritating, foul-smelling discharge. The discharge contains a mixture of bacteria.

Clinical Features

The patient complains of a foul-smelling discharge, and examination confirms both the discharge and the odour. In appearance, the discharge is thin, greyish and sometimes shows bubbles. A vaginal smear reveals the presence of 'clue' cells. Gram staining is usually negative but can be variable.

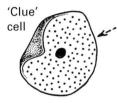

'Clue' cell

Vaginal squame showing stippling of cytoplasm due to adherent cocco-bacilli

Pus cells tend to be few in number. Lactobacilli are also scanty but frequently many other bacteria are present. The pH of the fluid is raised. Although the main complaint is of malodorous discharge, some patients will have pruritus, frequency, dysuria and dyspareunia.

Treatment

Oral metronidazole appears to be effective. Clindamycin vaginal cream may also be employed. Male partners should also be treated.

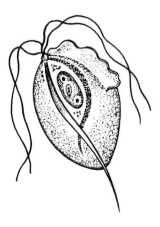

TRICHOMONAS VAGINALIS

T. vaginalis is a protozoan organism, which infests the vagina in women and the urethra, prepuce and prostate in men. It is a common cause of irritant vaginal discharge.

T. vaginalis is a single-cell organism about $20\mu \times 10\mu$, with four flagellae and an undulating membrane which gives it a characteristic jerky movement. It is transmitted mainly during sexual intercourse.

VAGINAL DISCHARGE

TRICHOMONAS VAGINALIS—(cont'd)

Clinical Features

In the acute phase, the patient complains of severe vaginal tenderness and pain, and an irritant discharge. The vagina is seen to be inflamed, sometimes with a patchy strawberry vaginitis, and there is a copious, offensive, frothy discharge. Frequently there is a burning sensation, pruritus, dysuria and dyspareunia. In the latent or dormant phases, there are no symptoms although the presence of the organism can be demonstrated, often in a cervical smear.

Incidence

T. vaginalis affects perhaps 18% of the female population. It is commonly found in patients with gonorrhoea and is associated with cervical dysplasia. No cause-and-effect relationship has been proved.

Diagnosis

Diagnosis is by observation of the motile organisms in a fresh smear diluted with saline and by laboratory culture.

Treatment

Always systemic and, if possible, including the patient's sexual partner. Metronidazole (Flagyl) 400 mg thrice daily for a week, or 2 g orally once daily.

Pathology

Passing from host to host during coitus, *T. vaginalis* attaches itself to the vaginal epithelium and multiplies rapidly, taking glycogen away from lactobacilli, which disappear. The vaginal pH rises to about 5.5, allowing the increase of bacterial pathogens that aggravate the infection and resulting discharge.

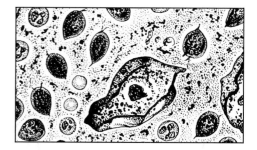

VAGINITIS

ATROPHIC VAGINITIS

This occurs at times when ovarian activity ceases with the onset of menopause, after surgical removal of the ovaries or following ablation by radiotherapy or chemotherapy.

Clinical Features

Symptoms consist of irritation and vaginal dryness. Discharge may occur if superimposed infection has occurred. Examination of the vaginal mucosa reveals a rash of petechial haemorrhages and there may be ulceration. Smears show rounded epithelial cells, with no glycogen, many polymorphs and bacteria. In neglected cases intravaginal adhesions may develop. Topical vaginal oestrogen quickly reverses the changes. This is available as creams or pessaries. There is also a silicon vaginal ring containing oestrogen for management of atrophic changes.

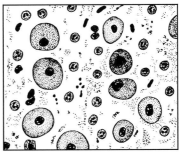

Vaginal smear of atrophic type, with numerous polymorphs, a mixed bacterial content and para-basal epithelial cells.

VULVOVAGINITIS IN CHILDREN

This is a less common condition and arises only in certain circumstances, for example, those given below.

  (a) Sexual interference.
  (b) Insertion of foreign bodies by a child herself.
  (c) Threadworm infestation.

With reference to the above points.

  (a) the changes will be those of physical damage to the tissues. Infection will depend to some extent on whether the person guilty of the offence is a carrier of a specific agent.
  (b) infection may arise from bowel commensals.
  (c) the diagnosis may be made by applying Sellotape (Scotch tape) to the vulva then pressing the tape onto a microscope slide for microscopic examination.

Many of the cases of vulvovaginitis may arise from the irritation caused by threadworms. Scratching will lead to maceration of the skin, which in turn will encourage bacterial contamination.

FOREIGN BODIES

Vaginitis due to foreign bodies is sometimes seen in adults. Tampons, contraceptive devices and supportive pessaries used for prolapse may be left, forgotten, *in situ*. These give rise to an offensive purulent discharge. Bacteriological investigation will give an indication of the type of infection and appropriate treatment following removal of the offending body.

OTHER CAUSES OF VAGINITIS

Secondary vaginitis may arise because of contamination of the vagina through fistulous openings (vesicovaginal or rectovaginal) following injury, surgical operations or tumour growth. Repeated attacks of infection may occur. Treatment is obviously repair of the fistula where this is possible.

In all cases of vaginal discharge, the possibility of malignant disease in the tract must be considered.

GENITAL HERPES

Herpes simplex virus (HSV) types 1 and 2 may affect the lower genital tract or the mouth. It is highly infectious – 80% of women in contact with male carriers become infected. The initial attack may be severe. There may be, in 50% of victims, less severe recurring attacks every 3 or 4 weeks and they represent a potential for wide dissemination to others in the immediate environment. The incubation period is short – 3–7 days.

CLINICAL FINDINGS

The disease affects the vulvovaginal and peri-anal regions but may be transmitted to the mouth. The patient complains of burning, itching and hyperaesthesia of the area and the skin shows evidence of acute inflammation – oedema and erythema. There is usually a vaginal discharge. If the peri-urethral area is involved, there may be dysuria and retention of urine.

The specific lesions start as small indurated tender papules which become vesicles and quickly break down to form shallow ulcers, 5 mm or more in diameter, with a yellowish grey slough in the base. These can be seen on the vulva and labia, but in some cases they are confined to the vagina and cervix and there may be no external evidence of the disease. In these circumstances the ulcers may be large and could be mistaken for carcinoma of the cervix. The inguinal nodes are enlarged. The infection is accompanied by general symptoms of malaise, headache and even encephalitis. Sacral ganglion involvement causes neuralgia.

The acute phase lasts for 4–5 days. The lesions heal over 8–10 days and then a latent period ensues during which the virus remains in the sacral ganglia. Further attacks may follow.

Infection of the neonate can lead to herpes encephalitis with a primary infection.

DIAGNOSIS

Clinical suspicion is confirmed by tissue culture isolation of virus or detection of virus antigen by immunofluorescence or ELISA techniques. Some degree of immunity may be conferred during recurrent attacks and a search for antibodies will help to differentiate primary from second attacks.

TREATMENT

Ice packs, local analgesia (2% lidocaine), non-steroidal analgesic creams, saline bathing and systemic analgesics help relieve acute local symptoms. Aciclovir 3% ointment, applied repeatedly, is effective only if commenced at the onset of signs and symptoms.

Oral antiviral agents such as aciclovir for 5 days may be commenced within 5 days of onset of a first episode. Antibiotics may be required if there is secondary infection. Antiviral agents do not eradicate the virus and recurrent episodes may occur.

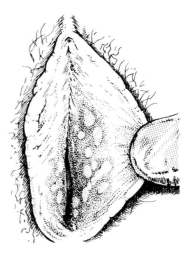

Chromatin at nuclear membrane

Eosinophilic inclusion bodies

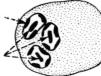

GENITAL WARTS

Genital warts are a common viral infection. They are caused by human papilloma viruses (HPVs) which are transmitted sexually, with more that 50% of contacts developing lesions. Numbers 6 and 11 are particularly associated with warts or condylomata. Infectivity is greatest just after appearance of a wart. Incubation varies from a few weeks to 9 months or more.

CLINICAL FINDINGS

A single warty growth quickly spreads to form multiple growths showing a tendency to fuse. They are pinkish with dry surfaces unless macerated and are of softer consistency than the ordinary skin wart. The growths develop in moist areas and especially during pregnancy. They affect the labia, peri-anal area, perineum and the lower part of the vagina, and may even spread to the thighs. Secondary infection may give rise to purulent discharge.

DIFFERENTIAL DIAGNOSIS

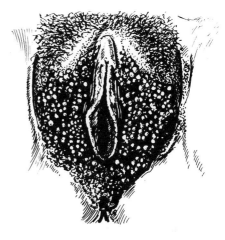

1. *Syphilitic condylomata.* These are more widespread and not confined to the genital area. They are also flatter and more rounded. Treponemes can be found in the tissue fluid. Serological tests will of course confirm the diagnosis.
2. *Benign papilloma.* This is commonly single and similar to ordinary skin warts.
3. *Verrucous carcinoma.* This is a locally malignant lesion, but vulval carcinoma is rare in premenopausal patients. Biopsy will differentiate the two conditions.
4. Sometimes, genital warts affect the cervix and can resemble carcinoma.

HISTOLOGY

The warts have a central core of connective tissue covered by a thick layer of prickle cells. Chronic inflammatory changes are present in the dermis.

TREATMENT

Podophyllotoxin, a cytotoxic agent, can be used. It is topically painted on the lesions. It is toxic if used systemically and may not be used in pregnancy.

Imiquimod cream is an alternative. It works by stimulating the immune response but is also unsuitable during pregnancy.

Cryo-cautery, electro-cautery and laser ablation can be employed. Lesions may recur and may also regress spontaneously.

BACTERIAL INFECTIONS

CHLAMYDIA TRACHOMATIS
This is a widespread gynaecological infection.

Clinical Features
The initial symptoms in women are often mild and may in fact be asymptomatic. Discharge may be present, varying from watery to frankly purulent according to the severity of the reaction to the disease. In severe cases, there is obvious cervicitis which looks like an infected erosion. Sometimes, there is a punctate haemorrhagic inflammation with microabscesses. Occasionally, there are few changes in the vagina and the first evidence of infection is the appearance of a salpingitis. It is an important cause of chronic pelvic inflammation.
A gelatinous exudate is formed in the Pouch of Douglas which proceeds to multiple adhesions and tubal occlusion.

It is an important cause of infertility. Ophthalmia neonatorum occurs if there is transmission to the neonate during delivery.

Reiter's syndrome with urethritis, arthritis and conjunctivitis is more common in the infected male.

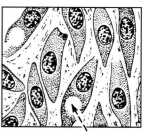

Chlamydia

It may spread to cause perihepatitis with so-called violin string adhesions to the parietal peritoneum. This is accompanied by acute pain in the upper right quadrant and is known as Fitz–Hugh–Curtis syndrome. It can be mistaken for cholecystitis or pancreatitis.

Diagnosis
Culture of *Chlamydia* requires sampling of endocervical cells, urethral cells or endosalpinx cells (salpingitis detected at surgery). They should be sent in special transport medium to an appropriate laboratory.

Nucleic acid amplification techniques are now commonly used to diagnose chlamydia from a vulval swab or a first-void urine sample, with 30% greater sensitivity than viral culture.

The organism can be seen under the microscope. It is intracellular. Staining by an immunofluorescence technique confirms the diagnosis. It multiplies like bacteria, but like viruses can only do so within cells. It contains both DNA and RNA.

Treatment
Azithromycin 1 g as a single dose or doxycycline 100 mg orally, twice a day for 7 days. Azithromycin and doxycycline are equally effective. The primary advantage of azithromycin is that it is administered in a single dose. Erythromycin should be given in pregnancy.

TROPICAL SEXUALLY TRANSMITTED INFECTIONS

LYMPHOGRANULOMA VENEREUM (LGV)
LGV is attributed to a strain of *Chlamydia*. This is rare in the developed countries.

Clinical Findings
The primary lesion is a small painless ulcer with raised irregular borders which may involve the labia, clitoris or urethra. It appears 1–3 weeks after infection. Several weeks later the inguinal and iliac lymph nodes enlarge, become soft and fluctuant and this is followed by rupture creating discharging sinuses. The lesions eventually heal with the creation of large fibrous scars. In the process, the urethra may be virtually destroyed and the rectum stenosed. The pelvic organs may be involved in the same way giving rise to intestinal obstruction and various fistulous communications.

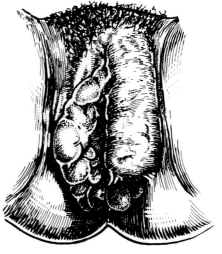

Histologically, the reaction is of granulomatous type. Lymph channels are often obstructed giving rise to elephantiasis of the vulva. The picture shows an advanced case of LGV.

Treatment: Tetracyclines, doxycyline or erythromycin is effective.

GRANULOMA INGUINALE
Granuloma inguinale is another tropical ulcerative condition, caused by *Klebsiella granulomatis*; this begins as a painless genital, inguinal or peri-anal nodule, which ulcerates. Local lymphatic glands enlarge, but do not ulcerate.

Prolonged antibiotic treatment is required.

CHANCROID
This lesion is due to infection by *Haemophilus ducreyii*. After a short incubation period, a red macule appears, which quickly changes to a pustule and then an ulcer. The ulcers are numerous and vary in size from millimetres to several centimetres. They are well defined with projecting margins but shallow with a greenish slough in the base. These ulcers are soft and painful. This, together with the short incubation period, helps to differentiate them from syphilitic lesions. The labia major, clitoris and peri-anal regions are affected. Two weeks later the local lymph nodes tend to enlarge and suppurate. There is usually secondary infection and the discharge is foul smelling.

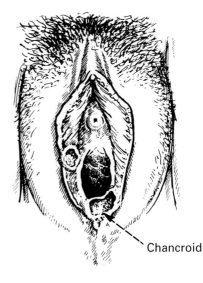

Chancroid

Treatment
Azithromycin, ceftriaxone or erythromycin may be used.

143

GONORRHOEA

Gonorrhoea in women carries a high risk of salpingitis and sterility, but early diagnosis is difficult to achieve. Symptoms are often mild or absent.

CLINICAL FEATURES
The classical history is of urethritis, vaginal discharge and menstrual upset of sudden onset, but any infection in the genital area, however it presents, may be gonococcal. After the acute phase, vaginal discharge will persist, followed in approximately 15% of cases by signs of pelvic inflammatory disease (PID).

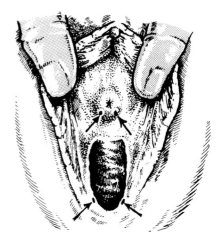

Systemic signs – conjunctivitis, dermatitis, arthritis – are rare in women.

EXAMINATION
The labia are held apart, and the urethra, Skene's ducts and Bartholin's ducts examined for signs of infection. Swabs are taken from the cervix which is the main reservoir of infection.

Diagnosis is a laboratory procedure. Intracellular diplococci may be seen with Gram staining, or the more time consuming immunofluorescent method. Alternative tests include nucleic amplification tests (NAATs) and nucleic acid hybridisation tests. NAATs are more sensitive than culture and can also be used as diagnostic/screening tests on non-invasively collected specimens (urine and self-taken vaginal swabs). Caution is required in interpretation of positive results as the specificity of NAATs is not 100%. Confirmation of a NAAT positive result by culture is advisable. This is also useful to assess for antibiotic sensitivities.

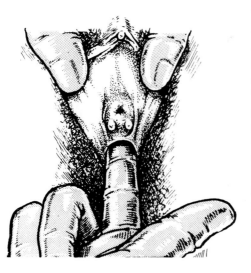

TREATMENT
Uncomplicated anogenital infection in adults: ceftriaxone 250 mg IM as a single dose or cefixime 400 mg oral as a single dose. Antimicrobial therapy should take account of local patterns of antimicrobial sensitivity to *Neisseria gonorrhoeae*. The chosen regimen should eliminate infection in at least 95% of those presenting in the local community. Alternative regimens may be required when an infection is known to be unresponsive to these antimicrobials.

SEXUAL PARTNERS
Partner notification should be pursued in all patients identified with gonococcal infection, preferably by a trained health adviser in genito-urinary medicine.

SYPHILIS

Syphilis is an uncommon disease in gynaecological practice, but any genital sore should come under suspicion. It is less uncommon in association with human immunodeficiency virus. Pregnant women continue to be screened for syphilis in the UK despite its very low levels, as transmission can occur to the fetus.

PRIMARY SYPHILIS

The chancre (a corruption of 'cancer') has an incubation period of about a month and its appearance is often accompanied by pyrexia and malaise. The most common site is the vulva and then the cervix, but infection can occur anywhere. The chancre is the point at which the treponema enters the body.

The typical chancre is about 1 cm in diameter and begins as a reddish papule which becomes ulcerated. It is painless and highly infective. The inguinal glands are markedly enlarged.

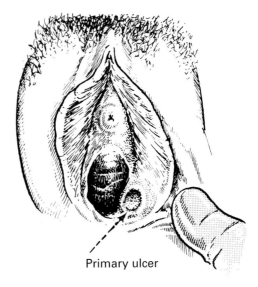

Primary ulcer

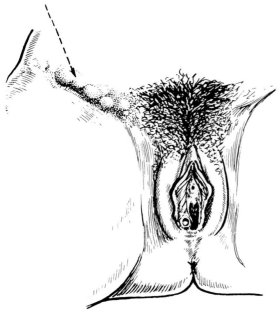

Diagnosis requires the identification of *Treponema pallidum* in the exudate of the chancre or in material aspirated from an enlarged gland. Treponemata are not easily recognisable in stained preparations and the dark-ground illumination of fresh specimens is used. Light is reflected off the edges of the organisms, making them easy to perceive and they are recognised by their shape and movement. *T. pallidum* must be distinguished from other treponemata.

SYPHILIS

DIAGNOSIS OF SYPHILIS

Positive identification of *T. pallidum* is difficult for various reasons including the failure, so far, to grow the organism *in vitro*. The usual method of diagnosis is by serological tests, which become positive 4–6 weeks after infection.

Enzyme immunoassay (EIA) tests which detect antitreponemal IgM and IgG antibodies are useful as screening tests. Confirmation is required in the context of a positive EIA.

These include TPHA (*Treponema pallidum* haemagglutination) and fluorescent treponemal antibody absorption. False positives can occur.

Fluorescent Treponemal Antibody
Principle of Fluorescent Treponemal Antibody tests (FTA)

1. Antihuman globulin (AHG) is combined with fluorescein.

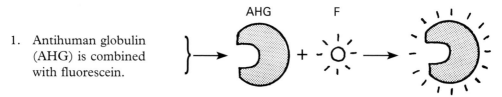

2. Dead treponeme is combined with test serum. If subject is infected, the treponeme acquires a coating of globulin antibody.

3. 1 and 2 are combined and the treponeme becomes fluorescent.

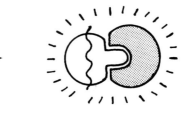

SYPHILIS

SIGNS AND SYMPTOMS OF SYPHILIS

Signs and symptoms of the spread of *T. pallidum* throughout the whole body appear usually about 2 months after the primary stage, and the disease may present in this phase to the gynaecologist.

There is likely to be a mild pyrexia and malaise, but the dominating signs are a generalised lymphadenopathy and mucocutaneous lesions. 'Snail track' ulcers appear on mucosal surfaces, and the skin develops a very wide variety of macular and papular rashes. In warm moist areas such as the breast flexures and the vulva, the papules become hypertrophic and flattened and present as 'condylomata lata', which are highly infective.

Diagnosis is by the demonstration of *T. pallidum* in the lesions and by serological tests.

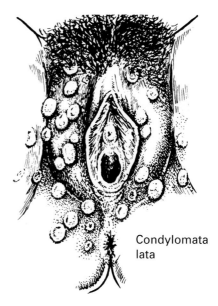

Condylomata lata

Treatment of Early Contagious Syphilis

T. pallidum is sensitive to many antibiotics, but reactions are common and care is required in treatment. Prolonged antibiotic treatment, mainly penicillin based, is required and long-term follow-up should be performed by an infectious disease specialist.

If not treated in the early stages, syphilis leads to a complex immune reaction and the patient can develop cardiovascular and neurological complications many months or years later.

TOXIC SHOCK SYNDROME

This is a very rare syndrome which can arise in women using tampons. It is caused by exotoxins produced by staphylococci which may be carried by the woman herself in various sites such as the vagina, cervix, perineum or nasopharynx.

Clinical Signs

There is a rapid onset of fever often with vomiting, diarrhoea, muscular aches and skin erythema. It can be a life-threatening condition.

Treatment should provide general supportive measures and antibiotic treatment, usually clindamycin.

PHYSIOLOGICAL VARIATION OF THE CERVIX

CERVICAL ECTOPY

Columnar epithelium appears on the cervical surface. This is usually because of physiological changes, for example, eversion which occurs as the cervix develops during puberty and the squamocolumnar junction becomes visible. This is physiological and no treatment is required. It is also common in pregnancy and while on the contraceptive pill.

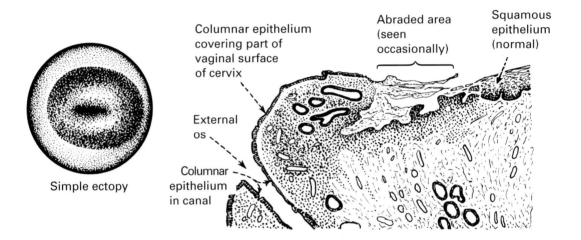

Women who have symptoms relating to an ectopy may opt for local treatment with the aim of ablating the columnar cells so that squamous cells develop. A number of techniques have been employed. The patient will experience a prolonged heavy discharge and the ectopy may recur.

PELVIC INFLAMMATORY DISEASE

Infection of the fallopian tubes usually involves the ovaries and peritoneum, and the combined infection is called pelvic inflammatory disease (PID). It results from ascending infection by micro-organisms from the vagina or cervix. Its incidence is closely related to that of sexually transmitted diseases and it is predominantly a disease of young, sexually active, women.

ACUTE PID

The following clinical features are suggestive of a diagnosis of PID: bilateral lower abdominal tenderness (sometimes radiating to the legs); abnormal vaginal or cervical discharge; fever (greater than 38°C); abnormal vaginal bleeding (intermenstrual, postcoital or 'breakthrough'); deep dyspareunia; cervical motion tenderness on bimanual vaginal examination and adnexal tenderness on bimanual vaginal examination (with or without a palpable mass).

BACTERIOLOGY

N. gonorrhoea and *C. trachomatis* are said to be the commonest pathogens, but anaerobic organisms are often found in pelvic abscesses.

DIFFERENTIAL DIAGNOSIS

Appendicitis

Signs are mainly right sided, and the menstrual cycle is undisturbed.

Diverticulitis

This is a disease mainly of older women and signs are left sided.

Torsion of Pedicle of a Cyst

There may be a history of intermittent pain over several months. A cyst should be palpable.

Tubal Pregnancy

A positive HCG pregnancy test should suggest ectopic pregnancy.

MANAGEMENT

In the Outpatient Setting

An intrauterine device, if in the uterus, should be removed. After swabs have been taken from the vagina and cervix, a broad spectrum antibiotic such as doxycycline, azithromycin or ampicillin should be given. This should be on the basis of one of the following regimens recommended by the Royal College of Obstetricians and Gynaecologists, UK (Greentop Guideline 32, Management of Acute Pelvic Inflammatory Disease):

- Oral ofloxacin 400 mg twice daily plus oral metronidazole 400 mg twice daily for 14 days
- Intramuscular ceftriaxone 250 mg single dose followed by oral doxycycline 100 mg twice daily plus metronidazole 400 mg twice daily for 14 days.

If acute signs and symptoms persist, an ultrasound should be carried out to search for abscess formation. Surgical intervention to drain abscesses may be required.

Referral to a genito-urinary medicine clinic is advisable. Without tracing and treatment of contacts, reinfection is likely. Acute PID may be relatively asymptomatic, but this does not preclude tubal damage, infertility and ectopic pregnancy. Ectopic pregnancy follows in almost 10% of subjects compared with a background rate of 1.5%.

PELVIC INFLAMMATORY DISEASE

CHRONIC PID

The patient complains of pelvic pain made worse during the periods, which are irregular and heavy. Dyspareunia is common. There is a 10-fold increase in hysterectomy after PID.

Examination

Some swelling may be felt, but often there is little to find except tenderness in the fornices.

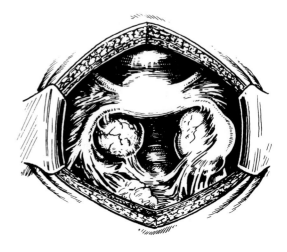

Pathology

All degrees of inflammation are met with, from salpingitis alone to a widespread inflammatory reaction involving all the pelvic tissues. It is rare to recover any organism in chronic PID, other than in the case of tuberculosis. The ascending infection first attacks the tubes which are sealed off by oedema and adhesions. The tubes either swell up with watery exudate forming a hydrosalpinx or pyosalpinx; or they become highly thickened and adherent to the ovary. The ovary may also be the seat of abscess formation, and the uterus and adnexa, normally mobile, become fixed by adhesions.

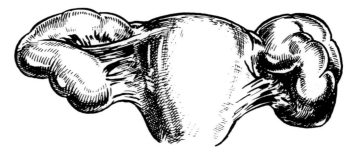

Blocked and distended tubes in PID

Treatment

The course of chronic PID is not predictable, and mild degrees may resolve spontaneously. Where possible, any infective agents should be identified and treated. Hydrosalpinx and any abscess formation must be relieved by laparotomy and drainage. In advanced cases however, the only effective treatment is operation to remove the uterus and tubes and perhaps the ovaries as well.

GENITAL TUBERCULOSIS

Tuberculosis is a rare disease in gynaecology. It attacks the fallopian tubes and the endometrium. Lesions elsewhere in the genital tract are uncommon.

CLINICAL FEATURES

The patient is usually a young woman seeking treatment for primary infertility or complaining of irregular menstruation or perhaps abdominal pain.

DIAGNOSIS

1. Histological evidence from curettings. This is the commonest method and it is assumed that the tubes are also infected.
2. Laboratory culture.
3. Biopsy from any suspicious ulcerated area in the vagina or vulva.
4. By laparoscopic inspection and biopsy.

Once evidence of genital infection is obtained, the respiratory and urinary tracts must also be investigated.

PATHOLOGY

This infection is blood borne, usually from a primary focus in the lung or kidney, and it infects the tubes, spreading thence to the endometrium.

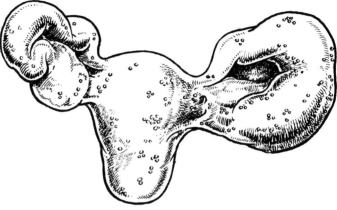

The tubes may appear normal (endosalpingitis) but usually display the distortion and swelling of chronic infection, and small pinhead tubercles appear on the serosa.

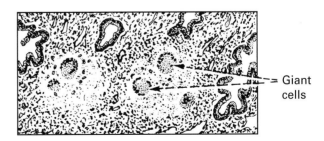

Giant cells

The endometrium also shows tuberculous follicles, best developed in the premenstrual phase. There may be debris in endometrial glands.

151

GENITAL TUBERCULOSIS

TREATMENT

Antituberculous Chemotherapy

A combination of rifampicin, isoniazid and ethambutol has been used effectively in recent years. This should be managed by an infectious disease specialist.

Surgery

Surgery may be required when chemotherapy has failed (about 5% of cases) or in combination with chemotherapy in older women. All infected tissue must be removed to avoid subsequent fistulous openings in the bowel or bladder.

Tuberculosis and Infertility

Failure to conceive is probably the most important consequence of genital tuberculosis, and 90% of women presenting with the disease will never have a pregnancy. There is also an increased chance of ectopic gestation.

HUMAN IMMUNODEFICIENCY VIRUS

TRANSMISSION

The following are the main modes of transmission of human immunodeficiency virus (HIV):

- Unprotected penetrative sex with someone who is infected.
- Injection or transfusion of contaminated blood or blood products, donations of semen (artificial insemination), skin grafts or organ transplants taken from someone who is infected.
- From a mother who is infected to her baby; this can occur during pregnancy, at birth and through breastfeeding.
- Sharing unsterilised injection equipment that has previously been used by someone who is infected.

The course of the disease is erratic, associated with progressive loss of immune resistance. Death is almost inevitable but may be delayed for years with appropriate antiviral treatment.

ACQUIRED IMMUNE DEFICIENCY SYNDROME (AIDS)

The progress of the disease can be roughly divided into six phases, but these phases are ill-defined, and variable in time of onset and duration:

1. Infection
2. Window period
3. Seroconversion
4. Asymptomatic period
5. HIV/AIDS-related illness
6. AIDS.

The duration of the different phases of HIV/AIDS is variable. It is not possible to predict the course of the disease in an individual. Factors affecting the course of HIV/AIDS include nutrition, emotional stress and access to health care. People infected with HIV can infect others at any phase of the disease.

Three conditions are particularly characteristic of the immunodeficiency state:

1. Kaposi sarcoma, usually an indolent growth in the skin, becomes aggressive.
2. Hairy leukoplakia of the tongue.
3. Lymphomas are common in AIDS patients and lymphoma of the brain is almost diagnostic.

HUMAN IMMUNODEFICIENCY VIRUS

INTERCURRENT INFECTIONS FREQUENTLY FOUND IN AIDS PATIENTS

Minor infections and infestations, which remain localised in normally immune persons and produce mild symptoms if any, spread rapidly and cause life-threatening clinical conditions in the AIDS patient whose immunity is seriously compromised.

Infective agents	Clinical results
Parasites *Pneumocystis carinii* *Cryptosporidium* *Strongyloides stercoralis* *Toxoplasma gondii*	Pneumonia Severe diarrhoea Severe diarrhoea Chorio-retinitis
Viruses Herpes J.C. virus	Pneumonia Leuco-encephalopathy
Bacteria Species usually causing minor lesions, e.g. skin spots	Septicaemia
Fungi *Cryptococcus neoformans*	Pneumonia, meningitis

PAEDIATRIC AIDS

Infection of the fetus or newborn from the mother can occur *in utero*, intrapartum or, through breastfeeding, post-partum. Zidovudine has been shown to reduce vertical transmission of HIV-1.

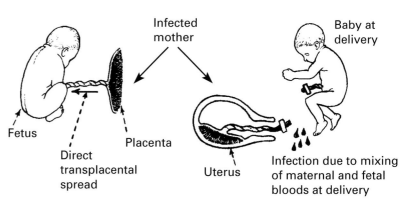

Infected mother

Baby at delivery

Fetus

Direct transplacental spread

Placenta

Uterus

Infection due to mixing of maternal and fetal bloods at delivery

TREATMENT

Specialised knowledge and experience are essential.

ANTIRETROVIRAL DRUGS ARE THE MAINSTAY OF TREATMENT

Combination therapy is used and for many patients can significantly control the disease within developing countries access to antiretroviral therapy may be limited. There is ongoing research to develop a vaccine.

CHAPTER 8

DISEASES OF THE VULVA

Vulval Dermatoses — 156
  Classification — *156*
  Lichen Sclerosus — *157*
Benign Tumours of the Vulva — 158
Vulval Intraepithelial Neoplasia — 159
  Vulval Intraepithelial Neoplasia (VIN) — *159*
  Paget's Disease of the Vulva (Adenocarcinoma
    In Situ) — *159*
Carcinoma of the Vulva — 160
  Aetiology — *160*
  Histology — *160*
  Clinical Features — *160*
  Lymphatic Spread — *161*
  Surgical Treatment — *162*
  Complications — *164*
  Radiotherapy and Chemotherapy — *164*
  Prognosis of Vulval Carcinoma — *164*
Diseases of the Urethra — 165
  Prolapse of the Urethral Mucosa — *165*
  Caruncle — *165*
  Urethrocele — *165*

VULVAL DERMATOSES

Vulval dermatoses is the term applied to non-infective non-neoplastic diseases of the vulval skin. Their management has evolved into a multidisciplinary approach involving specialist nursing staff, dermatologists and gynaecologists. Specialist clinics may have direct referrals, but the symptoms of itching, soreness and dyspareunia will usually take the patient in the first place to the gynaecologist.

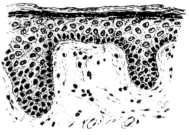

Normal vulva

CLASSIFICATION
The following classification is recommended by the International Society for the Study of Vulvar Disease (ISSVD – 2004).

Non-neoplastic disorders of the vulva
   lichen sclerosus
   lichen planus
   other dermatoses
Vulval intraepithelial neoplasia (VIN)
   VIN, usual type
      (i) warty
      (ii) basaloid
      (iii) mixed
   VIN, differentiated type
      Paget's disease

VULVAL DERMATOSES

LICHEN SCLEROSUS

Lichen sclerosus is a common condition found in postmenopausal women complaining of vulval itch. Premenopausal women may also be affected, as well as men and children. The aetiology is unknown, but it appears to be associated with autoimmune disorders.

It is most commonly seen in the vulvo-perineal skin of women, but can affect skin in any region of the body.

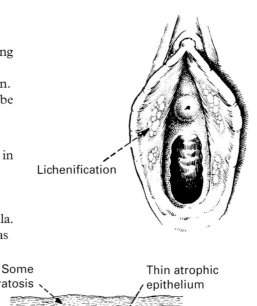

Lichenification

Appearance
The disease starts as a flat pinkish-white macula. As it progresses, there is atrophy of the labia as well as clitoral recession with loss of normal architecture. With further deterioration, labial fusion and perineal fissuring occur. Scratching may induce lichenification (thickening).

Some hyperkeratosis

Thin atrophic epithelium

Histology
There is atrophic thinning of the epidermis with some hyalinisation of the dermis. The keratinised layer is thickened, giving a whitened appearance ('leukoplakia').

Hyalinisation of dermis

Differential Diagnosis of Vulval Itch
Lichen planus, lichen simplex, candidiasis, VIN, psoriasis.

Management
Ultrapotent steroid such as clobetasol propionate (suggested regimen)
    Apply once daily 4 weeks.
    Apply alternate days for 4 weeks.
    Apply twice weekly for 4 weeks.
    NB maintenance/interval treatment with clobetasol at previous minimal effective frequency.
Soap substitute
There is an extremely limited role for vulval surgery in the management of this condition, unless there is suspected malignancy.

If asymptomatic, no treatment is required.

Malignant Associations
A recent estimate suggests that 5% of women with lichen sclerosus will develop invasive cancer.

157

BENIGN TUMOURS OF THE VULVA

The complaint is usually of a 'lump' or 'swelling' at the vaginal introitus. (In many cases, the patient may mistake prolapse of various types for tumour growth.)

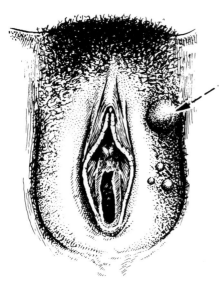

Cyst of Bartholin's gland This is the commonest simple tumour of the vulva. Caused by obstruction of the duct, the cyst often becomes infected and requires surgical treatment (see p. 133).

Sebaceous cyst of the vulva occurs in the hair-bearing vulval tissue. The cyst may become infected and cause pain. The cyst contains whitish, cheesy sebaceous material. If painful, it can be removed.

Vulval haematoma is a result of direct violence or wounding (it is most commonly found with childbirth). Treatment is by incision, evacuation and drainage if the patient is symptomatic.

Lipoma, fibroma and myoma are found rarely and can become sarcomatous. Treatment is by excision, following appropriate imaging assessment. Magnetic resonance imaging (MRI) is usually the imaging modality of choice.

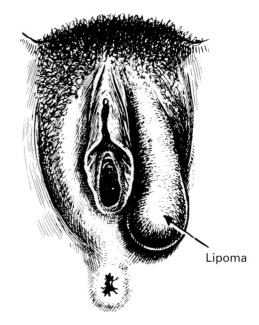

Lipoma

VULVAL INTRAEPITHELIAL NEOPLASIA

VULVAL INTRAEPITHELIAL NEOPLASIA (VIN)
There are two main types of VIN – usual and differentiated. Usual type is associated with oncogenic human papilloma virus (HPV), whereas differentiated type is not always associated with HPV infection; however, both can be precursors of vulval carcinoma.

HPV infection can infect all cloacal origin epithelium causing intraepithelial neoplasia. The site of epithelium affected dictates the term used to describe it: vaginal intraepithelial neoplasia (VAIN); anal intraepithelial neoplasia (AIN); and peri-anal intraepithelial neoplasia (PAIN). As such, intraepithelial neoplasia can often be a multifocal disease with histological features similar to that of cervical intraepithelial neoplasia (CIN). The malignant potential of VIN is thought to be less than that of CIN. However, the mechanism whereby it causes dyspaltic change is the same and can be reviewed on page 175.

VIN may present with vulval itch, burning or pain. However, it may be detected when abnormal skin is identified by the patient or when the patient is undergoing gynaecological examination for other reasons.

There is no distinct appearance, with the changes often being subtle. Lesions may be macular, papular with the abnormal area appearing mainly white but also red or pigmented in some cases. Diagnosis can be confirmed by biopsy.

Treatment of VIN
1. Careful observation only as spontaneous resolution can occur.
2. Wide local excision to achieve a clear margin, with or without plastic surgery.
3. CO_2 laser vaporisation.

Following treatment, patients should be seen regularly in the clinic as recurrent or new intraepithelial neoplasia can occur necessitating further treatment.

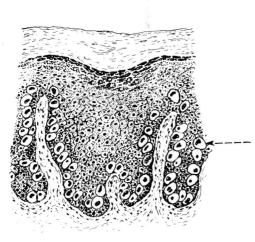

PAGET'S DISEASE OF THE VULVA (ADENOCARCINOMA *IN SITU*)
This malignant disease starts as an erythematous, irritant plaque which becomes eczematous (oedema and exudate) and spreads. The disease is multi-focal and the true margins are indistinct. To determine the margins, mapping biopsies from the periphery are required. Histology shows the characteristic Paget's cells – large round, clear-staining cells with large nuclei, often mitotic.

Thirty percent patients may have an underlying adenocarcinoma of the vulva, cervix, bladder, ovary, rectum or breast. Wide local excision of the lesion is the treatment of choice and plastic surgical reconstruction may be required.

159

CARCINOMA OF THE VULVA

Vulval cancer is very rare in young women.

Incidence
        1 per 100,000 women aged 25–44
        3 per 100,000 in those aged 45–64
        13.2 per 100,000 in women aged 65 and over (UK).

AETIOLOGY

The aetiology of squamous vulval cancer is related to the underlying vulval skin disorder.

The differentiated type is associated with underlying conditions such as lichen sclerosis and is not HPV related. The remaining squamous cancers are associated with oncogenic HPV infection. The mechanism for oncogenic HPV cancer induction can be reviewed on page 175.

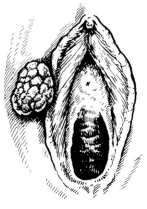

Squamous carcinoma

HISTOLOGY
Squamous carcinoma: 85%
Melanoma: 5%

CLINICAL FEATURES
The majority of patients with vulval cancer are over 60. The presenting features include vulval irritation and pruritus (70%), a vulval mass (60%) and bleeding (30%).

The diagnosis is often delayed, partly due to the patient's reluctance to seek medical help, and partly because of delay in performing a clinical examination once the patient presents.

Any lump on the vulva must be examined and if suspicious biopsied.

The inguinal lymph nodes may be enlarged, but absence of enlargement does not guarantee absence of lymphatic spread.

The FIGO staging of vulvar cancer 2009

Stage	Definition
Stage I 　　IA 　　IB	Confined to vulva. Tumour 2 cm or less maximum diameter. Stromal invasion no greater than 1 mm. No nodal metastases. As for IA, but stromal invasion greater than 1 mm.
Stage II	Tumour of any size with extension to adjacent perineal structures (lower 1/3 urethra, lower 1/3 vagina, anus). Negative nodes.
Stage III 　　III A 　　III B 　　III C	Tumour of any size with or without extension to adjacent perineal structures (1/3 lower urethra, 1/3 lower vagina, anus) with positive inguino-femoral lymph nodes. (i) With 1 lymph node metastasis ($\geq$5 mm), or (ii) 1–2 lymph node metastasis(es) (<5 mm). (i) With 2 or more lymph node metastases ($\geq$5 mm), or (ii) 3 or more lymph node metastases (b5 mm). With positive nodes with extracapsular spread.
Stage IV A	Tumour invades any of the following: (i) upper urethral and/or vaginal mucosa, bladder mucosa, rectal mucosa, or fixed to pelvic bone, or (ii) fixed or ulcerated inguino-femoral lymph nodes.
Stage IV B	Any distant metastasis, including pelvic lymph node.

CARCINOMA OF THE VULVA

LYMPHATIC SPREAD

1. To the superficial inguinal glands which lie along the inguinal ligament and the saphenous vein (vertical group). These nodes lie between the layers of the superficial fascia in relation to numerous superficial vessels.

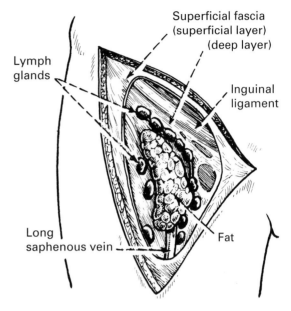

2. Then to the deep femoral nodes accompanying the femoral vessels, and from there to the external iliac, common iliac, and para-aortic glands.

3. This path is not invariably followed. The superficial nodes are occasionally bypassed. To detect aberrant pathways, techniques such as sentinel lymph node biopsy are being increasingly used. Using patent blue dye and radioactive tracer injection techniques, the primary drainage lymphatic pathway can be identified. This technique may also reduce the risk of lymphoedema.

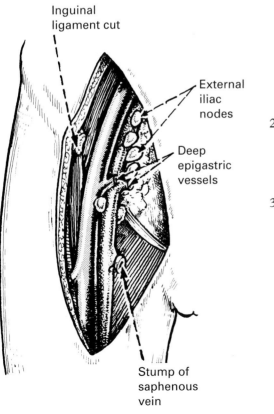

CARCINOMA OF THE VULVA

SURGICAL TREATMENT

Surgery is the optimum treatment for vulval cancer.

The conventional operation was radical vulvectomy with dissection of the superficial and deep inguinal glands and the external iliac glands. Such surgery increased the five-year survival for the disease.

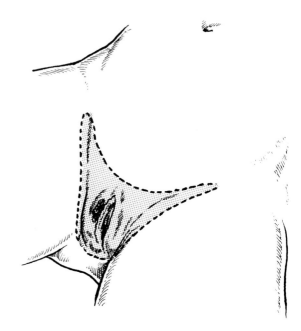

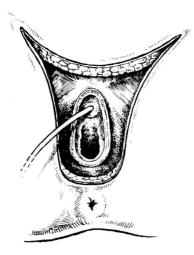

The whole vulva, skin and subcutaneous tissue are excised down to the periosteum.

The wound would be closed completely if possible, undercutting and mobilising skin if necessary. In this picture, closure is incomplete, but the small raw area would heal in a few weeks. Drains are shown, which remain in place for the first few days. Surgery for vulval cancer has evolved with the above illustrations providing a context for the need to improve and reduce morbidity.

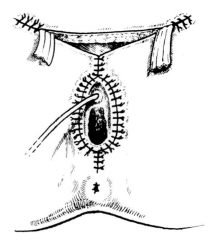

CARCINOMA OF THE VULVA

Radical vulvectomy with en bloc dissection and removal of the inguinal and iliac lymph glands is associated with significant morbidity. The following variations in technique have been introduced to reduce morbidity.

1. *Separate groin incisions*
   In vulval cancer, lymphatic metastases develop initially by embolisation. In early disease, there is no need to remove the lymphatic channels between the tumour and the groin nodes. Therefore, separate incisions can be used to remove the tumour and the nodes on the side(s) where lymphadenectomy is required. Such an approach is associated with lower morbidity than conventional surgery.

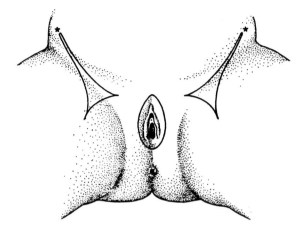

2. *Modified radical vulvectomy*
   If the primary tumour is small, and confined to one area, a more limited operation may be as effective as radical vulvectomy. In modified radical vulvectomy, the lesion and surrounding area are removed, leaving the remainder of the perineum intact. A 1–2 cm margin of healthy tissue should be removed along with the tumour.

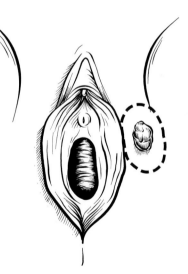

3. *Ipsilateral lymphadenectomy*
   If the tumour is confined to one side of the vulva only, at least 1 cm from a midline structure such as clitoris or anus, and the groin nodes appear clinically tumour free, ipsilateral lymphadenectomy may be sufficient to detect lymph node disease.

CARCINOMA OF THE VULVA

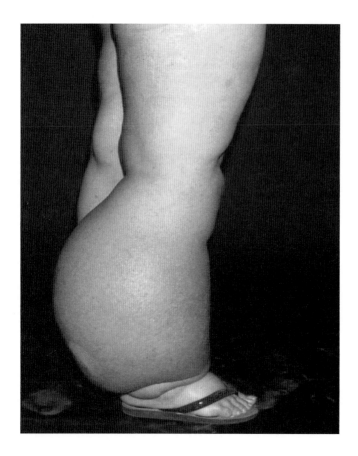

COMPLICATIONS
1. Wound breakdown and infection.
2. Thromboembolic disease.
3. Bleeding.
4. Lymphoedema.
5. Paraesthesia over the upper legs.
6. Impaired sexual function.
7. Psychological sequelae.

The incidence of wound breakdown and infection is reduced by the use of the three incision technique. The incidence of thromboembolic disease may be minimised by the use of low molecular weight heparin and thromboembolic disease stockings. The use of plastic surgery to restore normal anatomy, form and function of the tissues is very important in reducing morbidity and minimising sexual and psychological problems. Lymphoedema can also be treated using techniques such as massage and limb wrapping available with referral to specialist clinics.

RADIOTHERAPY AND CHEMOTHERAPY
Radiotherapy is useful for treatment of positive groin node disease after inguino-femoral lymphadenectomy. Preoperative chemoradiotherapy has been used for advanced tumours with impressive local response. It may reduce morbidity in advanced tumours, often facilitating surgical removal.

PROGNOSIS OF VULVAL CARCINOMA
Stage 1 93%
Stage 2 87%
Stage 3 62%
Stage 4 20–30%

Where a patient has involved groin nodes, survival is poorer.

DISEASES OF THE URETHRA

PROLAPSE OF THE URETHRAL MUCOSA

This forms a swelling round the meatus. Symptomatic urethral mucosal prolapse may be treated by cautery.

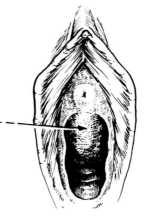

CARUNCLE

A small polypoid area arising from the lower end of the urethra. It is composed of a very vascular stroma and covered with squamous or transitional epithelium.

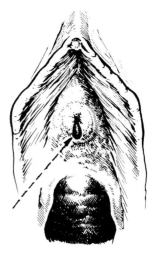

Clinical Features

Caruncles are red in colour because of their vascularity, and extremely sensitive. The patient is usually an elderly woman complaining of dysuria and bleeding.

Treatment

Caruncles can be excised and sent for histological examination if suspicious or symptomatic, although malignant change is rare. The base of the tumour on the urethral mucosa should be cauterised.

URETHROCELE

This is a descent of the urethra from its position under the pubic arch. It is sometimes a cause of stress incontinence and may exist by itself or more commonly with a cystocele.

Treatment is described in the section on prolapse.

165

CHAPTER 9

DISEASES OF THE VAGINA

Benign Vaginal Disease	168
Benign	*168*
Traumatic Epithelial Cysts	*168*
Vaginal Infections	*168*
Malignant and Premalignant Disease	169
Vaginal Intraepithelial Neoplasia (VAIN)	*169*
Carcinoma of the Vagina	170
Clinical Features	*170*
Site and Spread	*171*
Treatment	*171*
Plastic Surgery of the Vagina	172
Additional Procedures	*172*

BENIGN VAGINAL DISEASE

Vaginal diseases can manifest as benign, premalignant or malignant conditions

BENIGN
Vaginal cysts are not uncommon but are rarely large. They are found in the anterior or lateral walls of the lower third of the vagina and in the posterior wall of the upper third, are seldom larger than a walnut, are sometimes multiple, and may be mistaken for a cystocele. These cysts are occasionally a cause of dyspareunia but they usually cause no symptoms at all.

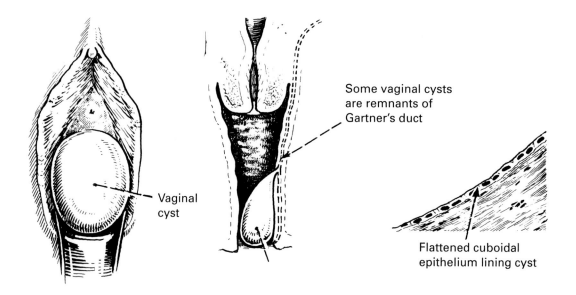

Some vaginal cysts are remnants of Gartner's duct

Vaginal cyst

Flattened cuboidal epithelium lining cyst

Treatment is by excision or marsupialisation.

TRAUMATIC EPITHELIAL CYSTS
Traumatic epithelial cysts (inclusion cysts) are found usually in the lower vagina and are caused by an infolding of epithelium at repair operations. If they cause any symptoms, they should be excised or marsupialised.

VAGINAL INFECTIONS
See pages relating to infection.

MALIGNANT AND PREMALIGNANT DISEASE

VAGINAL INTRAEPITHELIAL NEOPLASIA (VAIN)

This can be a very difficult condition to treat. It is rare, can affect any point on the vaginal wall and may progress to an invasive malignant disease. Its aetiology is likely to be due to human papilloma virus infection. The mature epithelium and a lack of metaplastic change may explain its reduced incidence when compared to cervical intraepithelial neoplasia.

It is often asymptomatic but symptoms may include irregular vaginal bleeding or discharge. Diagnosis is usually by colposcopy with directed biopsy, but it may also be detected incidentally in histology after a hysterectomy.

Treatment will depend on the age of the patient, previous treatment (some may have had a hysterectomy or treatment for cervical cancer), general health and desire to retain normal sexual function. Surgical excision (partial or total vaginectomy) and laser ablation have been employed and some authors report the use of topical 5-fluorouracil (5-FU) chemotherapy. Due to the rarity of this condition, treatment should be undertaken by a clinician with specialist skills in this area.

CARCINOMA OF THE VAGINA

Primary growths of the vagina are rare. The most common vaginal cancers are squamous cell carcinomas, however, adenocarcinomas, melanomas and sarcomas may also be seen. 30% of patients will have a history of CIN or of a carcinoma of the cervix.

Its aetiology is mixed, with oncogenic human papilloma virus being implicated in squamous carcinoma development. Although rare, VAIN is being diagnosed more frequently and it may proceed to cancer. Historically, intrauterine exposure to diethylstilboestrol (DES) has carried a risk of causing vaginal adenocarcinomas, but more commonly, vaginal adenosis. Metastatic deposits are also seen, especially as extensions from cervical cancer and endometrial carcinoma.

CLINICAL FEATURES

The patient is usually postmenopausal and asymptomatic. The most common symptoms are bleeding (60%), discharge (15%) and pelvic pain (10% or less). If the bladder is involved, patients may experience pain and dysuria.

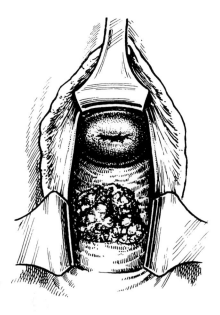

The tumour is not at first painful, and unless it appears in a woman who is still sexually active, it is not likely to present until it has penetrated the vaginal wall and caused bleeding. An early tumour can easily be missed if it is obscured by the blade of a speculum. The whole vagina should always be inspected, and a biopsy be taken from any unusual lesion.

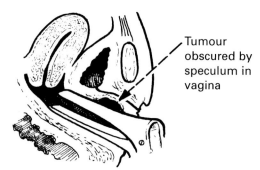

Tumour obscured by speculum in vagina

A thorough examination, including colposcopy, cystoscopy and proctosigmoidoscopy, may be indicated to detect its spread. In addition, magnetic resonance imaging (MRI) scans can provide information on local and regional disease.

CARCINOMA OF THE VAGINA

SITE AND SPREAD

The most common site of disease is the upper vagina. The disease can have a variety of appearances depending on its histology, such as a mass lesion, plaques of abnormal tissue or ulceration.

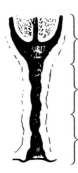

Upper third: approximately same drainage as the cervix.

Middle third: any pelvic lymphatic channel may be involved.

Lower third: approximately same drainage as the vulva.

Clinical staging		Five-year survival rates (%)
Stage I	Invasive. Confined to the vaginal mucosa.	75–90
Stage II	Invading paravaginal tissue, but not to the pelvic side wall.	45
Stage III	Extension to the pelvic side wall.	30–40
Stage IVa	Extension to mucosa of bladder or rectum.	$\not> 20$
Stage IVb	Extension beyond the pelvis.	$\not< 20$

Prognosis depends on the clinical stage of the disease.

TREATMENT

Treatment will be tailored to the patient; size and stage of the disease and psychosexual impact of the treatment will also be taken into consideration. If the disease is localised to the vagina in a fit patient, it may be treated by radical surgery (radical hysterectomy, vaginectomy, lymphadenectomy). More advanced disease and disease in the mid to lower third of the vagina may be treated with radiotherapy. Some authors are also exploring the use of chemotherapy (cisplatin and 5-FU) alongside radiotherapy.

The vaginal melanoma carries a poor prognosis, with radical excision and radiotherapy currently being employed in its treatment.

Sarcoma botryoides is a rare tumour of young children, presenting as grape-like masses with bleeding. Chemotherapy with vincristine, actinomycin D and cyclophosphamide gives good results.

PLASTIC SURGERY OF THE VAGINA

This is required when the patient is found to have a congenital absence of the vagina, is having the vagina removed as a part of radical cancer surgery, or distortion and contractures due to injury or genital mutilation. Such a situation is rare, but various operations have been devised. The small bowel has been used successfully in male to female sex change procedures.

The placement of a skin graft

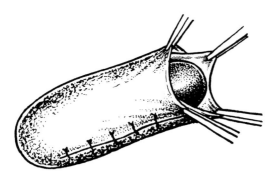

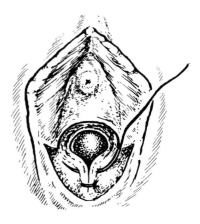

1. A plastic mould is covered with skin from the thigh. (This is done by a plastic surgeon.)

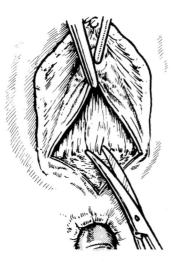

2. The space between the urethra/bladder and the rectum is opened up. A finger in the anus helps the surgeon to avoid damaging the rectum.

3. The mould and the graft are inserted and kept in place by suturing the split ends of the labia minora. The moulds can now be fashioned from inflatable plastic and in varying sizes. The vaginal orifice may need enlarging later on by the plastic surgeon.

The mould must be kept for a prolonged time, and once it is removed, the patient should use vaginal trainers or have regular sexual intercourse to prevent closure of the neovagina.

ADDITIONAL PROCEDURES
The techniques available to the plastic surgeon have allowed the evolution of a variety of procedures to create a neovagina. Some may raise myocutaneous flaps from the rectus abdominus muscle or the gracilis muscle.

CHAPTER 10

DISEASES OF THE CERVIX

Normal Cervical Epithelium 174
   Anatomy of the Cervix *174*
   Benign Squamous Metaplasia *174*
The Role of Human Papilloma
   Virus in Cervical Disease 175
   Risk Factors *175*
Screening for Cervical Cancer 176
   Screening Process *176*
Cervical Smears 177
   Interpretation of Cervical Smears *177*
Premalignant and Malignant
   Cervical Disease 178
   Dysplasia *178*
   Microinvasive Cervical Carcinoma *178*
   Risk of Progression of
     Cervical Intraepithelial
     Neoplasia *178*
Colposcopy 179
   Identification of Atypical
     Epithelium *179*
Treatment of Cervical
   Intraepithelial Neoplasia 180
   Ablative Techniques *180*
   Excisional Techniques *181*

Carcinoma of the Cervix 183
   Clinical Findings *183*
   Symptoms *183*
Carcinoma of the Cervix 184
   Squamous Cell Carcinoma *184*
   Spread *185*
Diagnosis of Cervical Carcinoma 186
Staging of Cervical Carcinoma 187
Radiotherapy and Chemotherapy
   in Cervical Carcinoma 189
   Brachytherapy *189*
   External Beam Therapy *189*
   Complications *189*
Surgery for Cervical Carcinoma 190
   Microinvasive Cervical Carcinoma *190*
   Radical Hysterectomy and Node
     Dissection *190*
   Radical Surgery for Cervical
     Cancer *192*
   Treatment of Cervical Carcinoma:
     Surgery or Radiotherapy? *193*
   Prognosis *193*

NORMAL CERVICAL EPITHELIUM

ANATOMY OF THE CERVIX
The cervix constitutes the lower third of the uterus.

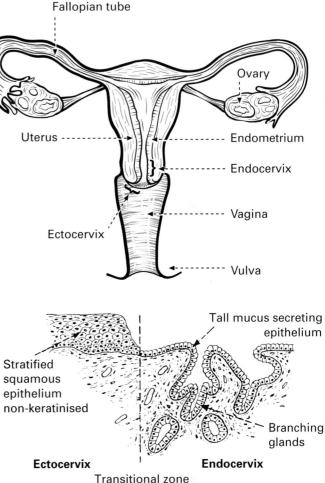

It is in two parts, the endocervix and the ectocervix. Before puberty, the dividing line between the endo- and ectocervix is sharp, and is determined by the character of the lining epithelium: the ectocervix is covered with squamous epithelium and the endocervix is covered with columnar epithelium.

BENIGN SQUAMOUS METAPLASIA
Stratification well defined with:

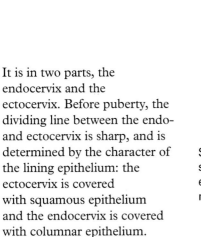

Squames at surface

Oval polygonal cells for several layers

Basal cells usually a single layer at right angles to the surface

Under the influence of oestrogen (e.g. at puberty, during pregnancy or when the combined pill is taken), the cervix enlarges, so that the columnar epithelium of the endocervix can be seen on the ectocervix. This region, formerly the endocervix, which is now anatomically the ectocervix, is known as the 'transformation zone'. The transformation zone is a dynamic area that responds to changes in endogenous or exogenous oestrogen. As it undergoes changes, it becomes a squamous metaplasia, which is a benign condition. The transformation zone is important as it is susceptible to infection with the human papilloma virus (HPV), which is known to lead to possible dysplastic change, and this in turn may lead to cervical cancer.

THE ROLE OF HUMAN PAPILLOMA VIRUS IN CERVICAL DISEASE

RISK FACTORS

Human Papilloma Virus (HPV) Infection

HPV infection is now known to be the viral agent required for the development of, initially, cervical intraepithelial neoplasia (CIN), and, ultimately, a cervical carcinoma. Approximately 80% of women will be infected with at least one of the more than 100 genotypes of HPV. 70–90% of women infected with HPV will clear the infection spontaneously within 1–3 years.

HPV is a DNA virus that can integrate into the human genome, and each genotype has a number. The most prevalent HPV genotypes in cervical carcinoma are 16 and 18. They are responsible for at least 70% of all cervical cancers.

The HPV genome encodes early (E) proteins that are responsible for viral regulation, cell transformation and late (L) proteins that make the viral capsule. HPV infects the basal cells and the expression of genes E6, E7 in high risk genotypes allows them to act as oncogenes via a variety of mechanisms to cause unregulated cell growth that may lead to dysplasia and cancer. Two tumour suppressor proteins that are affected by the E6/E7 gene products are p53 and retinoblastoma.

Suggested co-factors that may increase the likelihood of developing cervical cancer include: smoking, low socioeconomic status, immunosuppression (e.g. HIV infection, organ transplant), multiple sexual partners and combined oral contraceptive pill use for more than 10 years.

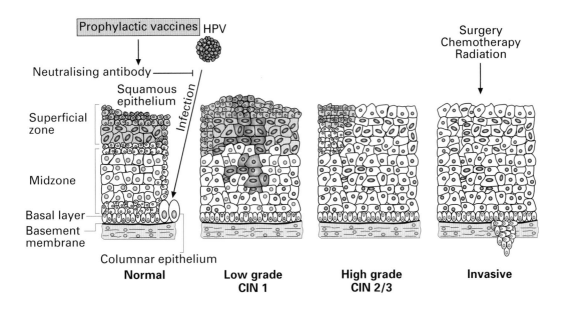

SCREENING FOR CERVICAL CANCER

Screening for cervical intraepithelial neoplasia (CIN) can be done by performing cervical smears and offering subsequent colposcopic assessment if significant dyskaryotic change is found. Treatment of CIN significantly reduces the incidence of and mortality associated with cervical cancer. For these reasons, many countries, including the UK, have set up a national screening programme.

SCREENING PROCESS

The Cervical Smear

A cervical smear is taken by a trained healthcare professional, often in their local practice. The cervix is visualised using a speculum. A wooden spatula or small plastic broom is placed in the cervical canal and rotated through 360°. The superficial layer of cells overlying the squamocolumnar junction is removed. If a wooden spatula is used, it is then smeared on a slide and fixed. If the broom is used, it is placed into a vial of liquid fixative (liquid-based cytology – LBC). Both methods then stain the specimen using Papanicolou's method and the cells are examined under a microscope. The LBC technique is automated once the sample is sent for processing and this method produces cleaner specimens for analysis, thus reducing the number of unsatisfactory slides. If abnormal cells, dyskaryosis, are identified, the patients are referred for colposcopy.

In Scotland, the current cervical screening programme includes the following:

- All women between 20 and 60 years are invited for a smear test every 3 years.
- Immunocompromised/immunosuppressed women are offered annual screening.
- A national electronic database records and monitors the cervical smear process from the point of invitation to the completion of a colposcopic assessment. This is the Scottish Cervical Call-Recall System (SCCRS).

An abnormal smear is usually an indication for colposcopy (see p. 179).

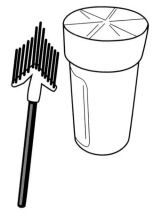

Cervix brush and pot

CERVICAL SMEARS

INTERPRETATION OF CERVICAL SMEARS

Smears are reported in the following categories:

Normal
Inflammatory changes
Borderline nuclear change
Mild dyskaryosis
Moderate dyskaryosis
Severe dyskaryosis
Invasion suspected
Glandular abnormality

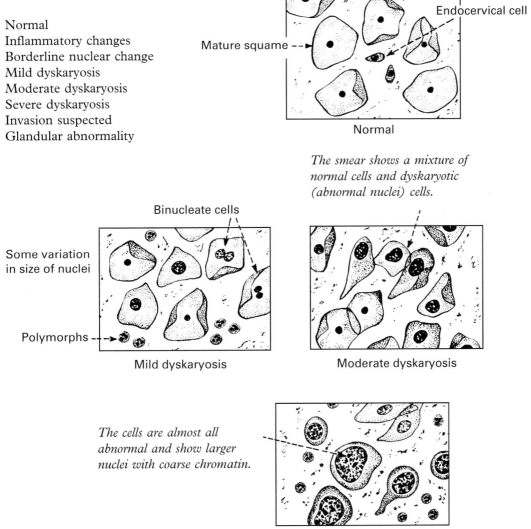

Normal

The smear shows a mixture of normal cells and dyskaryotic (abnormal nuclei) cells.

Mild dyskaryosis

Moderate dyskaryosis

The cells are almost all abnormal and show larger nuclei with coarse chromatin.

Severe dyskaryosis

In general, the more severe the dyskaryosis, the more likely the patient is to have high grade CIN. However, even in women with a mildly dyskaryotic smear, the incidence of high grade CIN can be 50%.

A referral for colposcopy is made for all women with, moderate or severe dyskaryosis. A repeat smear is justified in women with inflammatory or borderline nuclear changes. However, if these abnormalities persist, colposcopy is indicated. Colposcopy is also indicated if there are three or more abnormal smear tests of any grade in a 10-year interval.

177

PREMALIGNANT AND MALIGNANT CERVICAL DISEASE

DYSPLASIA

Dysplasia occurs when the epithelium shows changes such as nuclear enlargement, increased nucleocytoplasmic ratio and abnormal mitoses. It is regarded as the first step in a series of changes that may lead to *cervical intraepithelial neoplasia (CIN)* and subsequently to invasive carcinoma. The pathological features of mild, moderate and severe dysplasia are shown. In practice there can be inter- and intra-observer variation between these categories.

CIN 1 ≡ low grade dysplasia

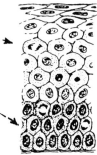

Upper two thirds stratified squames i.e. normal

Cells of basal third have high nucleocytoplasmic ratio; pleomorphic nuclei in layers at this level.

CIN 2 ≡ high grade dysplasia

Upper half of epithelium shows stratification and maturation

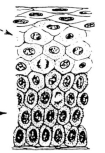

Abnormal basal cells occupy lower half

CIN 3 ≡ high grade dysplasia

(1) There may be one or two layers of stratified epithelium on surface.

(2) Remainder is immature with large nuclei.

(3) Abnormal mitoses are common.

MICROINVASIVE CERVICAL CARCINOMA

The histological appearance of an early cervical invasion with spread through the basement membrane is shown here.

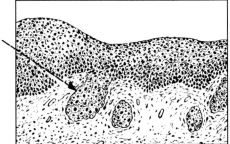

RISK OF PROGRESSION OF CERVICAL INTRAEPITHELIAL NEOPLASIA

CIN has the potential to develop into a malignant cervical disease but it may also regress or persist as CIN without undergoing any malignant change. The risk of developing cervical cancer following dysplasia is 10–20%. The risk is also influenced by the grade of CIN, oncogenic potential of the HPV type, and environmental factors such as smoking and the immune status of a patient.

COLPOSCOPY

Colposcopy means binocular inspection of the cervix with magnification.

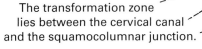

The transformation zone lies between the cervical canal and the squamocolumnar junction.

The colposcopist recognises two kinds of epithelium, the 'native' epithelium which may be squamous or columnar; and the metaplastic squamous epithelium which arises in the physiological transformation zone.

IDENTIFICATION OF ATYPICAL EPITHELIUM

Following the insertion of a speculum, the cervix is swabbed with 3% or 5% acetic acid. This dehydrates cells and the abnormal areas with larger and denser nuclei reflect light, appearing white. The vascular pattern within the white area can also be examined. Any changes are described with terms such as mosaicism and punctation. Trained colposcopists establish areas of abnormality and perform a small biopsy. Those patients with a high grade smear and an abnormal colposcopic appearance may be offered treatment at their first visit. Other patients requiring treatment will usually return as an outpatient.

Patients can find the whole process stressful and this is taken into account when seeing patients in the clinic and arranging management for the patient.

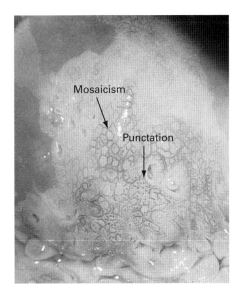

TREATMENT OF CERVICAL INTRAEPITHELIAL NEOPLASIA

There is a high rate of spontaneous regression within the first 2 years after a diagnosis of low grade CIN (CIN1). For this reason, the majority of CIN1 cases are usually kept under review to establish if the changes regress cytologically and colposcopically.

High grade CIN (CIN2/3) has a lower rate of regression and is associated with a malignant transformation rate of up to 22%. Treatment is therefore offered to women with high grade CIN. This is usually done as an outpatient, under local anaesthetic, but some women may require admission for a general anaesthetic. The method of treatment chosen will depend on training, availability of technique and the need to minimise morbidity.

ABLATIVE TECHNIQUES

All these techniques destroy abnormal cervical tissue. In contrast to the excisional methods, there is no tissue for analysis after treatment and any occult invasive disease may not be recognised. Hence it is essential to have:

Excluded invasive disease by colposcopically directed biopsy, prior to treatment.
No discrepancy between cytology/colposcopy/histology.
No evidence of microinvasion/invasion.
No evidence of a glandular lesion.
Satisfactory colposcopy.

Morbidity with these techniques is often lower compared to the excisional techniques and there is less bleeding and no increased risk of adverse pregnancy outcomes such as preterm delivery and preterm rupture of the membranes.

Cold Coagulation

This involves the application of a probe, heated to 120°C, to the cervix, for between 20 and 30 s over one to five applications, depending on the size of the area to be treated. This simple technique can be performed under local anaesthetic, it is inexpensive and it has been shown to adequately treat CIN.

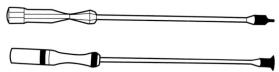

Cold coagulator probes

CO₂ Laser

This is a precise method that vaporises tissue to a depth of 7 mm. However, it is an expensive technique that requires significant training and attention to safety issues.

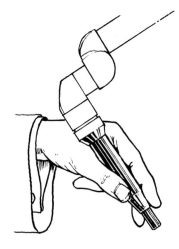

TREATMENT OF CERVICAL INTRAEPITHELIAL NEOPLASIA

Cryosurgery
This allows destruction of affected tissue to a depth of 3–5 mm. It is a rapid treatment but it may not treat the cervix to an adequate depth to destroy all CIN. For this reason this technique is not employed.

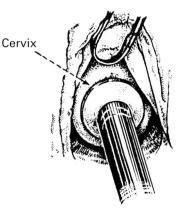

Cervix

EXCISIONAL TECHNIQUES
Excisional techniques have a major advantage over ablative methods in that tissue is obtained and can be examined histologically. The diagnosis can be confirmed and the completeness of excision can be assessed.

Many operators prefer to perform excisional techniques on all patients. However, increasingly, in response to the data concerning pregnancy-related morbidity, some individuals are more selective and offer excision rather than ablation when they

1. Suspect invasive disease
2. Are treating a glandular abnormality
3. Cannot visualise the squamocolumnar junction
4. Are managing a patient with previous cervical surgery

The following techniques are currently in use:

Large Loop Excision of the Transformation Zone (LLETZ)
This has become one of the most popular methods for treating premalignant cervical disease. A thin wire loop is used to excise the transformation zone using a blended diathermy current. It is also known as a LEEP (Loop Electrosurgical Excision Procedure). Ball diathermy is applied for haemostasis at the treated the excision base.

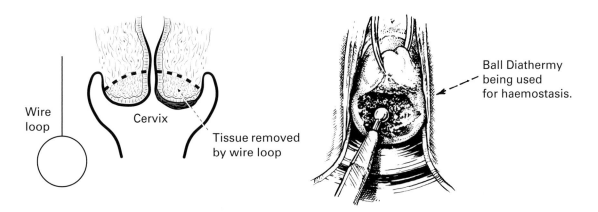

Wire loop

Cervix

Tissue removed by wire loop

Ball Diathermy being used for haemostasis.

181

TREATMENT OF CERVICAL INTRAEPITHELIAL NEOPLASIA

Knife Cone Biopsy

This technique was extremely popular prior to the introduction of LLETZ. However, it requires a general anaesthetic and is now less commonly used. Complications include bleeding, infection, and cervical stenosis or incompetence during a subsequent pregnancy.

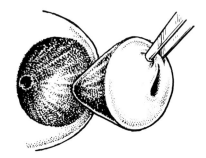

Laser Cone Biopsy

In a laser cone biopsy, a cone of tissue is removed as above. However, the procedure may be done under local anaesthesia. The costs of the equipment and the training required have reduced its potential popularity. Laser does have the advantage that co-existing VAIN may be treated at the same time.

Follow-Up

The above techniques are effective in treating CIN but recurrence can occur in 5% of the patients. All women who have had CIN should be followed up with increased smear cytology surveillance for a minimum of 5–10 years; there is regional variation within the UK.

CARCINOMA OF THE CERVIX

Worldwide, carcinoma of the cervix is the commonest malignancy of the female genital tract. Its incidence varies from country to country and is significantly reduced where there is an organised screening programme. In developed countries, such as the UK, cervical cancer is the twelfth most common malignancy in females.

CLINICAL FINDINGS

The cervix becomes very indurated; necrosis and ulceration commonly follow quickly.

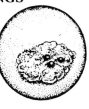

Later, a large fungating mass is produced. Sloughing may leave an excavated crater.

The tumour may form a proliferating growth which protrudes into the vagina – a 'cauliflower', 'exophytic', 'everting' growth. This tumour type bleeds easily and soon becomes ulcerated.

Sometimes the spread is in the substance of the cervix – called 'excavating', 'endophytic', 'inverting' growth. The cervix becomes stony, hard and enlarged – the 'barrel-shaped' cervix.

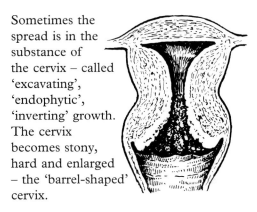

SYMPTOMS

Cervical cancer may present with no symptoms or may be detected at the microscopic stage through a screening programme. If symptoms are present, then, they may include:

1. *Irregular vaginal bleeding.* It is not often due to carcinoma but the possibility must be kept in mind. The bleeding may be due to intermenstrual bleeding, postcoital bleeding or postmenopausal bleeding.
2. *Vaginal discharge.* The growth may become infected and produce offensive discharge.
3. *Symptoms of advanced disease.* Pain, bladder/bowel pressure symptoms, haematuria and cachexia.

CARCINOMA OF THE CERVIX

The two commonest cancers are squamous cell carcinomas and adenocarcinomas. 70% are squamous cell carcinomas and 15% are adenocarcinomas with the remainder being the less common types.

SQUAMOUS CELL CARCINOMA
The appearances are typical, but cell nests are absent and keratinisation is rarely seen.

Adenocarcinoma
This less common form of cervical malignancy usually arises from the columnar epithelium of the endocervix.

The appearances in this form are typical of adenocarcinomas in other organs.

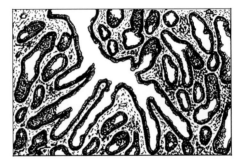

Low power. Tubular processes spread out from the lumina of the glands. The characteristic pattern is an aggressive adenomatous formation with very little fibrous stroma.

Many indeterminate patterns are seen on microscopic examination. Sometimes, both glandular and squamous malignant cells appear together – an adenocanthoma – and squamous metaplasia is common.

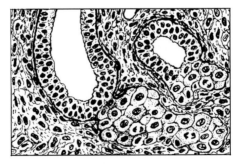

High power appearance of squamous epithelium, which appears to originate by metaplasia of the columnar epithelium.

CARCINOMA OF THE CERVIX

SPREAD

Direct spread into adjacent tissues such as the vagina or parametrium can occur. In postmenopausal women, it can also lead to a uterine outlet obstruction and pyometra. Its spread to the parametrium may induce pain and tenderness.

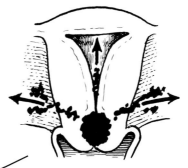

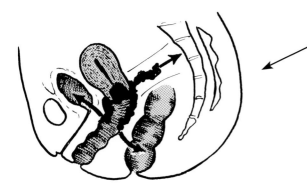

Spread downwards into the vaginal wall, if not diagnosed or treated, may involve the bladder or rectum and lead to the formation of fistulae. A backwards spread along the uterosacral ligaments can lead to an involvement of the sacral plexus causing intractable sciatic pain that can be felt in the hip or the leg.

Lymphatic spread also occurs and may precede direct spread. This is why lymphadenectomy is still important in the assessment of cervical cancers. From the cervical lymphatics, the spread is usually along the paracervical lymph tract to the iliac and obturator nodes. Blood borne spread is less likely to occur in early stage disease but may be significant in advanced disease. Ovarian involvement is rare.

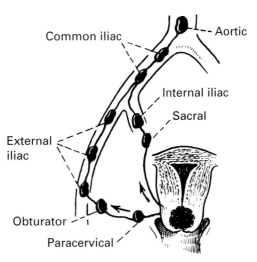

DIAGNOSIS OF CERVICAL CARCINOMA

Biopsy is necessary for histological confirmation of the carcinoma. If the growth is early, some normal tissue should be removed as well, and a diagram provided to show the pathologist from where the biopsy was taken. It should be no bigger than necessary and a punch biopsy, millimetres in size, may be sufficient. LLETZ biopsy can be performed for diagnosis but is generally not performed in the presence of evidence of malignant growth that is visible to the naked eye. Very occasionally, what appears to be a definite malignant lesion turns out to be benign.

Some differential diagnoses include:

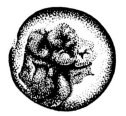

Cervicitis with ectopy, the commonest cervical lesion and, if florid, can be most misleading.

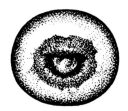

Mucous cervical polyps, when infected, can present with a very suspicious appearance. (But all polyps require examination.)

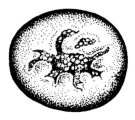

Tuberculosis is rare in the cervix. There is nearly always a history of genital tuberculosis.

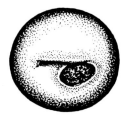

A primary chancre (syphilis) can appear in the cervix and is ulcerated, hard and indurated. In the United Kingdom, this is rare.

STAGING OF CERVICAL CARCINOMA

Each growth is allocated to a stage according to the extent of spread (FIGO).

Stage IA Microscopic Cervical Cancer.
Stage 1A1
Stromal invasion ≤3.0 mm in depth and ≤7.0 mm in horizontal spread.
Stage 1A2
Stromal invasion ≤5.0 mm in depth and ≤7.0 mm horizontal spread.

Stage IB The growth is confined to the cervix.
Stage 1B1
Clinically visible lesion ≤4.0 cm dimension.

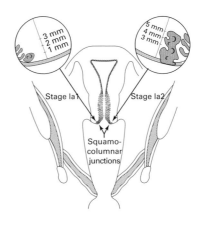

Stage 1B2
Clinically visible lesion >4 cm in greatest dimension.

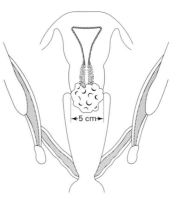

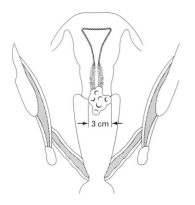

Stage II Tumour invades beyond the uterus but not to pelvic wall or to lower third of the vagina.
IIA Without parametrial invasion.
IIA1 Clinically visible lesion ≤4 cm greatest dimension.
IIA2 Clinically visible lesion >4 cm greatest dimension.

IIB Extension into the parametrium but not as far as the pelvic wall.

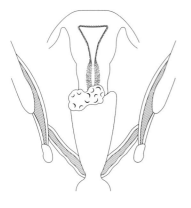

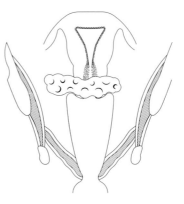

STAGING OF CERVICAL CARCINOMA

Stage III Extension to lower third of vagina or to pelvic wall.

IIIa Carcinoma involving the lower third of the vagina.

IIIb Carcinoma extending to the pelvic side wall and/or hydronephrosis due to tumour.

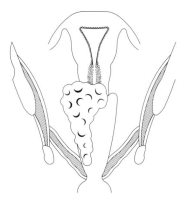

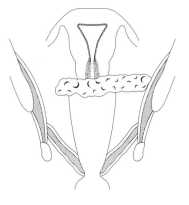

Stage IV Extension through vagina into bladder or outside the pelvis.

IVa Carcinoma involving adjacent organs.

IVb Carcinoma extending to distant organs.

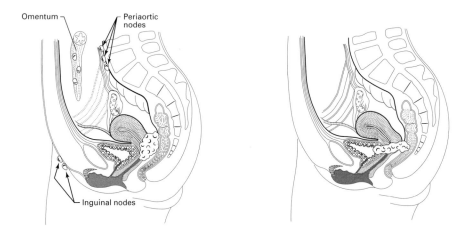

Staging is clinicopathological and, currently, imaging that demonstrates hydronephrosis due to tumour involvement can be used for staging purposes. Whilst magnetic resonance imaging (MRI) is commonly available in developed countries, it is less so in developing countries. Therefore, although MRI is useful in assessing the local spread of disease and may be used in clinical decision, it is not included in the FIGO staging.

RADIOTHERAPY AND CHEMOTHERAPY IN CERVICAL CARCINOMA

Chemotherapy combined with radiotherapy is equivalent in terms of treatment efficacy, compared to radical surgery, for early stage cervical cancers. The choice of treatment will depend upon patient fitness, size of tumour and likelihood of requiring adjuvant treatment based on preoperative factors; the aim being to deliver the most effective combination of treatments to minimise morbidity.

Chemotherapy given along with radiotherapy has been shown to improve treatment outcomes, with chemotherapy given at the same time as radiotherapy further sensitising tumours to radiotherapy. A haemoglobin >11 g/dl will also increase efficacy.

The radiotherapy is delivered by two modes – external beam therapy and brachytherapy (delivered close to tumour site).

BRACHYTHERAPY

Hollow carriers are placed in the uterus and vaginal fornices under general anaesthesia. Radioactive sources can then be loaded into these tubes for treatment at a later date. Intracavity therapy allows high doses of radioactivity to be targeted to the cervix. The activity falls with increasing distance from the source, therefore the tissues around the cervix (bladder, bowel, etc.) receive a lower dose.

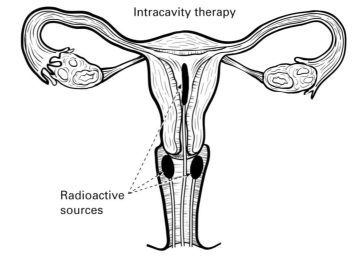

Intracavity therapy

Radioactive sources

EXTERNAL BEAM THERAPY

External beam therapy is applied to the pelvis to control spread outside the cervix. The total radiotherapy dose is divided into smaller doses or fractions that are delivered over short daily treatments, usually as 20–25 fractions. Treatment, therefore, lasts for 4–5 weeks.

COMPLICATIONS

Short term	Long term
Diarrhoea	Persistent bowel and bladder symptoms
Urinary frequency	Radiation menopause
Nausea	Vaginal stenosis/scarring/dryness
Vulval inflammation	Late secondary tumours

SURGERY FOR CERVICAL CARCINOMA

MICROINVASIVE CERVICAL CARCINOMA
This may be treated with a LLETZ biopsy or if the patient has completed her family, by a simple hysterectomy.

RADICAL HYSTERECTOMY AND NODE DISSECTION
This consists of removal of the uterus, upper 2 cm of the vagina, the tissues/ligaments adjacent to the cervix (parametrium) and the lymph glands overlying the iliac vessels and the obturator nerve at the sides of the pelvis. It can be performed abdominally, vaginally or laparoscopically, with robots being increasingly used for laparoscopic dissection.

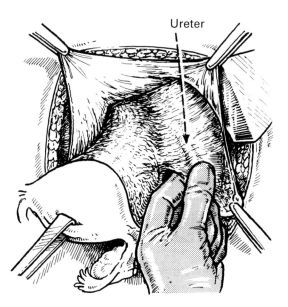

The broad ligament is opened up and the ureter dissected off the uterus and cervix. This is a vascular area. This diagram shows the ureter being identified by palpation but it is also directly visualised and dissected.

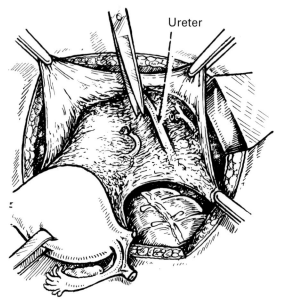

The ureter is identified at the common iliac division and followed downwards. The ureter has to be mobilised to protect it, but this does lead to the possibility of a fistula due to avascular necrosis.

The ureter has been dissected clearly down to the bladder and the uterine vessels, divided at their origin, form the internal iliac artery.

SURGERY FOR CERVICAL CARCINOMA

RADICAL HYSTERECTOMY AND NODE DISSECTION—(cont'd)

After division of the ligamentous attachments (uterosacral and cardinal) of the uterus, the vagina is transected. The vaginal opening may then be over sewn around its margin to provide haemostasis and allow fluid to drain. This will seal within a short time following surgery.

In this description the hysterectomy is shown first, followed by the lymphadenectomy; but many surgeons carry out the lymphadenectomy first followed by the block dissection of the radical hysterectomy.

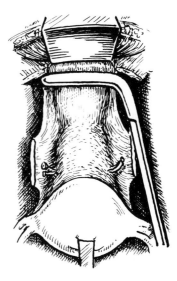

The vagina is severed below the Wertheim clamp in this example but similar clamps may also be used.

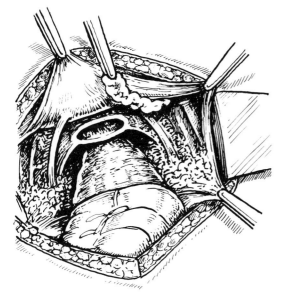

Dissecting out the fatty tissue and glands from the obturator fossa.

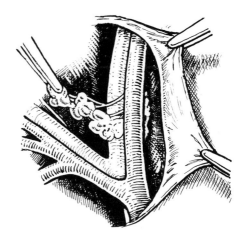

Dissecting out the external iliac glands. (Other accessible groups of nodes are also removed.)

SURGERY FOR CERVICAL CARCINOMA

RADICAL SURGERY FOR CERVICAL CANCER

Special Circumstances

Fertility sparing surgery

Removal of the uterus leads to loss of fertility and many women in the age range for the development of cervical cancer may not have any children or have completed their family. Daniel Dargent, Lyon, France, has developed a technique for a radical vaginal excision of the cervix and retaining the uterine body. This technique has the potential to preserve fertility. Lymph node spread is assessed by laparoscopic lymphadenectomy. This is now an accepted technique and is being performed in specialist centres. Pregnancies have been recorded but there are potential pregnancy-related complications such as pre-term labour, pre-term rupture of the membranes and late miscarriages.

Exenteration for relapsed disease

Localised, central, pelvic relapsed carcinoma can be salvaged by radical excision of the pelvic tumour. Due to the proximity of the bladder and the rectum to the vagina, such surgery may involve – in addition to removal of the vagina – removal of the bladder (anterior exenteration), bowel (posterior exenteration) or both (total exenteration). This is a long and complex procedure that may require urinary diversion, colostomy formation and the creation of a new vagina.

Surgical complications of surgical treatment for cervical cancer

Early	Late

Haemorrhage
Infection
Damage to ureters or
    bladder
Venous thromboembolic
    disease
	Atonic bladder
	Lymphoedema
	Ureteric/bladder
	    fistulae (1–2%)

SURGERY FOR CERVICAL CARCINOMA

TREATMENT OF CERVICAL CARCINOMA: SURGERY OR RADIOTHERAPY?
Early stage cervical cancer is normally treated by surgery up to and including Stage 1B1. Later stage cervical cancer (Stage 1B2 onwards) is usually treated by chemo-radiotherapy.

The advantages of the two treatment types are shown below.

Advantages of Surgery
Ovarian function is retained.
Normal vaginal function is retained.
Avoidance of the effect of radiotherapy on the bladder and bowel.

Advantages of Chemo-Radiotherapy
As effective as surgery for treatment.
Suitable in women who are unfit for surgery or do not wish surgery.
May allow avoidance of surgery where, at diagnosis, there is strong indication that it will be required.

PROGNOSIS
5-Year Survival Figures According to Stage
Palliative care
In women with advanced cancer, it may be unrealistic to seek to cure the disease with surgery, radiotherapy or chemotherapy. In some women, these procedures may be performed palliatively, to reduce symptoms.

The care of patients with advanced or terminal disease is now a specialty in itself, and help should be sought from palliative care specialists at an early stage. Such specialists are invaluable in minimising symptoms, including pain, whilst maximising the quality of life.

CHAPTER 11

DISEASES OF THE UTERUS

Uterine Polyps 196
   Endometrial Polyp 196
   Placental Site Trophoblastic
     Tumour 196
Fibroids 197
   Fibroids (Leiomyoma) 197
   Pressure Symptoms 198
   Diagnosis 199
   Complications 199
   Treatment 200
Endometrial Hyperplasia 201
   Clinical Findings 201
   Simple Hyperplasia 201
   Complex Hyperplasia 201
   Atypical Hyperplasia 201
   Aetiology 202
   Investigation 202
   Treatment 202
Carcinoma of the Endometrium 203
   Presentation 203
   Diagnosis 203
   Histology 204
Staging of Endometrial Carcinoma 205
Spread of Endometrial Carcinoma 206

   Local Spread 206
   Lymphatic Spread 206
Aetiological Factors in Endometrial
   Carcinoma 207
Prognosis of Endometrial
   Carcinoma 208
Treatment of Endometrial
   Carcinoma 209
   Stage I 209
   Stage II 209
   Stage III/IV 209
Recurrence of Endometrial
   Carcinoma 210
   Sites 210
   Treatment for Recurrence 210
Sarcoma of the Uterus 211
   Clinical Features 211
   Histological Appearances 211
   Endometrial Stromal Sarcomas 212
   Carcinosarcoma (Malignant Mixed
     Mesodermal Tumour) 212
   Leiomyosarcoma 212

UTERINE POLYPS

ENDOMETRIAL POLYP

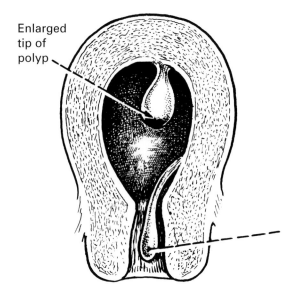

Enlarged tip of polyp

Symptoms

Symptoms are heavier but regular periods, postmenopausal bleeding, and irregular bleeding on hormone replacement therapy (HRT).

Cramping pain occurs as the uterus tries to expel the polyp.

Intermenstrual bleeding – usually occurs due to congestion or necrosis, but a malignant change must always be considered.

The polyp may be visible in the external os and there may be more than one polyp. Endometrial polyps may be identified by transvaginal scan but hysteroscopy will allow direct visualisation.

PLACENTAL SITE TROPHOBLASTIC TUMOUR

This is due to the survival of chorionic tissue from a recent pregnancy. The tissue remains adherent to the uterine wall and enlarges with the accretion of fibrin and fibrous tissue. This can produce either high or low grade disease.

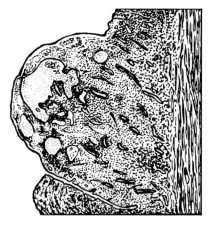

Symptoms

Menorrhagia and intermenstrual bleeding may present some time after the pregnancy has terminated or miscarried. Examination can reveal an enlarged uterus.

Treatment

All polyps must be removed and submitted to pathology. The final treatment will depend upon the histology, malignant potential and patient's symptoms. Surgery, including hysterectomy, may be required in some cases, especially where malignant transformation is known or is suspected.

FIBROIDS

FIBROIDS (LEIOMYOMA)

Fibroid is the gynaecological term for
a leiomyoma of the uterus or, occasionally,
of the cervix.

It is a circumscribed tumour of non-striped
muscle with supporting fibrous tissue. ➝

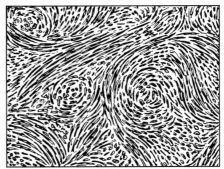

Fibroids develop in the myometrium and are not
encapsulated, but they develop a false capsule of
compressed myometrial tissue.

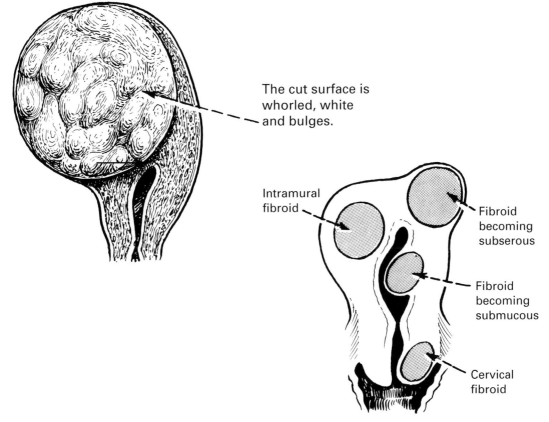

The cut surface is
whorled, white
and bulges.

Intramural
fibroid

Fibroid
becoming
subserous

Fibroid
becoming
submucous

Cervical
fibroid

The location of the fibroid describes the type.

They are sometimes conglomerate and multiple, and vary in size from tiny (millet seed) to
large, which may be many centimetres in diameter.

Some fibroids develop a long pedicle and present as polyps.

197

FIBROIDS

Fibroids are common tumours found in 15–20% of women. They may make the uterus bulky and irregular and may enlarge the cavity so that there is a greater area of endometrium to be shed at menstruation. Menstruation tends to be heavy but the cycle is usually regular. Fibroids are associated with infertility and nulliparity.

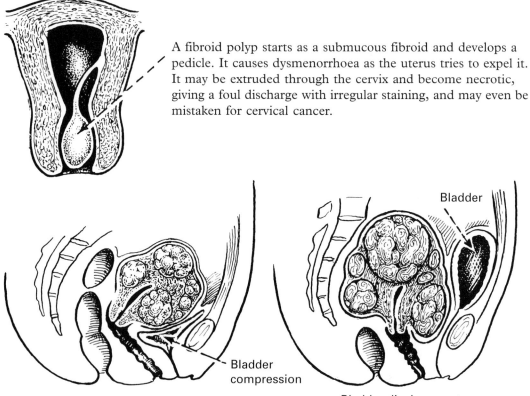

A fibroid polyp starts as a submucous fibroid and develops a pedicle. It causes dysmenorrhoea as the uterus tries to expel it. It may be extruded through the cervix and become necrotic, giving a foul discharge with irregular staining, and may even be mistaken for cervical cancer.

Bladder

Bladder compression

Bladder displacement

PRESSURE SYMPTOMS

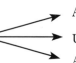

The bulk of fibroids in the uterus gives

→ A palpable abdominal tumour

→ Urinary frequency

→ A growth filling the pelvis leading to bladder displacement, retention and overflow and difficulty with defecation.

FIBROIDS

DIAGNOSIS

Symptoms and Signs

Menstrual disorders, pressure related symptoms and abdominal distension are all potential symptoms. A palpable mass per abdomen and/or on bimanual examination may be elicited during examination. The mass is usually firm, smooth and can be irregular.

Investigations

Patients may be anaemic if suffering from menorrhagia and investigations for this should be undertaken with full blood count and possibly assessment of ferritin, folate and B12 levels, where appropriate.

The suspicion of a fibroid on clinical assessment should be confirmed with imaging. Imaging will assess the size, site and nature of the fibroid. While rare, some fibroids can show signs of malignant change (leiomyosarcoma). Ultrasound will suffice for the assessment of most but further information may be gained by the use of magnetic resonance imaging (MRI), especially when the nature of the mass is being considered.

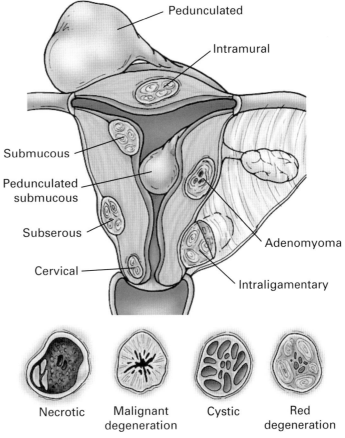

COMPLICATIONS

Sarcomatous change. This is rare but can occur, and large or complex asymptomatic fibroids must be kept under observation if not being removed surgically.

Degeneration. Fibroids tend to outgrow their blood supply and are subject to various forms of degeneration. *Necrobiosis* ('red degeneration') occurs in pregnancy and is a cause of pain. Usually, this remits and no treatment is needed.

Hyaline, mucoid, cystic degeneration. These changes may produce soft or hard fibroids, confusing the diagnosis. *Torsion of the pedicle.* This can arise in the case of a polypoid subserous fibroid, and will give rise to acute abdominal symptoms. If the torsion is subacute and the blood supply is gradually reduced, the fibroid may develop a new vascularity through adhesions (parasitic tumour).

199

FIBROIDS

TREATMENT
Conservative management.
  Small, asymptomatic fibroids need not be treated.

Medical treatment
  Gonadotropin releasing hormone (GnRH) analogues may give 50% reduction in 6 months, but rapid return to former size may follow cessation of therapy. Treatment for longer than 6 months can lead to osteoporosis.

Surgical treatment
  Uterine artery embolisation – radiologically guided arterial embolisation
  Myomectomy – conserving the uterus but removing the fibroid *may* preserve fertility.
  Hysterectomy – removal of uterus with the fibroids.

Myomectomy
The approach to the tumour is made through the uterine wall following an injection of a vasopressor to minimise blood loss. The fibroid is shelled out by sharp and blunt dissection. The false capsule may make the plane of dissection difficult to identify. It can be performed by open or laparoscopic techniques.

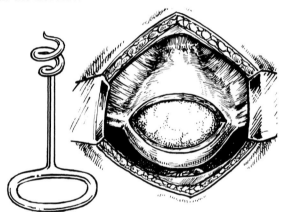

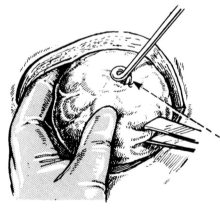

Myoma screw can be used to steady fibroid

The resultant cavity is obliterated by buried sutures and the uterine wall flapped over to bring the suture line as low on the uterine wall as possible to reduce the risk of adhesions to the bowel.

The disadvantages of myomectomy are possible blood loss and the recurrence of fibroids. Hysterectomy is the treatment of choice unless the patient wishes to retain fertility potential.

ENDOMETRIAL HYPERPLASIA

Being less accessible than lesions of the vulvar, vaginal or cervical epithelium, endometrial premalignant conditions are less easily diagnosed and followed up. Any hyperplastic condition raises the question of development of cancer and assessment of risk is important. Hyperplasia and carcinoma may coexist.

Endometrial hyperplasia may be classified as simple, complex or atypical.

CLINICAL FINDINGS

Most patients are in the 3rd and 4th decades of life, but hyperplasia is not confined to these age groups. It may be found in association with anovulation in teenage girls and in postmenopausal women. Heavy and/or irregular vaginal bleeding are the presenting symptoms but its severity or frequency is not related to the degree of pathological change.

SIMPLE HYPERPLASIA

This is the most common type. The endometrium has a characteristic appearance, often termed 'Swiss cheese' or cystic glandular hyperplasia.

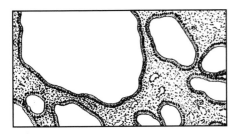

At low power magnification the pattern is a mixture of glands of varying sizes, a significant proportion of them being cystic. There is no crowding of the glands which are lined by cubical or columnar epithelium. Mitotic figures are present in small numbers. A similar gross picture may be seen in atrophic endometria but the mitotic activity is absent. Other associated pathology is rare.

COMPLEX HYPERPLASIA

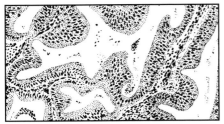

In this grade of hyperplasia the most striking feature is the quite obvious hyperplasia – crowding of glands so that they are back-to-back, the epithelium is stratified and mitoses are relatively frequent. There is, however, no epithelial atypia.

ATYPICAL HYPERPLASIA

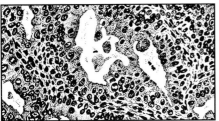

At this stage nuclear atypia is present. Intra-glandular polypoid formations and abnormal mitotic figures are seen. Severe cases may be indistinguishable from a carcinoma and adjacent areas of endometrial carcinoma may occur.

ENDOMETRIAL HYPERPLASIA

AETIOLOGY

Exogenous or endogenous unopposed oestrogens are primarily implicated in the pathogenesis of hyperplasia. Anovulatory cycles in perimenopause, obesity, polycystic ovarian disease, oestrogen secreting ovarian tumours (granulosa cell tumours), tamoxifen therapy (selective oestrogen receptor modulator) and unopposed oestrogen hormone replacement therapy can cause hyperplasia of endometrium.

INVESTIGATION

Imaging of the uterus with ultrasound to assess the endometrium is indicated. To obtain a diagnosis, an endometrial biopsy, with or without hysteroscopic assessment, will be required. Investigation will usually be in an outpatient setting but inpatient general anaesthetic assessment may also be needed.

TREATMENT

This depends principally on the types of hyperplasia. The age of the patient and a desire to retain fertility are factors to be considered.

Simple hyperplasia, with 1% risk of progression to carcinoma requires no routine follow-up. Symptomatic patients can be treated with progestogenic agents such as oral preparations or, increasingly, with the levonorgestrel releasing intrauterine device (IUD) (Mirena®). Recurrent abnormal bleeding would, of course, merit investigation.

Complex hyperplasia is not thought to merit hysterectomy. Progestin therapy, such as levonorgestrel releasing IUD, is again indicated for symptomatic management. Subsequent care after diagnosis can reasonably be dictated by the presenting symptoms.

Atypical hyperplasia, with estimated risks of co-existence of, or progression to, endometrial carcinoma of between 20% and 50% merits hysterectomy and a bilateral salpingo-oophorectomy in most cases. Women who wish to remain potentially fertile may be treated with oral progestogens or by levonorgestrel releasing IUD but long-term data is lacking. Recurrence on cessation of therapy has been reported and long-term surveillance with repeated endometrial sampling is mandatory.

Hysteroscopy

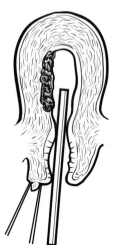

Endometrial biopsy

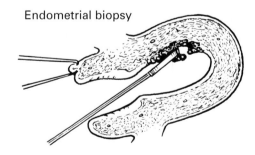

CARCINOMA OF THE ENDOMETRIUM

One of the commonest gynaecological cancers, it occurs most often in postmenopausal women (up to 80% of cases) with less than 5% diagnosed under 40 years of age. Its association with obesity, diabetes and polycystic ovarian syndrome is common. Postmenopausal American women may run a 1 in 1000 risk of endometrial carcinoma each year. There is no effective screening programme, but postmenopausal bleeding may be a cardinal symptom prompting urgent investigation.

PRESENTATION

The usual presenting symptom of endometrial carcinoma is *postmenopausal bleeding* which carries a 10% risk of associated malignancy. However, patients may also present in the perimenopause with frequent, irregular bleeding or before the menopause with irregular vaginal bleeding. An awareness of the risk factors will prompt appropriate investigation. Pyometra also carries a high risk of underlying carcinoma

Increased risk is associated with obesity, nulliparity, late menopause, tamoxifen, polycystic ovarian disease, oestrogen secreting tumours.

DIAGNOSIS

Patients presenting with postmenopausal bleeding should be reviewed urgently and investigated with an abdomino-pelvic ultrasound including a transvaginal ultrasound. This will allow an assessment of the ovaries and the endometrium. Where the endometrial thickness is measured to be less than 3 mm in women not on HRT and less than 5 mm in women taking HRT, there is an extremely low incidence of endometrial cancer and the patient can be reassured. Recurrent bleeding should prompt further investigation.

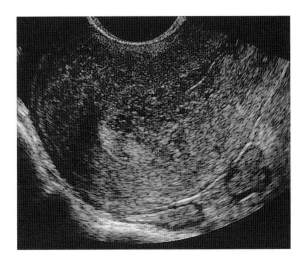

Transvaginal scan showing thickened endometrium

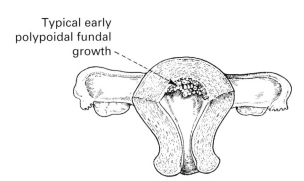

Typical early polypoidal fundal growth

Patients with abnormal scans and all women with irregular bleeding on tamoxifen should undergo hysteroscopy and endometrial biopsy. In addition, careful inspection of the cervix, vulva and vagina should be undertaken to exclude these as a source of bleeding due to malignant change.

CARCINOMA OF THE ENDOMETRIUM

HISTOLOGY

Distribution of Subtypes

Endometrioid	85%
Adenosquamous	4%
Serous carcinoma	4%
Clear cell	3%

The majority of tumours are adenocarcinoma and they are divided into three groups according to the degree of glandular differentiation.

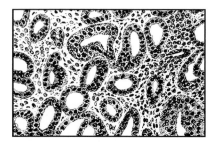

Grade 1 – Well differentiated.

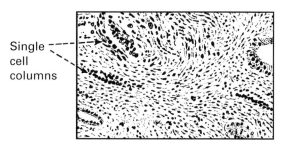

Single cell columns

Grade 2 – Moderately differentiated. Gland forms are much less prominent and many of the deposits consist of infiltrating single cell columns or solid masses.

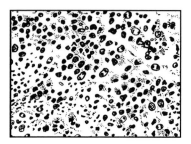

Grade 3 – Poorly differentiated. This type consists of solid masses of malignant cells of varying sizes and shapes with little or no stroma. Mitoses are numerous.

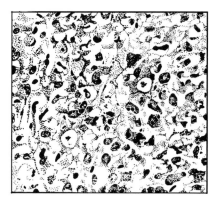

Clear cell carcinoma
This tumour has a poor prognosis and is included with the Grade 3 adenocarcinomata. It occurs mainly in the elderly.

STAGING OF ENDOMETRIAL CARCINOMA

The classification given below is that of the International Federation of Gynecology and Obstetrics (FIGO 2009).

Stage I Growth confined to
A Inner half of the uterus
B Growth into the outer half of the uterus

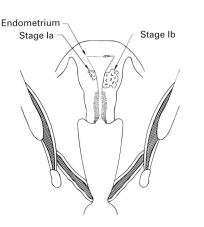

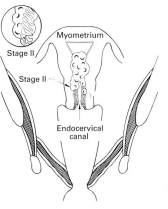

Stage II
The growth has extended to the cervix.

Stage III
The growth has extended to
A Serosa and/or adnexa
B Vagina
C Pelvic or paraaortic lymph nodes

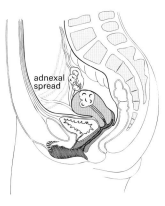

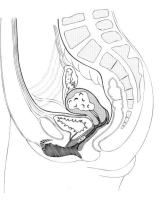

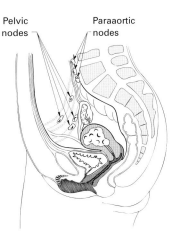

Stage IV
The growth has invaded

(a) the rectum or bladder or
(b) structures beyond the pelvis.

Histological grading, G1, G2 or G3 is applied to Stages I, II and III only.

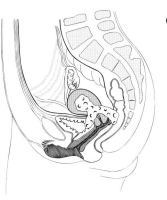

SPREAD OF ENDOMETRIAL CARCINOMA

Magnetic resonance imaging is preferable to an ultrasound for the assessment of myometrial invasion and pelvic spread. To assess distal metastases, a computerised tomography (CT) scan of the chest, abdomen and pelvis may also be of value.

LOCAL SPREAD
Invasion of the myometrium and cervix is the commonest spread. It may produce considerable uterine enlargement.

LYMPHATIC SPREAD
Lymphatic spread is more likely to occur when the tumour is poorly differentiated and the uterine wall is deeply invaded. The incidence of pelvic nodal metastases is in the region of 10%.

Most metastases occur in the adjacent structures and in the peritoneum. In advanced cases, distant metastases do occur, most commonly in lung, but occasionally in liver, vertebrae or other bones and in the supraclavicular lymph nodes.

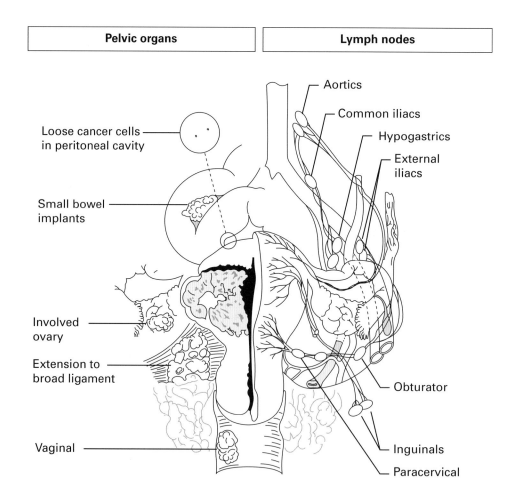

| Pelvic organs | Lymph nodes |

AETIOLOGICAL FACTORS IN ENDOMETRIAL CARCINOMA

There are two suggested types of endometrial carcinoma, based on aetiology.

Type 1 – arising in patients with a background history of oestrogen excess.

Type 2 – arising without evidence of oestrogenic stimulation.

Type 1 tumours would appear to have a better prognosis with a better differentiation pattern and a less invasive component. They would appear to be derived from a hyperoestrogenic stimulus. Type 2 tumours, including serous and clear cell cancers, arise from a atrophic type endometrium and have a more aggressive phenotype with greater invasion, poorer differentiation, more metastatic disease and, as such, they carry a poorer prognosis. Type 2 tumours have been associated with abnormalities in tumour suppressor genes.

Obesity, in particular, appears to be a developing issue in terms of the risk of endometrial carcinoma. Obese patients convert peripheral androgens to oestrogens via the action of the aromatase enzyme in adipose cells. Countries where the incidence of obesity is rising have started to also see an increase in the incidence of endometrial carcinoma. In some countries, it is now the commonest cancer of the female genital tract, overtaking ovarian carcinoma.

Hereditary non-polyposis colorectal cancer (Lynch II) syndrome is an inherited mutation in DNA mismatch repair genes. In those affected, the endometrial carcinoma occurs more frequently, together with breast and colon cancer.

PROGNOSIS OF ENDOMETRIAL CARCINOMA

The overall 5-year survival rate is approximately 80%. Fortunately, over 80% of cases are diagnosed at Stage I. The survival is affected by multiple prognostic factors including:

Stage at diagnosis

Histological grade

Depth of myometrial invasion

Lympho-vascular space involvement (LVSI)

Non-endometrioid type

5-year survival rates according to clinical staging are as follows:

Stage	5-year survival (%)
I	85
II	75
III	45
IV	25

Assessing 5-year survival rates according to International Federation of Gynecology and Obstetrics (FIGO) histological grading is reported as follows:

Grading	5-year survival (%)
G1	92
G2	90
G3	81

Using both methods on similar cases, we find that the 5-year survival rates for Stage I are the only ones altered significantly:

Stage and histology	5-year survival (%)
I, G1 and 2	80
I, G3	60

TREATMENT OF ENDOMETRIAL CARCINOMA

This is essentially *surgical*, with postoperative adjuvant *radiotherapy* added when unfavourable prognostic features are found at surgery. Adjuvant therapy for endometrial cancer is a contentious, evolving field. To date, it provides improved local control but without improved survival. Many believe that the addition of adjuvant chemotherapy may add a survival advantage and research is underway.

Progestogen therapy is probably only of value in recurrent disease, but has been studied in early stage, well-differentiated, disease where fertility preservation is an issue and in patients not fit for radical therapy. If a woman is unfit for surgery then radiotherapy may be used alone, but it is less effective.

STAGE I
Surgery for total abdominal hysterectomy and bilateral salpingo-oophorectomy without partial removal of vagina is the treatment of choice. Peritoneal saline washings are taken for cytology on opening the abdomen during surgery and the abdominal contents are carefully examined. The procedure can also be performed laparoscopically with equivalent 5-year survival and a lower operative morbidity. Evidence from randomised trials does not support lymphadenectomy as a therapeutic intervention.

STAGE II
Stage II carries a prognosis that is similar to Stage I, and is usually treated as for Stage I and diagnosed by pathology. Where preoperative assessment suggests obvious cervical involvement then a radical hysterectomy with pelvic lymphadenectomy may be undertaken.

STAGE III/IV
Treatment of this stage is designed to control tumour growth and alleviate symptoms. Treatment will depend upon tumour burden at the preoperative assessment and imaging. Many cases may only be identified as Stage III, following surgical management. Surgery, radiation therapy, chemotherapy and adjuvant progestogen therapy all have a place.

RECURRENCE OF ENDOMETRIAL CARCINOMA

The majority of recurrences appear within 3 years of treatment. Early recurrence has a poor prognosis.

SITES
Recurrence can be local but endometrial carcinoma can also recur outside the pelvis. Vault recurrence is less common after adjuvant vaginal vault irradiation but distal recurrence is found more frequently if vault irradiation has been performed.

TREATMENT FOR RECURRENCE
Where recurrence is localised to the central pelvis, its salvage with radiotherapy and/or surgery can be successful. *Progestogens* have been used as part of a combined primary treatment, as well as for recurrent or metastatic growths. Between 15% and 50% of recurrences will respond to therapy. Tumour response is especially noted in those patients with progesterone receptors in the tumour. Medroxyprogesterone acetate is most commonly employed and the addition of tamoxifen may improve the response. *Chemotherapy* also has a place in recurrent disease. Combination treatment with adriamycin and cisplatin gives response rates between 20% and 40%.

SARCOMA OF THE UTERUS

These are rare tumours and include:
Endometrial stromal sarcomas
Leiomyosarcomas
Carcinosarcomas

This group of cancers has undergone changes in nomenclature and even now some consider that uterine sarcomas are best described as high or low grade uterine sarcomas. They share a common presentation with other uterine cancers, with irregular and/or postmenopausal bleeding.

CLINICAL FEATURES

The patient is usually over 50 years old and presents with a complaint of fairly heavy bleeding of recent origin, accompanied by pain. Pelvic examination reveals a large intrauterine mass with friable tissue palpable through the os. The tumour may originate from the vagina in younger women and from the cervix in the child; but these are, indeed, very rare conditions. Sarcomatous change may occur in 0.1% of fibroids.

HISTOLOGICAL APPEARANCES

Tumour tissue may infiltrate the whole myometrium and fill the uterine cavity or arise from a pedicle. This type often presents as a cervical or vaginal polyp. The tissues of origin are the connective tissue and muscle of the myometrium or leiomyoma, or the endometrial stroma.

These are composed of undifferentiated round- or spindle-cell masses. In children, striated muscle is often a feature and a characteristic polypoidal growth occurs – sarcoma botryoides.

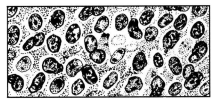

High power appearance of round-cell sarcoma

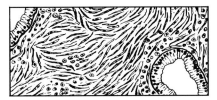

Low power view of spindle-cell sarcoma

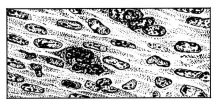

High power view of smooth muscle sarcoma

SARCOMA OF THE UTERUS

ENDOMETRIAL STROMAL SARCOMAS
These are tumours of the endometrial stromal cells and form two groups:

Low Grade Stromal Sarcomas
The clinical course is often uncomplicated and cure may follow surgery. They can recur, often years later, and recurrence up to 25 years later has been reported.

High Grade Stromal Sarcoma
This type of stromal tumour shows numerous mitoses and is infiltrative from the start. There is early recurrence and widespread metastases occur even if there has been little local invasion of the myometrium. The prognosis is poor.

CARCINOSARCOMA (MALIGNANT MIXED MESODERMAL TUMOUR)
In this variant, both epithelial and stromal elements are malignant. It forms a soft polypoid mass that is usually haemorrhagic. Microscopically, most of the growth is sarcomatous but there are foci of carcinoma – adeno, squamoid, undifferentiated or various mixtures of these. The prognosis is poor. Treatment is surgical with hysterectomy, bilateral salpingo-oophorectomy and pelvic lymphadenectomy.

LEIOMYOSARCOMA
Usually these cases do not present with postmenopausal bleeding and are found in patients thought to have a uterine fibroid. Fibroids of a very large size or those which increase rapidly in size should be suspected as having a higher chance of malignant change.

Treatment is usually hysterectomy and bilateral salpingo-oophorectomy. It is often not suspected at diagnosis. If detected postoperatively, then CT scan of chest, abdomen and pelvis should be undertaken to look for metastases. 10% of cases at diagnosis may have pulmonary metastases. Haematogenous spread is most common.

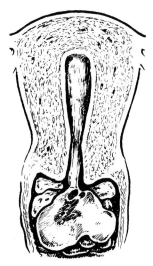

Pelvic examination, in this case, would suggest a cervical origin.

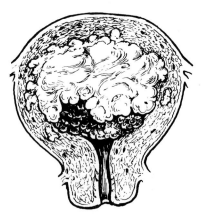

A diffuse infiltrating sarcoma.

CHAPTER 12

PROLAPSE AND UROGYNAECOLOGY

Retroversion of the Uterus	214	Genuine Stress Incontinence	238
Symptoms and Treatment of		*Symptoms*	238
Displacement	215	*Genuine Stress Incontinence*	238
Uterovaginal Prolapse	216	Other Incontinence Mechanisms	239
Vaginal Prolapse	218	*Overflow Incontinence*	239
Anterior Prolapse	218	*Neurological Disease*	239
Prolapse of the Posterior Wall	219	*Other Symptoms and Signs*	
Clinical Features of Prolapse	220	*Associated with Incontinence*	239
Differential Diagnosis of Prolapse	221	The Urethral Syndrome	240
Pessary Treatment	222	Investigation of Incontinence	241
Alternative-Shaped Pessaries	222	*Examination*	241
Indications for Pessary Treatment	222	*Demonstrations of Stress*	
Anterior Colporrhaphy (and Repair		*Incontinence*	241
of Cystocele)	223	Urodynamic Investigation of	
Anterior Repair	223	Bladder Function	242
Manchester Repair	225	*Cystometry*	242
Posterior Colpoperineorrhaphy		*Abnormal Cystometry*	242
(Including Repair of		Indications for Urodynamic	
Rectocele)	227	Assessment	243
Repair of Enterocele	228	*Other Investigations*	243
Vaginal Hysterectomy	229	Treatment of Stress Incontinence	244
Indications	229	*Conservative Treatment of Stress*	
Operative and Postoperative		*Incontinence*	244
Complications	230	*New Surgical Developments in the*	
Late Complications	230	*Treatment of Stress Incontinence*	244
Urogynaecology	231	Surgical Treatment of Stress	
The Anatomy of the Urinary Tract	231	Incontinence	245
Blood Supply of the Ureter	233	Marshall–Marchetti–Krantz	
Histology of the Ureter	233	Urethropexy	246
Physiology of Micturition	234	Burch's Colposuspension Operation	247
Intravesical Pressure	234	*Stamey Needle Suspension*	
Intraurethral Pressure	234	*Procedure*	247
Innervation of Bladder and Urethra	235	Sling Procedures	248
Mechanism of Voiding	236	Treatment of Detrusor Instability	249
Detrusor Instability	237	*Bladder Retraining*	249
Symptoms	237	*Drug Treatment*	249

RETROVERSION OF THE UTERUS

An alteration from the usual anteverted position of the uterus often with a change in the curve of the uterine axis. Most of the so-called displacements are merely variations of the normal and are of little clinical significance.

Anteverted Uterus
The uterus is approximately at right angles to the vagina and has a slight forward curve.

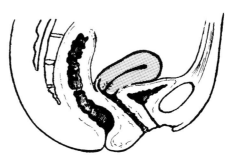

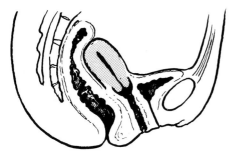

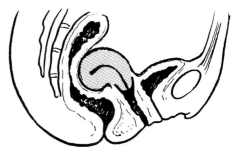

Retroversion
The long axis of the uterus is directed backwards. The uterus is displaced backwards and this is simply a physiological variation for the vast majority of women. It occurs in approximately 20–30% of women.

Retroflexion
This is a variation of retroversion but the uterus is curved backwards. The cervix may remain in the normal position but is usually positioned as in retroversion.

RETROVERSION OF THE UTERUS

Causes of Displacement

Displacement may be due to the presence of some other condition such as a cyst or fibroid or endometriosis.

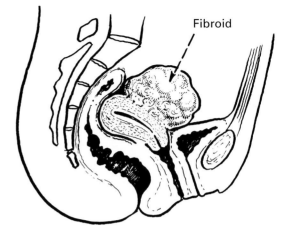

Fibroid

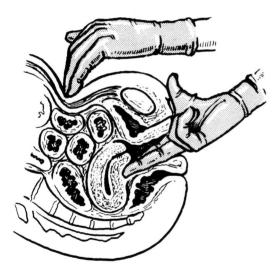

Diagnosis is by bimanual palpation. The vaginal hand palpates a mass in the Pouch of Douglas, the abdominal hand detects the absence of a uterine corpus in the expected place. The possibility of pelvic pathology should be considered and ultrasound may be used to confirm the clinical findings.

SYMPTOMS AND TREATMENT OF DISPLACEMENT

Consequences of Uncomplicated Displacement

Usually none. However, if there is pelvic pathology present, the woman may complain of deep dyspareunia. If such pain occurs, it can easily be reproduced by pressing with the examining fingers. It is quite possible for the patient to present with a complaint of dyspareunia and to have a retroverted uterus which has nothing to do with her complaint.

215

UTEROVAGINAL PROLAPSE

Herniation of the genital tract through the pelvic diaphragm.

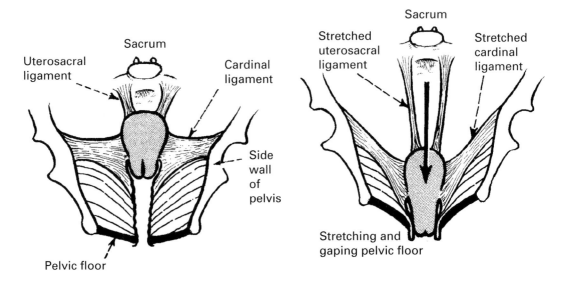

The uterus and vagina are held in the pelvis by the cardinal and uterosacral ligaments and by the pelvic floor musculature, mainly the levatores ani.

When these ligaments and muscles become ineffective, the uterus and vagina descend (prolapse) through the gap between the muscles.

The causes of prolapse are the following:

- The stretching of muscle and fibrous tissue which occurs with childbirth and damage to the innervation of the pelvic floor.
- Age and menopausal changes lead to changes in connective tissue support.
- Increased intra-abdominal pressure, for example, chronic cough, heavy manual work; congenital predisposition to stretch the ligaments.
- Distortion of pelvic anatomy by previous surgery, for example, vault prolapse after hysterectomy or entercoele after colposuspension.

The incidence of this condition in the United Kingdom has been greatly reduced because of smaller families and higher caesarean section rates.

UTEROVAGINAL PROLAPSE

The uterus gradually descends in the axis of the vagina taking the vaginal wall with it. It may present clinically at any level, but is usually classified as one of three degrees.

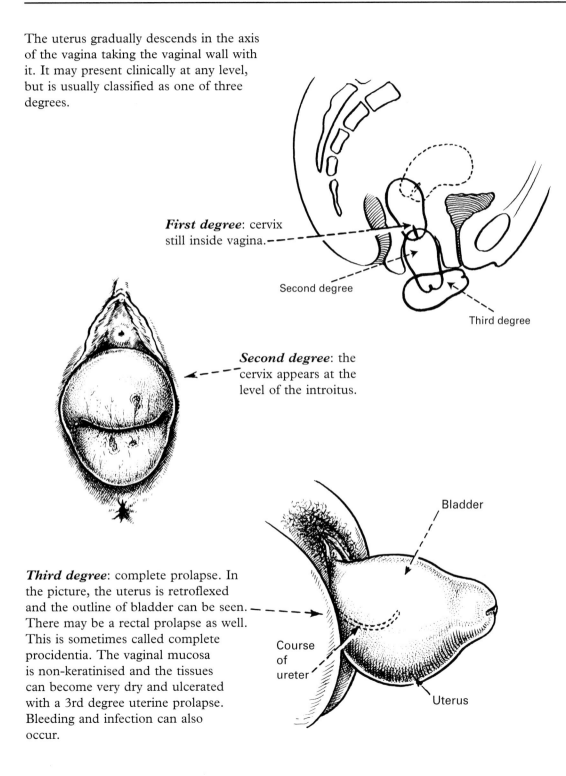

First degree: cervix still inside vagina.

Second degree

Third degree

Second degree: the cervix appears at the level of the introitus.

Bladder

Third degree: complete prolapse. In the picture, the uterus is retroflexed and the outline of bladder can be seen. There may be a rectal prolapse as well. This is sometimes called complete procidentia. The vaginal mucosa is non-keratinised and the tissues can become very dry and ulcerated with a 3rd degree uterine prolapse. Bleeding and infection can also occur.

Course of ureter

Uterus

VAGINAL PROLAPSE

The prolapse involves the vaginal walls and the related viscera. Prolapse of several sites may co-exist and a uterine prolapse may also be present.

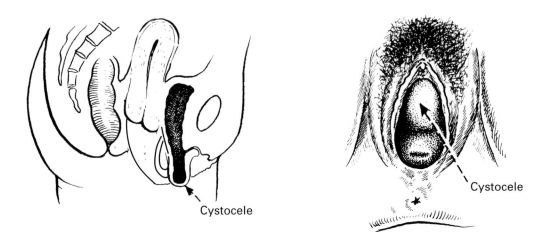

ANTERIOR PROLAPSE

When the upper part of the anterior wall prolapses, there is an underlying failure of the investing fascia, and the bladder base also descends. This is called a cystocele.

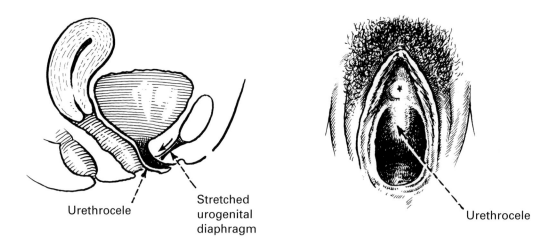

Sometimes the lower part of the vaginal wall prolapses and the urethra also descends. This is called a urethrocele.

VAGINAL PROLAPSE

PROLAPSE OF THE POSTERIOR WALL

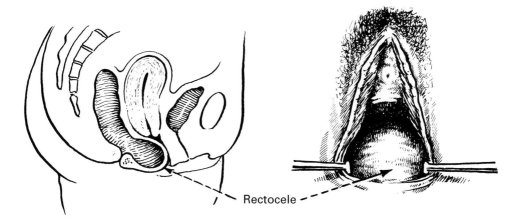

Rectocele

If the prolapse is at the level of the middle third of the vagina, the rectovaginal septum is often involved and rectum prolapses with vaginal wall. This is called a rectocele. If the lowest part of the vagina prolapses, the perineal body is involved rather than the rectum.

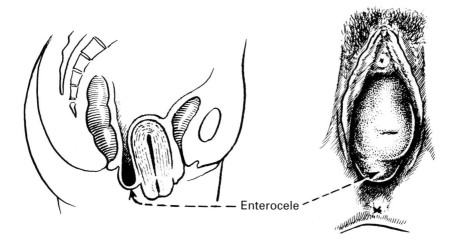

Enterocele

If the upper part of the posterior vaginal wall prolapses, the Pouch of Douglas is elongated and small bowel or omentum may descend. This is called an enterocele. Enterocele is often associated with uterine prolapse, as in the picture.

Where the uterus has been removed, prolapse of this region is known as a vault prolapse. This is a difficult condition to treat. The technique depends on suspending the vaginal vault from fixed ligaments within the pelvic and often requires insertion of a non-absorbable mesh.

219

CLINICAL FEATURES OF PROLAPSE

- *Asymptomatic*. It is not uncommon for women to palpate a prolapse, for example, during washing or attempting to insert a tampon. For some women, simple reassurance that there is no sinister cause is all that is required. It can also be identified during routine smear, etc., and if asymptomatic no treatment is required.
- 'Something coming down' within the vagina is the commonest symptom. It tends to be worse when the woman has been on her feet and it disappears when she lies down.
- *Backache*. Some women will experience a dragging feeling or bearing down sensation. This is sometimes resolved with treatment of the prolapse, but mechanical back pain is very common and it may be unrelated to prolapse.
- *Coital problems*. This is relatively unusual but the woman may admit to difficulties with intercourse, only on direct questioning.
- *Increased frequency of micturition*. This can be due to anatomical changes that make it difficult to empty the bladder fully. Detrusor instability is also common in older women and may co-exist. A careful urinary history should be taken including fluid and caffeine intake.
- *Stress incontinence*. This is by no means always present. Sometimes, it is found that reduction of the prolapse causes stress incontinence.
- *Difficulty in voiding urine and defecating*. The patient may find that it is impossible to initiate micturition except by pushing up the cystocele with her finger. In the same way, the rectocele must be pushed back to allow emptying of the rectum.

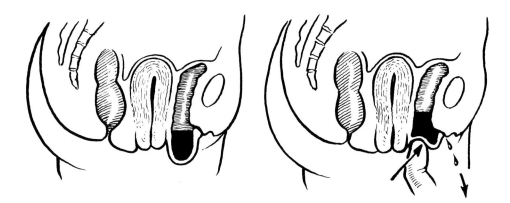

The onset may be gradual or quite sudden and is commoner after the menopause when the genital tract tissues begin to atrophy.

DIFFERENTIAL DIAGNOSIS OF PROLAPSE

Prolapse should be confirmed by vaginal examination. The following conditions resemble prolapse on superficial examination; however, careful examination will detect the difference.

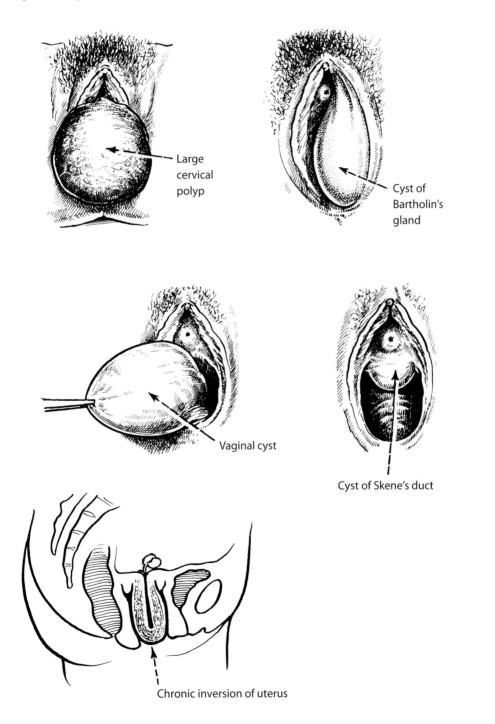

Large cervical polyp

Cyst of Bartholin's gland

Vaginal cyst

Cyst of Skene's duct

Chronic inversion of uterus

221

PESSARY TREATMENT

There are a number of different shapes of vaginal pessaries, the simplest to insert is a ring pessary. This is usually made of semi-rigid plastic and is inserted into the vagina so that the vaginal walls are stretched and they cannot prolapse through the introitus.

The pessary is compressed into a long ovoid shape, lubricated and gently pushed into the vagina, where it resumes its circular shape and takes up a position in the coronal plane. It must not be too tight; and correct fitting is learnt by experience. To an extent, pessary fitting is trial and error and the woman should be warned that the pessary may dislodge. A point of contact should be given so that she can be seen again without delay if this is the case.

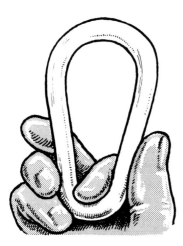

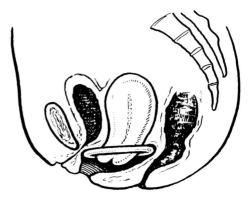

ALTERNATIVE-SHAPED PESSARIES

The 'shelf' pessary can be particularly useful for uterine prolapse but it is slightly less malleable and insertion can be more difficult.

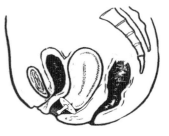

INDICATIONS FOR PESSARY TREATMENT

- The patient prefers a pessary. Pelvic surgery with its unavoidable risks should only be applied to a willing patient.
- The prolapse is amenable to pessary support. If the perineal muscles are very deficient they will not hold a pessary and the pessary will fall out. If too big a ring is required, the vaginal wall or cervix will prolapse through it. Posterior vaginal wall prolapses are poorly supported by pessaries.
- The patient is not fit for surgery.
- The patient wishes to delay operation temporarily (e.g., another pregnancy is anticipated).

Plastic rings should be changed once or twice a year, and if it has been properly fitted, the patient will be unaware of its presence in her vagina even during coitus. An ill-fitting pessary is ineffective and may cause dyspareunia and discomfort. If it is too tight or left too long, ulceration of the vaginal wall will occur, and malignant change has been reported. Vaginal oestriol cream or vaginal oestradiol tablets (0.025 mg) help prevent atrophic vaginitis.

ANTERIOR COLPORRHAPHY (AND REPAIR OF CYSTOCELE)

Surgical restoration of the normal anatomy is the purpose of treatment. Reconstitution of the fibrous 'scaffolding' of the pelvic organs aims to allow the musculature to function efficiently

Cystocele and rectocele are dealt with by anterior and posterior colporrhaphy. Uterine prolapse may require vaginal hysterectomy. Cervical amputation or Manchester repair may be adequate if the cervix is hypertrophied and the uterus is well supported. Each 'repair' must be adapted to the extent of the prolapse and this may often be fully appreciated only at examination under anaesthesia. Women should be counselled regarding the possible surgical consequences prior to surgery and consent should reflect this.

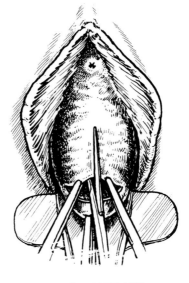

ANTERIOR REPAIR

1.   Opening up the anterior vaginal wall.

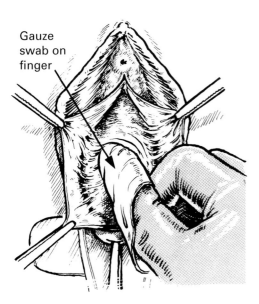

Gauze swab on finger

2.   Mobilising cystocele from vaginal walls.

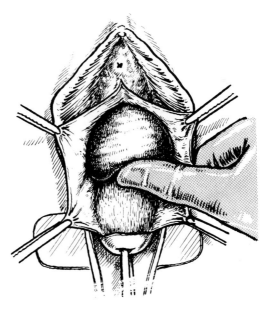

3.   Mobilising cystocele from cervix.

223

ANTERIOR COLPORRHAPHY (AND REPAIR OF CYSTOCELE)

ANTERIOR REPAIR—(cont'd)
The next step is obliteration of the cystocele protrusion by tightening the fascial layer between it and the vaginal wall, a layer which is often very difficult to identify.

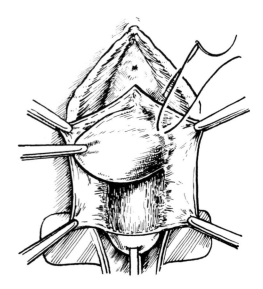

4. Placing the tightening sutures as far laterally as possible.

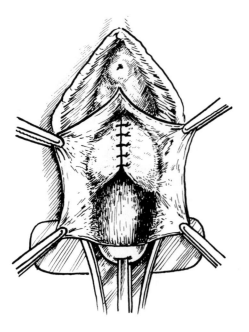

5. Obliteration of the cystocele completed.

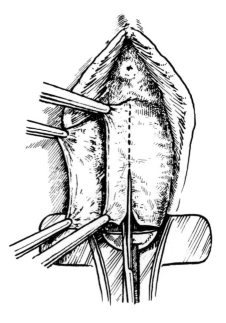

6. Removing redundant vaginal wall. This is followed by closure with interrupted absorbable sutures.

MANCHESTER REPAIR

This involves at the least some shortening of the transverse cervical ligaments and usually amputation of the elongated supravaginal cervix. It is often done in conjunction with anterior and posterior repairs.

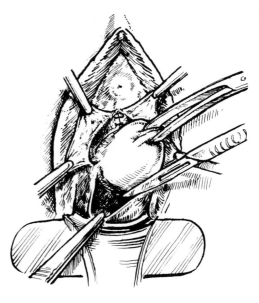

1. The cystocele has been repaired. The cervix is being stripped of vaginal wall.

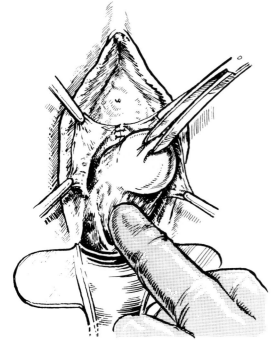

2. Posterior vaginal wall being stripped back.

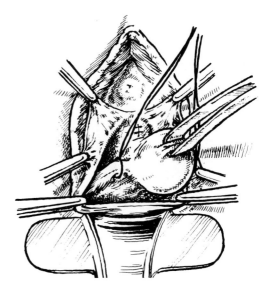

3. Elongated transverse cervical and uterosacral ligaments are sutured and divided.

225

MANCHESTER REPAIR

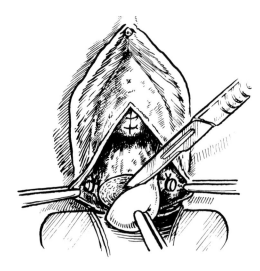

4. Amputation of cervix.

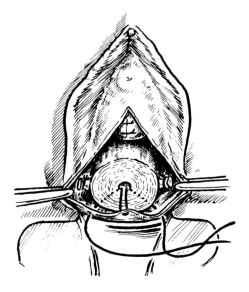

5. Covering the posterior stump with vaginal wall.

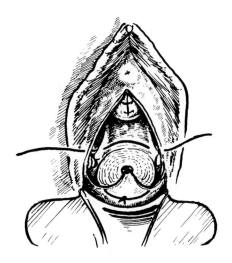

6. Tying the transverse cervical ligaments in front of the cervix and so shortening them and raising the uterus. (This is the so-called Fothergill suture: sometimes two are put in.)

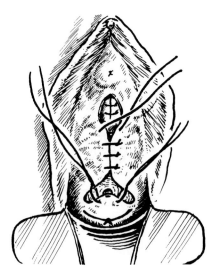

7. Covering cervical stump and closing the vaginal wall. On release of the cervical stump, the uterus returns to the pelvis.

POSTERIOR COLPOPERINEORRHAPHY (INCLUDING REPAIR OF RECTOCELE)

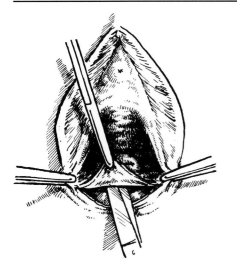

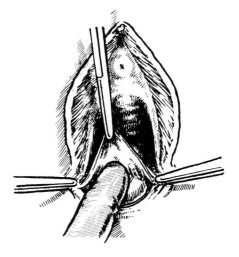

1. Mobilisation of the posterior vaginal wall.

2. Separating rectocele from posterior vaginal wall.

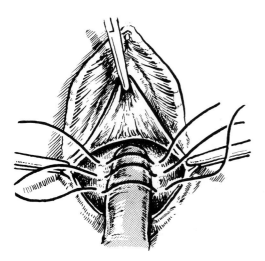

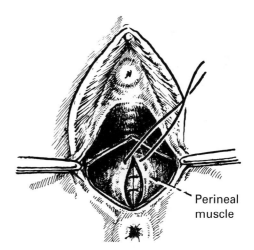

Perineal muscle

3. Obliterating the rectocele by tightening the fascial layer (cf. obliterating the cystocele).

4. Excess vaginal skin is removed. The perineal muscles are sutured over the obliterated rectocele. The skin and vagina are closed.

REPAIR OF ENTEROCELE

An enterocele is a prolapse of the Pouch of Douglas peritoneum in between the upper vagina and rectum, and must be distinguished from a rectocele. Repair of enterocele is often combined with repair of uterine prolapse which is not shown here.

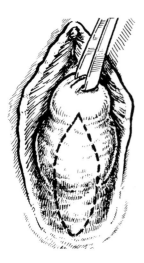

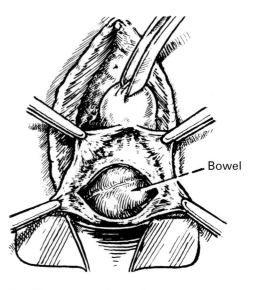

Bowel

1. Dotted lines show the area of vaginal wall which will be removed.

2. The enterocele sac is identified and opened.

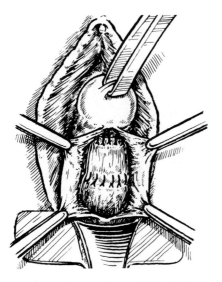

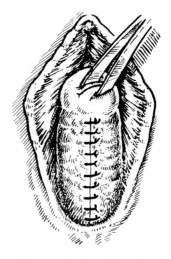

3. Once the sac is mobilised the neck is sutured up as far as possible to obliterate the enterocele.

4. The vaginal wall is closed in the usual way.

VAGINAL HYSTERECTOMY

INDICATIONS

- When the uterine prolapse is significant.
- When hysterectomy is required for a non-malignant uterine condition – menorrhagia.

It may be difficult to remove the ovaries by the vaginal route and laparoscopically assisted vaginal hysterectomy may facilitate this.

Appropriate access is required to the remove the uterus. The blood supply has to be divided from the uterus and the pedicles secured. The bladder has to be mobilised so that it is not injured during the procedure. Access may be limited by a number of factors, for example, an enlarged fibroid uterus or if there is pelvic adhesion related to endometriosis. This procedure is always easier in women who have had vaginal deliveries.

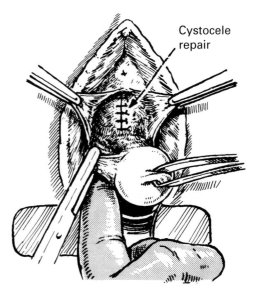

Cystocele repair

1. The bladder has been mobilised. The uterine ligaments are put on the stretch and divided.

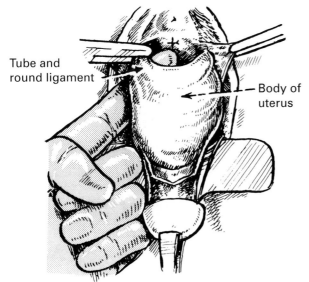

Tube and round ligament

Body of uterus

2. Uterovesical pouch has been entered. Broad ligament structures are put on the stretch and divided. The uterus is then removed.

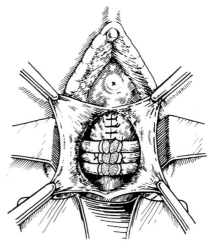

3. The lateral pedicles are sutured together to support the Pouch of Douglas. The vaginal vault is closed.

VAGINAL HYSTERECTOMY

OPERATIVE AND POSTOPERATIVE COMPLICATIONS

Selection of Patients
- Neither youth nor age is a contraindication, but the patient must be reasonably fit, with adequate cardiorespiratory and renal function. Oestradiol vaginal cream may be used to treat atrophic vaginitis prior to surgery.
- The prolapse should be symptomatic.

Perioperatively
- Bleeding pedicles are more difficult to control than during abdominal surgery. The parametric structures should be clamped, divided and ligated in small rather than large bites.
- With the uterus gone, there is a risk of distorting the ureters if the bladder fascia is tightened too much during repair of the cystocele.

Postoperatively
If uncomplicated, the recovery following vaginal surgery is usually associated with less pain and more rapid mobilisation than with abdominal surgery. There is a higher risk of vault haematoma with vaginal hysterectomy when compared to abdominal hysterectomy. This may become infected; however, this usually responds to antibiotics and usually discharges per vaginam. Insertion of a vaginal pack at the end of the procedure is often performed to provide local pressure and reduce the risk of haematoma. A urinary catheter is required when a pack is used.

LATE COMPLICATIONS

Recurrence of prolapse
This is a relatively common problem. The prolapse that returns within the first months of a repair may be due to a break down or herniation within the primary repair. There may have been a history of postoperative infection. In the long term, women who have undergone pelvic floor repair are at an increased risk of prolapse. It is likely that the fundamental weakness of the fibrous supports of the pelvic floor continues but it may also be that a repair in one area of the pelvic floor transits pressure to another area of the pelvis.

Urinary incontinence
Urinary symptom can appear for the first time after a pelvic floor repair. This is often due to an underlying problem when the anatomy returns to normal.

Dyspareunia
The surgeon must enquire before the operation about the patient's sexual activity and must be careful to leave a functional vagina where this is required (although this may make support of the prolapse more difficult). Occasionally, dyspareunia may be caused by vaginal adhesions.

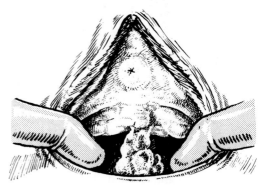

Vaginal wall adhesions

UROGYNAECOLOGY

THE ANATOMY OF THE URINARY TRACT

The Ureters

The ureter enters the pelvis retroperitoneally by crossing over or near the bifurcation of the common iliac artery.

The ureter is itself crossed by the ovarian vessels and is near the fold of peritoneum which forms the infundibulo-pelvic ligament.

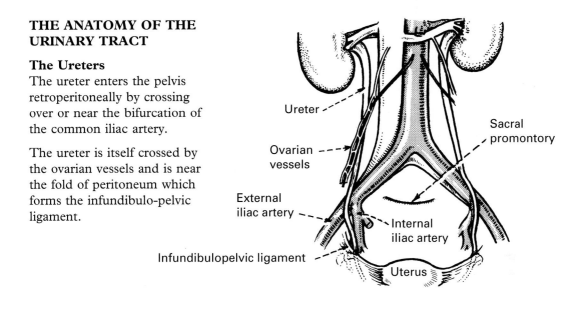

It passes down and medially behind the ovarian fossa and is in close relation to the internal iliac artery. In the healthy subject, its shape can be made out beneath the peritoneum and peristatic movements can be observed (vermiculation).

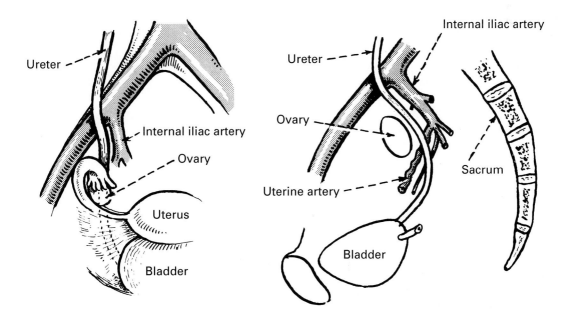

231

UROGYNAECOLOGY

The ureter then passes beneath the base of the broad ligament, through the transverse uterine ligament and into the bladder. In this parametrial part of its course, it lies alongside the vaginal fornix and passes under the uterine artery.

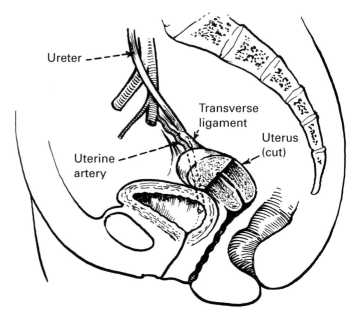

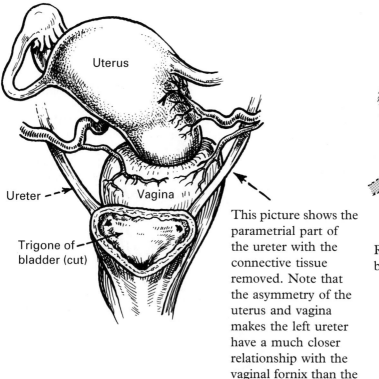

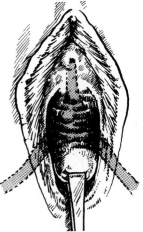

This picture shows the parametrial part of the ureter with the connective tissue removed. Note that the asymmetry of the uterus and vagina makes the left ureter have a much closer relationship with the vaginal fornix than the right.

Relationship of bladder base to vagina

BLOOD SUPPLY OF THE URETER

The ureter is supplied by branches from the main arteries with which it is in relation, principally the renal and ovarian arteries. The pelvic vessels are variable and because the blood enters mostly at the upper and lower ends, the peri-ureteric anastomoses are important.

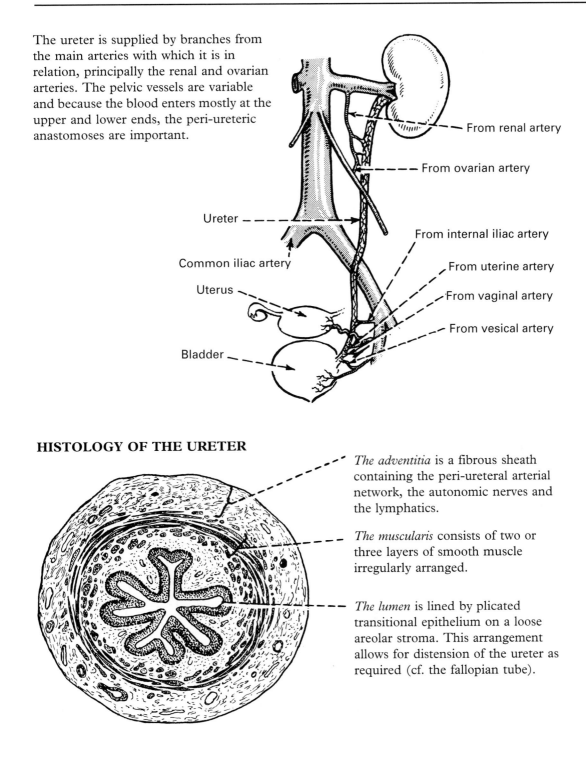

From renal artery

From ovarian artery

Ureter

From internal iliac artery

Common iliac artery

From uterine artery

Uterus

From vaginal artery

From vesical artery

Bladder

HISTOLOGY OF THE URETER

The adventitia is a fibrous sheath containing the peri-ureteral arterial network, the autonomic nerves and the lymphatics.

The muscularis consists of two or three layers of smooth muscle irregularly arranged.

The lumen is lined by plicated transitional epithelium on a loose areolar stroma. This arrangement allows for distension of the ureter as required (cf. the fallopian tube).

PHYSIOLOGY OF MICTURITION

Incontinence of urine is very common in women. The assessment and treatment call for an understanding of bladder and urethral physiology.

INTRAVESICAL PRESSURE
The bladder displays the phenomenon of adaptation to increased urinary volume. Pressure remains below 10 cm H_2O until over 500 ml of urine are contained.

INTRAURETHRAL PRESSURE
Urethral pressure is maintained by the 'internal sphincter' made up of longitudinal and circular plain muscle and elastic tissue; and an 'external sphincter' which contributes striated muscle.

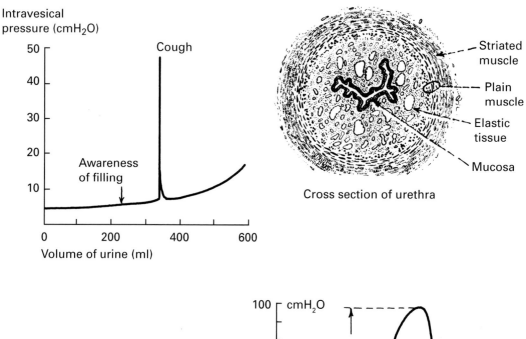

Cross section of urethra

A 'urethral pressure profile' shows the changes in pressure along the length of the urethra. This is normally much greater than the intravesical pressure, thus ensuring continence.

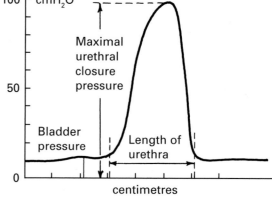

234

PHYSIOLOGY OF MICTURITION

INNERVATION OF BLADDER AND URETHRA

There is an intercommunicating sympathetic, parasympathetic and somatic supply. The parasympathetic stimulates detrusor contraction, and the sympathetic fibres (chiefly through the alpha receptors) stimulate contraction of the bladder neck and urethra.

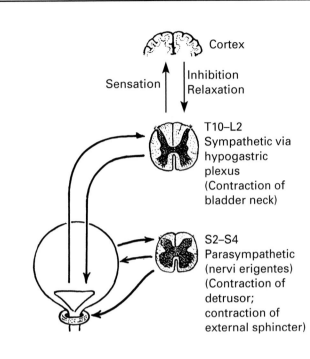

Cortex

Sensation

Inhibition
Relaxation

T10–L2
Sympathetic via hypogastric plexus
(Contraction of bladder neck)

S2–S4
Parasympathetic (nervi erigentes)
(Contraction of detrusor; contraction of external sphincter)

The striated muscle has been shown to have a dual autonomic/somatic supply via the pelvic plexus. In normal urethral closure, all the components of the sphincter mechanism must function together and the striated muscle has more to do than merely contract voluntarily when the desire to micturate must be resisted.

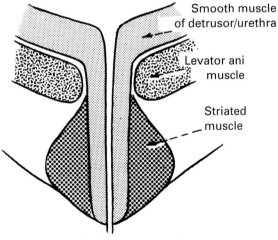

Smooth muscle of detrusor/urethra

Levator ani muscle

Striated muscle

Diagram of urethral closure mechanism

MECHANISM OF VOIDING

Cystometry recording
demonstrates the timing of events.

1. Intra-abdominal pressure
   increase. (Measured with a
   vaginal or rectal probe.)

2. Detrusor contracts.
   (Intravesical pressure
   increase.)

3. Sphincter relaxes.
   (Electromyogram of anal
   sphincter.)

4. Urine flow begins.

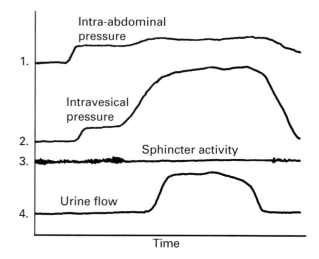

The urethra and bladder neck are maintained in the closed state by the trigonal condensation of muscle (the base plate) and the urethral sphincter (plain and striated muscle).

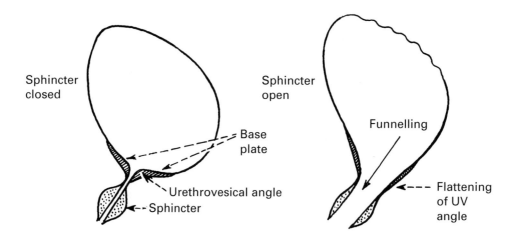

When cortical inhibition is withdrawn, the detrusor contracts and the bladder neck relaxes (funnelling). The sphincter also relaxes and urine is voided. As the flow continues, the bladder neck moves downwards and backwards and the urethrovesical (UV) angle is obliterated.

DETRUSOR INSTABILITY

For most women with this condition, it may be associated with neurological conditions, for example, multiple sclerosis and stroke.

The normal bladder does not contract unless voiding is desired. For reasons that are poorly understood, patients with detrusor instability experience detrusor contractions at other times. This can occur spontaneously but may also be provoked, for example, with coughing. The mechanism is altogether different from that of genuine stress incontinence, but some women will have both pathologies.

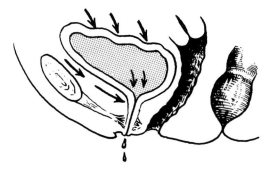

SYMPTOMS

The patient experiences an irresistible and sudden desire to micturate (urgency). Detrusor instability is the commonest cause, but it may also be due to inflammatory disease of the bladder without detrusor contraction. All forms of bladder pathology must be considered including calculus and carcinoma. There is usually an associated complaint of frequency.

GENUINE STRESS INCONTINENCE

SYMPTOMS

When a sudden increase in intravesical pressure is caused by a contraction of the detrusor muscle or by an increase in intra-abdominal pressure as by coughing or straining, the stimulus is usually applied to the intra-abdominal urethra as well, and there is no leakage of urine. If urine does escape, the symptom is called *stress incontinence*.

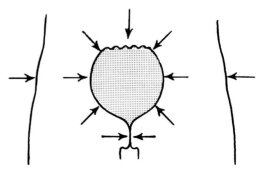

GENUINE STRESS INCONTINENCE

(alternatively named urethral sphincter incompetence)

Involuntary leakage occurring in the absence of a detrusor contraction. This leakage is attributed to weakness and displacement of the bladder neck so that it cannot respond normally to a sudden increase in intra-abdominal pressure. The cause is likely to be a pelvic floor weakness as a result of parturition and/or oestrogen deficiency.

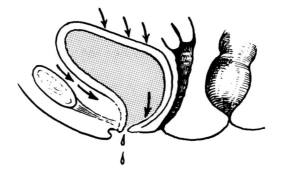

OTHER INCONTINENCE MECHANISMS

Fistula incontinence is described in Chapter 14 Complications of Gynaecological Surgery.

OVERFLOW INCONTINENCE

Retention of urine is relatively unusual in women; however, it can occur after surgery and is particularly common after regional anaesthesia. Spasmodic detrusor contractions force a little urine into the urethra and the stretched muscle takes several days to regain its tone.

When obstruction to outflow occurs gradually, as from pressure by a pelvic tumour or an incarcerated retroverted gravid uterus, the detrusor has time to hypertrophy and, for a time, forces urine out; but eventually the bladder becomes atonic and painless, and urine dribbles out only when the intra-abdominal pressure is raised.

NEUROLOGICAL DISEASE

Failure of detrusor inhibition is the commonest symptom and is the cause of senile incontinence. It is also a symptom, although not usually the presenting one, of multiple sclerosis. Full sensation is present, but the incontinence is of the urgency type and cannot be resisted.

Failure of bladder sensation is a result of diseases which interrupt the posterior columns of the cord, for example, tabes, syringomyelia and occasionally multiple sclerosis. Chronic overdistension leads to an atonic bladder and overflow incontinence, and infection is a common complication.

OTHER SYMPTOMS AND SIGNS ASSOCIATED WITH INCONTINENCE

Frequency

Increased frequency of micturition may arise from any source of irritation including infection, detrusor instability, tumour or incomplete emptying. It is usually diurnal – during waking hours only – but in severe cases will awaken the patient from her sleep. It is one of the earliest symptoms of pregnancy.

Urgency

This is defined as a desire to void urine before the bladder contains 50 ml of urine. True urgency occurs in the absence of a detrusor contraction, and is often associated with infection. Severe urgency leads to 'urge incontinence'.

Dysuria

This means pain associated with micturition and indicates an infection either of the bladder and urethra, or of the vulval and perineal epithelium which is irritated by the dribbling of urine.

Nocturia

Requiring to pass urine during the night.

THE URETHRAL SYNDROME

The urethral syndrome includes complaints of frequency, dysuria, urgency and a sensation of incomplete emptying in a patient in whose urine no evidence of infection can be demonstrated. The cause is not known and there are several views.

Urinary infection is strictly defined as being present only when 10^4 or more typical urinary pathogens are grown per ml of freshly voided mid-stream urine and it may be that the urethral syndrome is simply a condition caused by fewer than the usual number of organisms, or by organisms which cannot be cultured in the media used for conventional organisms. Clinically, these patients must be regarded as suffering from a possible urinary tract infection and investigation should be persevered with. Even if no evidence of infection is obtained, empirical antibiotic treatment may be of benefit. In menopausal women, topical oestrogens will treat atrophic changes in the urethral epithelium which can predispose to infection.

INVESTIGATION OF INCONTINENCE

It is useful to distinguish between genuine stress incontinence and detrusor instability as their treatment is different although it is important to remember that some women will have dual pathologies.

History and clinical examination are useful but investigation of bladder function may be required particularly where surgical intervention is being considered.

Incontinence may be due to the following:

1. *Genuine stress incontinence*

Usually occurs after one or more pregnancies.

Urine appears only after effort (stress) such as coughing, laughing or running for a bus.

Usually only small quantities of urine are passed, whether the bladder is full or not.

2. *Detrusor instability*

Complaints of urge incontinence and frequency, especially at night (nocturia).

May pass large volumes of urine when bladder muscle contracts.

Stress incontinence combined with urgency incontinence due to bladder infection or cystocele is quite common. Continuous incontinence suggests fistula (p. 292).

The social effects of urinary incontinence should be considered when planning treatment.

EXAMINATION
Signs of infection (urethritis) and scarring from previous surgery are looked for, and the usual bimanual and speculum examinations are performed (Chp. 5).

DEMONSTRATIONS OF STRESS INCONTINENCE
The patient is asked to strain and cough and, if stress incontinence is present, small amounts of urine will be observed escaping from the urethral meatus. Unfortunately, this test is really valid only in the erect position when observation of the meatus becomes almost impossible.

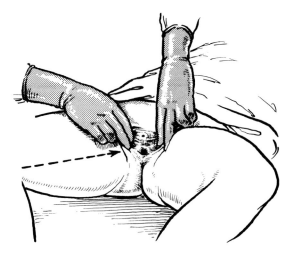

URODYNAMIC INVESTIGATION OF BLADDER FUNCTION

This means an investigation of bladder movements and tensions during different levels of filling, and involves measurement of bladder activity (cystometry) and urethral flow (uroflowmetry).

CYSTOMETRY

The bladder pressures are continuously recorded as the bladder is filled. In twin channel cystometry, the intra-abdominal pressure is simultaneously recorded by a transducer in the rectum or vagina. The detrusor pressure is calculated by subtracting abdominal pressure from intravesical pressure.

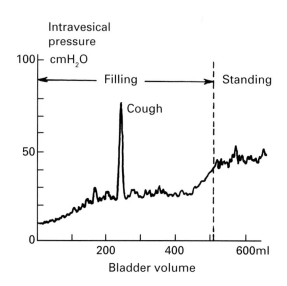

ABNORMAL CYSTOMETRY

If detrusor contractions are seen in the filling phase (up to 400 ml infused into bladder), a diagnosis of detrusor instability can be made.

In stress incontinence, leakage on acts such as coughing occurs in the absence of a rise in detrusor pressure.

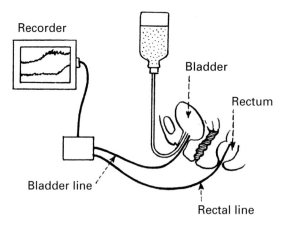

INDICATIONS FOR URODYNAMIC ASSESSMENT

These investigations are invasive, but their application would be justified in the presence of the following indications:

1. Continuing difficulty in distinguishing genuine stress incontinence from detrusor instability.
2. After failure of surgery to relieve a complaint of incontinence.
3. Where there are other complicating factors such as neurological disease.
4. Where difficulty in voiding urine is complained of or is suspected. Such a condition may be met with after pelvic surgery and leads to incomplete emptying and perhaps retention overflow.
5. Some clinicians would advocate urodynamic assessment prior to surgical treatment for stress incontinence. The purpose of this is to assess for underlying detrusor instability which may be exacerbated by surgery.

OTHER INVESTIGATIONS

Bacteriological Culture of Urine
This must be carried out in every case.

Fluid Balance Chart
The patient is asked to record the volume of oral fluid intake and urine output over the course of a week. Recordings of urine production should include the volume and the time of each micturition. Any episodes of incontinence should also be recorded. This procedure is useful for identifying the patient with an excessive oral intake. An estimate of the patient's normal bladder capacity can also be made.

Neurological Disease
This possibility must always be borne in mind and the gynaecologist should test for reflexes in the usual manner. Where there is doubt, the patient must be referred to a neurologist.

Endocrine Diseases
Diseases such as diabetes mellitus and insipidus may present with frequency of micturition.

TREATMENT OF STRESS INCONTINENCE

General measures:
The following should be treated if present:

1. Chronic urinary tract infection
2. Obesity
3. Chronic cough.

CONSERVATIVE TREATMENT OF STRESS INCONTINENCE

1. *Physiotherapy – pelvic floor exercises*
   Pelvic floor exercises may be of value, especially in the puerperium. The best results are achieved when the patient has input from a physiotherapist with an expertise in pelvic floor exercises. Repeated contraction of the pelvic floor will strengthen the muscle tone. A number of techniques are used to achieve this including vaginal cones and biofeedback. This is where the woman's pelvic floor strength is measured to enable her to be aware of her own pelvic floor tone.

2. *Mechanical devices to occlude urethra or support the bladder neck*
   These devices are usually placed within the vagina and efficacy is variable. Urinary tract infection, expulsion of the device and patient discomfort are reasonably common.

NEW SURGICAL DEVELOPMENTS IN THE TREATMENT OF STRESS INCONTINENCE

1. *Peri-urethral injections*
   Substances such as collagen or subcutaneous fat are injected around the urethra using a vaginal approach. This procedure is suitable for frail patients. Cure rates of up to 80% have been reported in the short term but this is reduced in longer follow-up.

2. *Artificial urinary sphincters*
   Implantation of an artificial urinary sphincter may be considered as a last resort in the treatment of stress incontinence.

SURGICAL TREATMENT OF STRESS INCONTINENCE

All operations attempt to elevate the bladder neck above the pelvic floor and behind the symphysis so that increases in intra-abdominal pressure will compress the urethra and not force it downwards. There are three conventional methods, each with several variations.

1. *Anterior colporrhaphy*
    This procedure may be useful in women with coexisting anterior vaginal wall prolapse, but the rate of objective cure for stress incontinence is less than 40%.

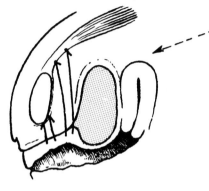

2. *Urethropexy*
    The bladder neck is approached through a suprapubic incision and elevated by suturing the paraurethral tissues to adjacent structures such as the rectus sheath or the ilio-pectineal ligament.

    These operations are more difficult than vaginal urethroplasty, especially in obese women. Some operators employ a laparoscopic technique.

3. *Urethral sling operations*
    A sling of synthetic material, sutures or tendon is passed under the urethra and attached to the rectus muscles or adjacent ligaments. This requires a combined vaginal-suprapubic approach and is the most difficult of the three methods.

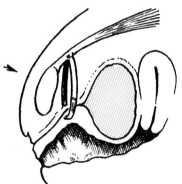

The urethropexy operations are probably most likely to be successful when the incontinence is due to urethral inadequacy and not detrusor instability.

MARSHALL–MARCHETTI–KRANTZ URETHROPEXY

The urethrovesical junction is made to adhere firmly to the anterior vaginal wall by suturing the vaginal tissue to the back of the symphysis pubis.

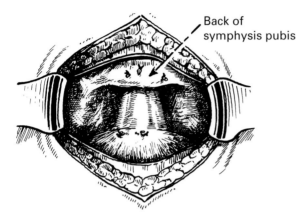

Back of symphysis pubis

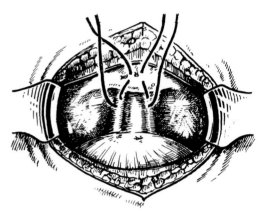

1. The urethrovesical junction is exposed in the space of Retzius. Adhesions are divided and all bleeding points picked up. The urethra must be dissected to within 1 cm of the external meatus.

2. A Foley's catheter in the bladder helps to identify the urethrovesical junction. Sutures pick up vaginal tissue on either side and suture it to the pubic periosteum.

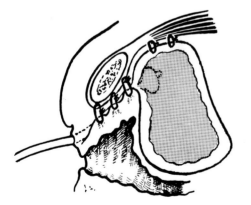

Bleeding from paravesical blood vessels is common and a drain can be useful to reduce the risk of a pelvic collection.

Periosteitis is sometimes a late complication and the operation is difficult in the presence of excessive obesity. If too acute an angle is produced, the patient may have difficulty in emptying her bladder.

BURCH'S COLPOSUSPENSION OPERATION

This operation elevates the anterior vaginal wall, bringing the urethra up with it.

1. Through a suprapubic incision, the bladder neck area is mobilised from the paravaginal fascia. This procedure may be accompanied by a good deal of bleeding which can be controlled by tightening the sutures.

2. The paravaginal fascia (and some vaginal tissue as well) is sutured on each side to the inguino-pectineal ligaments, using four or five sutures.

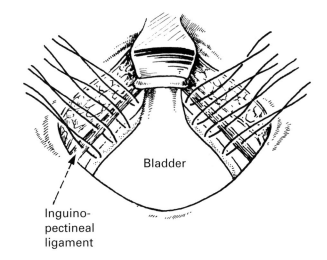

Bladder

Inguino-pectineal ligament

The wound is closed with drainage as for the Marshall operation, and the possible complications are similar. Suprapubic operations can be difficult when the patient is very obese. This procedure may now be performed laparoscopically by appropriately trained surgeons.

STAMEY NEEDLE SUSPENSION PROCEDURE

The Stamey procedure is one of a number of needle suspension procedures. They are less invasive than conventional colposuspension. A long Stamey needle is passed through a small incision above the pubis on each side, *behind the pubic bones,* into the vaginal lumen. A nylon suture is attached to the vaginal wall and tied to the rectus sheath, to elevate the vagina and bladder base.

A cystoscope is passed to ensure that the needle has not entered the bladder after each pass of the Stamey needle.

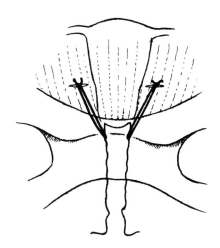

SLING PROCEDURES

Slings can be made from either the patient's own tissues (abdominal fascia) or synthetic material. These materials are placed under the urethra to achieve compression when the intra-abdominal pressure increases.

The synthetic materials are meshes, which are non-absorbable and permanent. They are inserted vaginally either side of the urethra. They can be a source of infection and can occasionally erode through tissues.

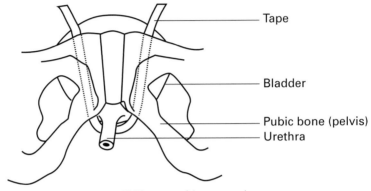

Tape

Bladder

Pubic bone (pelvis)
Urethra

TVT: retropubic approach

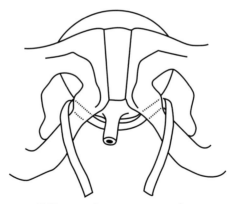

TVT: transobturator approach

TREATMENT OF DETRUSOR INSTABILITY

BLADDER RETRAINING

Women with symptoms suggestive of detrusor instability should be advised to cut out bladder stimulants such as caffeine and alcohol.

This may be done as an inpatient or an outpatient, although inpatient treatment is more effective. The patient is instructed to void only at defined intervals (to start with, this is normally 1.5 h). When the patient can achieve continence between scheduled voiding, the interval is increased gradually. A normal fluid intake should be allowed. Support and enthusiasm from medical and nursing staff is required for this procedure to be effective.

DRUG TREATMENT

Antimuscarinic agents (oxybutynin, tolterodine). These agents act by blocking parasympathetic stimulation of the detrusor muscle. Improvement is seen in 70% of patients who can tolerate the drug.

Non-compliance is common, because of the anticholinergic side effects of dry mouth, blurred vision, tachycardia, drowsiness and constipation.

Tricyclic Antidepressants (Imipramine)

These drugs are useful if nocturia is a significant compliant. Anticholinergic side effects may be a problem.

Oestrogen

Although few trials have formally evaluated the efficacy of oestrogens, they appear to have a role in postmenopausal women.

CHAPTER 13

DISEASES OF THE OVARY AND FALLOPIAN TUBE

Clinical Features of Ovarian Tumours 252
Symptoms Due to Size 252
Pressure Symptoms 252
Differential Diagnosis 255
Ascites 255
Uterine Fibroids 256
Pelvic Inflammation 257
Rectus Sheath Haematoma 257
The Obese Abdominal Wall 257
Broad Ligament Cysts 258
Ectopic or Transplanted Kidney 258
Retroperitoneal Tumours 258
Ovarian Cyst Accidents 259
Complications of Ovarian Tumours 259
Clinical Features 259
Differential Diagnosis 259
Management 259
Rupture of Ovarian Cyst 260
Benign and Malignant Ovarian Tumours 262
Clinical Features 262
Investigation 262
Histological Classification 263
Risk Factors for Ovarian Cancer 264
Carcinoma of the Ovary 264
Ovarian Cancer Risk Factors 264
Epithelial Ovarian Tumours 265
Serous Cystadenoma 265
Serous Cystadenocarcinoma 265
Mucinous Cystadenoma 266
Mucinous Cystadenocarcinoma 266
Germ Cell Ovarian Tumours 267
Clinical Features 267
Treatment 267
Germ Cell Ovarian Tumours –
Undifferentiated 268
Teratomata 269
Other Ovarian Tumours 270
Hormone-Producing Tumours 271
Oestrogen-Producing Tumours 272

Fibroma 272
Androgen-Producing Tumours 273
Other Hormone-Producing Tumours 275
Carcinoid (Serotonin-Producing
Tumour) 275
Struma Ovarii (Thyroid Type Tumour) 275
Choriocarcinoma of the Ovary 275
Hormone Production by Non-Functioning
Tumours 275
Surgical Treatment of Ovarian Tumours 276
Treatment of Ovarian Cancer 277
Spread of Ovarian Cancer 277
Incision 278
Inspection 278
Organs Removed 278
Cytology 278
Staging of Ovarian Cancer 279
Principles of Chemotherapy 281
Malignant Tumour Growth 281
Mode of Chemotherapeutic Action 281
Chemotherapeutic Agents in Ovarian
Cancer 282
Chemotherapy Toxicity 282
Present Prognosis for Invasive
Epithelial Ovarian Cancer 282
Broad Ligament Cysts 283
Broad Ligament Cysts (Parovarian
Cysts) 283
Diagnosis 284
Operation 284
Cysts of Kobelt's Tubules,
Hydatids of Morgagni,
Fimbrial Cysts 284
Carcinoma of Fallopian Tubes 285
Pathology 285
Clinical Features 285
Clinical Staging 285
Treatment 285

CLINICAL FEATURES OF OVARIAN TUMOURS

SYMPTOMS DUE TO SIZE

Ovarian tumours are often large by the time the doctor is consulted because of the lack of any specific symptoms. Menstrual function is usually normal, and any irregularity is attributed to perimenopausal change. The patient may have noticed that her clothes are getting tight and have attributed this to weight gain or, if the abdominal swelling has coincided with amenorrhoea, she may believe herself to be pregnant.

PRESSURE SYMPTOMS

There are commonly increased frequency of micturition, gastrointestinal symptoms and a dull pain in the lower abdomen. Very large tumours may cause shortness of breath, peripheral oedema or varicosities in the legs.

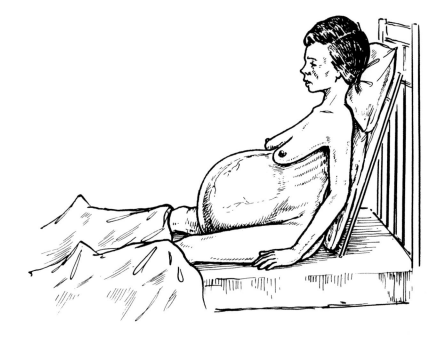

CLINICAL FEATURES OF OVARIAN TUMOURS

Small tumours remain in the pelvis and will only be detected on bimanual examination or by ultrasound.

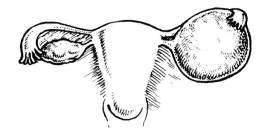

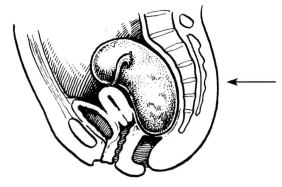

Larger tumours fill the pelvis and usually lie between the uterus and the sacrum. If the patient is not too obese, the uterus can be distinguished on palpation as separate from the tumour.

A tumour occupying the abdomen causes a midline swelling and is usually tense.

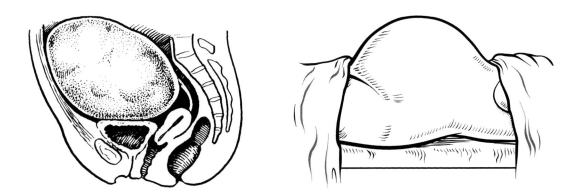

Little can be done at this stage to classify the tumour or exclude a malignancy. Further information can be gained by undertaking imaging and tumour marker assessment including CA125 and CEA (AFP, and B-HCG are included in younger patients).

CLINICAL FEATURES OF OVARIAN TUMOURS

If the patient is very thin, irregularities may be palpated and sometimes two tumours may be suspected.

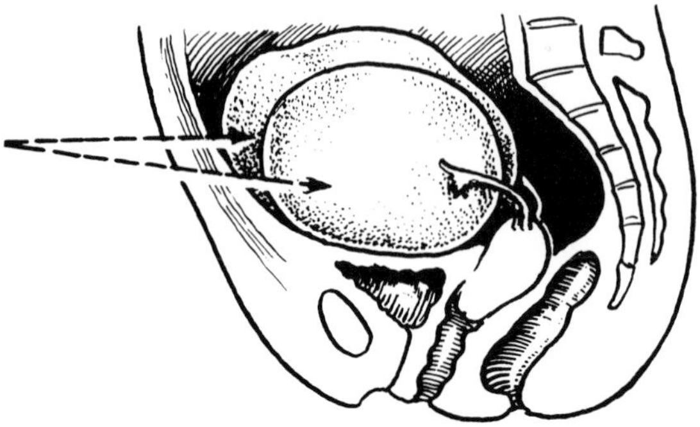

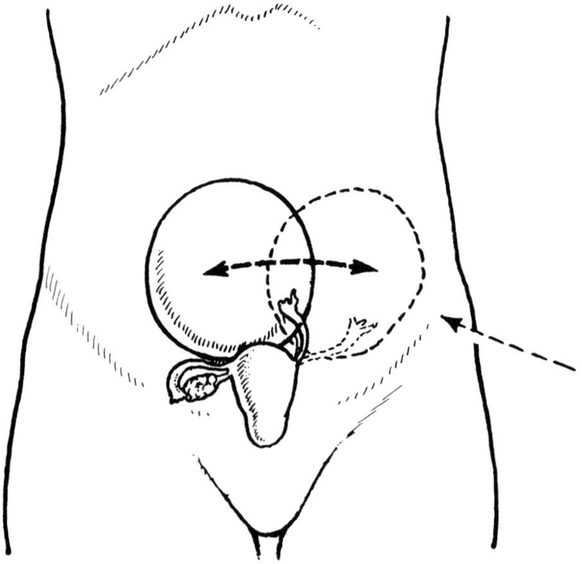

Some tumours of moderate size may have a long pedicle composed of the attenuated broad ligament and the fallopian tube, which allows the tumour to be displaced from side to side or to occupy a high abdominal position. Such cysts are at increased risk of torsion.

Omental adhesions

Cyst

The upper pole can usually be distinguished and the lower pole can be palpated per vaginam. Adhesions, inflammation and displacement of pelvic organs may all exist along with a tumour, making examination difficult.

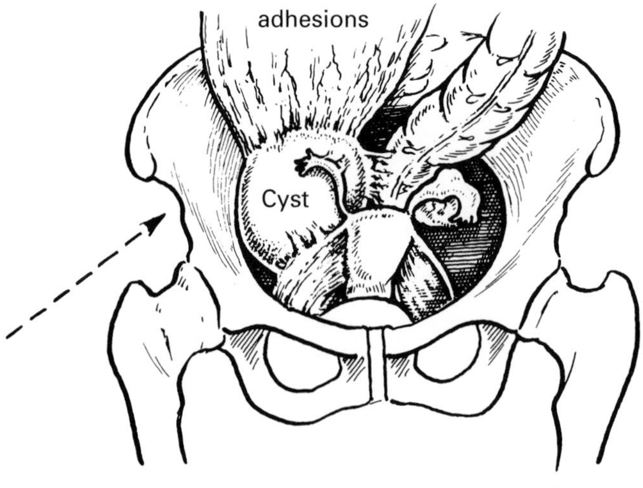

DIFFERENTIAL DIAGNOSIS

An experienced examiner will recognise an ovarian tumour mainly because ovarian tumour is, in the circumstances, the most likely diagnosis. All abdominal swellings should be subjected to further imaging with a combination that may include ultrasound, computerised tomography (CT) and magnetic resonance imaging (MRI) scan examination.

Two very obvious mistakes must be avoided.

1. The midline swelling due to a full bladder.

2. The 16-week pregnancy. The gravid uterus at this stage has a very soft isthmic region, which can resemble the pedicle of a cyst.

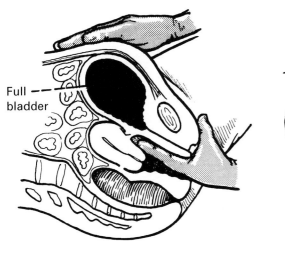

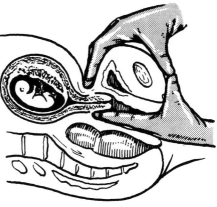

ASCITES

A fluid thrill may be elicited from an ovarian cyst, and ascites and tumour may coexist; but as a rule, the distinction should be easily made. The presence of ascites raises the suspicion of cancer.

(See 'Shifting dullness', page 77.)

With ascites
The bowel floats on the fluid. The percussion note is resonant over the top of the swellings and dull over the flanks.

With ovarian cyst
Percussion note is dull over the top of the swelling and resonant in the flanks.

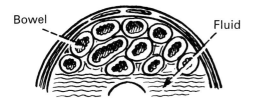

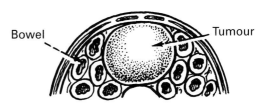

DIFFERENTIAL DIAGNOSIS

UTERINE FIBROIDS

A large midline intramural fibroid may be indistinguishable from a solid ovarian tumour until the abdomen is opened and an entirely different surgical problem encountered.

An ovarian tumour will displace the uterus forwards or downwards where it may, sometimes, be identified on vaginal examination.

An intramural fibroid will obscure the uterus. The cavity is often elongated.

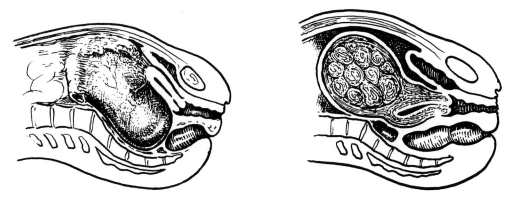

Ultrasound examination should be able to distinguish between a fibroid and an ovarian cyst; but many ovarian tumours are solid, and some fibroids undergo cystic degeneration. Vaginal ultrasound gives a more detailed picture of the pelvic contents and a more precise diagnosis.

DIFFERENTIAL DIAGNOSIS

PELVIC INFLAMMATION

The swelling palpated *per vaginam* may be due to an adherent mass of the uterus, the tubes, 'chocolate' ovarian cysts, and the bowel.

A pyosalpinx may give the same sensation.

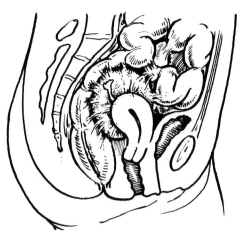

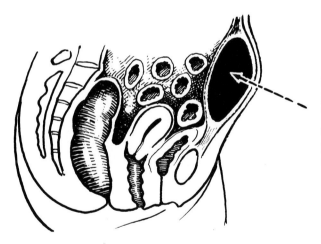

RECTUS SHEATH HAEMATOMA

This rare condition presents as a fixed abdominal mass, accompanied by pain, and usually follows sudden exertion such as severe coughing.

THE OBESE ABDOMINAL WALL

The obese patient may be convinced she has a tumour although she is only putting on weight (phantom tumour). Palpation is difficult; but the percussion note in the lower half of the abdomen will be resonant.

Mesenteric cyst
Hydatid cyst
Pancreatic cyst
Large hydronephrotic kidney
}
These are all rarities in the UK but must be considered if the physical signs are equivocal and especially if the swelling is not in the midline. Modern imaging techniques should differentiate.

257

DIFFERENTIAL DIAGNOSIS

BROAD LIGAMENT CYSTS

The distinction is not likely to be made before laparotomy, even with imaging, if the intact ovary is observed on the back of the swelling.

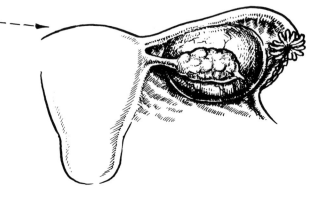

ECTOPIC OR TRANSPLANTED KIDNEY

These abnormalities are rare, but as they are usually detected for the first time on bimanual examination, they must be borne in mind. The ectopic kidney can lie anywhere in the pelvis and derives its blood supply from the iliac vessels. The ureter often runs a tortuous course.

RETROPERITONEAL TUMOURS

Retroperitoneal, in the surgical sense, means behind the peritoneum of the posterior abdominal wall. Such tumours are rare but may arise from any connective tissue, a lipoma being the commonest. Examination reveals a fixed tumour. The tumour may displace the ureter and is in close relation to the large vessels.

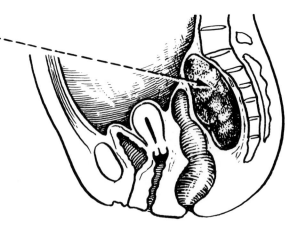

OVARIAN CYST ACCIDENTS

COMPLICATIONS OF OVARIAN TUMOURS

Torsion of the Pedicle
(Axial rotation)

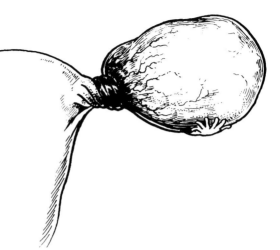

This is the commonest complication and may occur with any tumour except those with adhesions. The thin-walled veins of the pedicle are obstructed first while the arterial supply continues. As a result there is haemorrhage into the tumour and into the peritoneum, and if not treated, significant infection may occur.

CLINICAL FEATURES

Subacute
The patient complains of recurrent abdominal pain which passes off as the pedicle untwists. There is a rise in pulse and temperature during the bleeding, and over a period, anaemia develops.

Acute
The signs and symptoms are those of an acute abdominal condition. The problem becomes one of a differential diagnosis to exclude those conditions in which a laparotomy is not needed and those in which a laparoscopy may be useful.

Pain tends to be intense and continuous.

DIFFERENTIAL DIAGNOSIS
'Surgical conditions' (i.e. those conditions commonly seen and dealt with by a general surgeon).

Acute appendicitis
Inflammatory bowel disease
Obstruction of bowel
Diverticulitis/diverticular abscess

MANAGEMENT
Patients presenting with an acute abdomen should first be stabilised. Once stabilised, investigations to establish wellbeing and potential causes may then be undertaken with blood tests and imaging. In cases where there is no resolution with conservative treatment, then, a diagnostic laparoscopy and/or a laparotomy may be needed. If the ovulation bleeding is greater than usual the woman may show quite, marked signs of peritonism. The corpus luteum may thereafter become exaggeratedly cystic and mislead the examiner.

OVARIAN CYST ACCIDENTS

RUPTURE OF OVARIAN CYST

Rupture may be either traumatic or spontaneous and may occur in the following conditions:

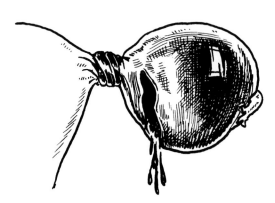

1. Following torsion of a pedicle.

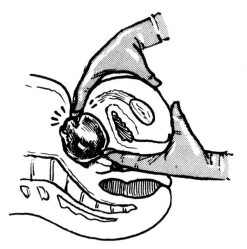

2. During bimanual examination.

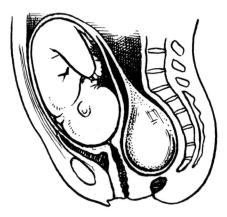

3. During labour when the cyst is impacted within the pelvis.

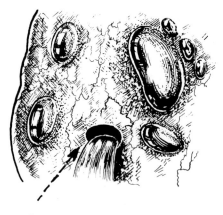

4. Spontaneous rupture. This is not uncommon, especially with malignant cysts, where the epithelial tissue outgrows the connective tissue.

OVARIAN CYST ACCIDENTS

Differential Diagnosis for an Ovarian Cyst Accident

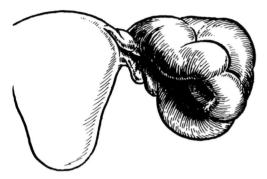

Acute pelvic inflammation with
tubo-ovarian abscess.

Signs of infection are more marked.
A cyst which has undergone rotation is
usually larger than the diffuse swelling of
pelvic inflammation.

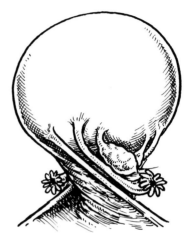

Torsion of a fibroid
Normal organs very rarely, if ever, develop
axial rotation, but a uterus, enlarged by a
fibroid, may do so.

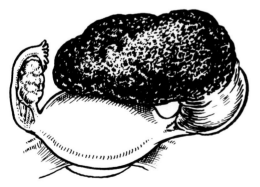

Ectopic pregnancy
The swelling is usually small although
extremely tender and the history usually
suggestive; but in a young woman this
condition must always be considered.

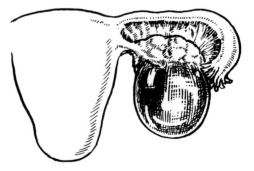

Ovulation bleeding

BENIGN AND MALIGNANT OVARIAN TUMOURS

Ovarian cysts can grow to a significant size before causing any symptoms. Ovarian cancer has been described as the 'silent killer' as approximately 60% of women present with advanced disease. While many patients, in retrospect, do have symptoms, they are non-specific and do not at first seem to be due to ovarian disease.

CLINICAL FEATURES

The patient usually has non-specific symptoms and appears well. Symptoms may include abdominal pain, bloating, changes in bowel habits, urinary symptoms and pelvic symptoms. Not unsurprisingly, many women are initially misdiagnosed with irritable bowel syndrome and/or are initially referred for general surgical review. However, referral from primary care was not found to be significantly delayed and did not have an impact on survival.

INVESTIGATION

Once a pelvic mass is suspected it should be investigated with tumour markers, as previously discussed. Imaging with ultrasound will delineate complex features (ascites, bilateral masses, thick septa, metastatic deposits, solid areas) and allow the calculation of a *risk of malignancy index* (RMI). This is calculated as below:

Score	Menopausal status	Ultrasound
1	Premenopausal	1 abnormality
3	Postmenopausal	2 or > abnormality

$$RMI = CA125\ VALUE \times MENOPAUSAL\ SCORE \times ULTRASOUND\ SCORE$$

Using a cut-off value of 200, the RMI has an 80% positive predictive value for ovarian malignancy. CT scanning will provide further information on the extent of disease. Using both the RMI and CT findings, patients can then be referred directly to specialist gynaecological oncology surgeons.

BENIGN AND MALIGNANT OVARIAN TUMOURS

HISTOLOGICAL CLASSIFICATION

Ovarian tumours can arise from the ovarian epithelium, stroma or the germ cells. The embryonic coelom, from which the epithelium develops, also gives rise to the Müllerian duct from which develop the structures of the genital tract; and it is this common origin which accounts for the great variety of epithelial patterns encountered.

Epithelial Tumours

Serous cystadenoma or cystadenocarcinoma.
Mucinous cystadenoma or cystadenocarcinoma.
Endometrioma or endometrioid carcinoma.
Clear cell carcinoma.
Brenner tumour.

Sex Cord Stromal Tumours

Fibroma or sarcoma.

Oestrogen-producing:
    Granulosa cell tumour.
    Thecoma.

Androgen-producing:
    Sertoli-Leydig cell tumour (arrhenoblastoma).
    Hilar cell tumour.
    Lipoid cell tumour.

Germ Cell Tumours

Dysgerminoma.
Teratoma.
Gonadoblastoma.
Yolk sac tumour.
Carcinoid hormone-producing
Thyroid tumour choriocarcinoma

There is one well-known secondary tumour of the ovary, the Krükenberg tumour, which is secondary to a Gastric carcinoma. This term is now being widely used to describe metastases to the ovary from other cancers such as breast and colon cancers.

RISK FACTORS FOR OVARIAN CANCER

CARCINOMA OF THE OVARY

In developed countries, women have a lifetime risk of about 1.4% for developing ovarian cancer, which is slightly greater than the risk of cervical or endometrial cancers, but well below the 13% lifetime risk of breast cancer.

5–10% of ovarian cancers are related to genetic factors such as BRCA gene mutations or the Lynch syndrome of familial breast, colorectal and ovarian cancers. The induction of ovulation with Clomiphene for more than a year carries a 10-fold increased risk of ovarian cancer. Long-term oral contraceptive use reduces the incidence of ovarian cancers.

BRCA 1

The mutation is located on chromosome 17. Those affected carry a 30–60% risk of developing ovarian cancer. Survivors of breast cancer have a 13% risk of developing ovarian cancer within 10 years.

BRCA 2

The mutation is located on chromosome 13. Those affected carry a 20% risk of developing ovarian cancer. Survivors of breast cancer have a 7% risk of developing ovarian cancer within 10 years.

If family members are identified as having a mutation, then, they may be offered risk reducing surgery such as prophylactic bilateral salpingo-oophorectomy.

OVARIAN CANCER RISK FACTORS

Increased	Decreased
Low parity	High parity
Infertility	Combined contraceptive pill
Endometriosis	Breastfeeding

Ovarian metastases from extra-genital tumours are not uncommon. The commonest sites of primary growth are the breast, stomach and the large intestine. They usually occur in functioning ovaries and their importance lies in the fact that these metastases grow to a large size while the primary growth is small and give rise to no clinical manifestations. The metastases usually reproduce the histological characteristics of the primary cancer.

EPITHELIAL OVARIAN TUMOURS

SEROUS CYSTADENOMA

It can be a unilocular or a multilocular cyst. They are the most common benign epithelial tumours and form 40% of all epithelial tumours. They are bilateral in 10% of cases. They show one of three structures:

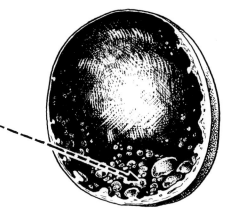

(1) A simple cystic form with a smooth surface and a smooth lining.
(2) A cystic structure with intracystic papillary formations. The latter may be sessile buttons or pedunculated, frond-like projections.
(3) An adenomatous form where many of the loculi are small and the papillary structures are solid and complex.

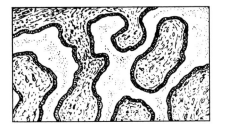

Microscopically, the tumour has a fibrous capsule. Septa support the cysts which are lined by cuboidal epithelium and contain thin serous fluid.

SEROUS CYSTADENOCARCINOMA

This is by far the commonest primary carcinoma, and in over half the cases, it is bilateral. The cysts are always of the papillary type and the epithelium burrowing through the capsule produces papillary processes on the serous surface. Extension of the growth to the pelvis and adjacent organs fixes the tumour. It commonly spreads across the peritoneal surface tissues becoming densely adherent, but at times, it can invade tissues directly. Ascites are frequently present.

EPITHELIAL OVARIAN TUMOURS

MUCINOUS CYSTADENOMA

It is a unilocular or multilocular cyst of an ovary lined by a tall columnar epithelium, resembling that of the cervix or the large intestine. They can be large and may reach immense proportions, occupying the whole peritoneal cavity and compressing other organs.
It may occur at any age.

The surface of the cyst is often completely smooth and round, but may be slightly nodular, due to the projecting loculi.

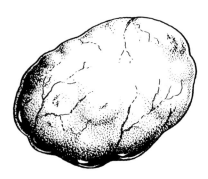

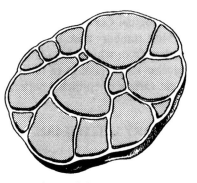

The cut surface of the cyst is multilocular and has a mosaic pattern.

Microscopically, the tumour has an outer fibrous capsule from which the septa extend to support the walls of the cysts. The latter are lined by tall columnar epithelium with basal nuclei and contain a gelatinous glycoprotein or mucin.

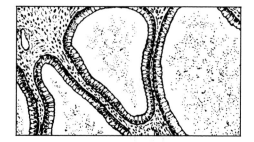

The signs and symptoms are similar to those generally associated with any non-functioning ovarian tumour. Rupture may occur and seeding of the epithelium on the peritoneal surface may cause a pseudomyxoma peritonei.

Pseudomyxoma Peritonei

This rare condition, occasionally, but not inevitably, follows the rupture of a mucinous cystadenoma (page 260). The epithelial cells get implanted on the peritoneum and continue to secrete mucin. The abdominal cavity is eventually filled with the jelly, while the secreting cells spread over the parietal and the visceral peritoneum. The disease develops slowly over several years and may require multiple operations to strip the mucin plaques. Current research is focusing on hot intraperitoneal chemotherapy. This disease is, commonly, chronically progressive.

MUCINOUS CYSTADENOCARCINOMA

This is only a third as common as the serous variety. Malignancy in a mucinous cyst is characterised by the formation of areas of solid carcinoma in the wall. The cells are columnar, show mitoses and tend to form glandular structures.

GERM CELL OVARIAN TUMOURS

Germ cell tumours may be:

Undifferentiated	Dysgerminoma
	Gonadoblastoma
Differentiated	Embryonal
	Teratomas
	Extra-embryonal
	Yolk sac tumour
	Choriocarcinoma

CLINICAL FEATURES

97% of these tumours are benign but they comprise 20% of all ovarian tumours. Patients are usually young, in the 20–30 year-old age group. They may present with an acute abdomen as the pelvic masses undergo torsion or rupture. In some, the pain can be of a more chronic nature. However, many women are often diagnosed incidentally, while undergoing investigations for other reasons.

TREATMENT

This will depend upon the age of the patient, the extent of the disease and fertility wishes. Where fertility is not an issue, then usually, bilateral salpingo-oöphorectomy and hysterectomy are indicated. Where fertility preservation is an important issue, evidence supports the strategy of unilateral salpingo-oöphorectomy with thorough assessment. All disease should be cyto-reduced at a laparotomy to the smallest possible level.

Disease is staged as for an ovarian carcinoma. If the disease is greater than Stage 1A, then postoperative chemotherapy is indicated to reduce the risk of recurrence and provide patients with a good long-term outcome or even a cure.

GERM CELL OVARIAN TUMOURS

GERM CELL OVARIAN TUMOURS - UNDIFFERENTIATED

Dysgerminoma

This is the only solid ovarian tumour of characteristic appearance. Usually ovoid with a smooth capsule, it is of rubbery consistency and greyish colour. It is most common in the younger age groups and is bilateral in 20%. About 70% of the cases are Stage 1A at diagnosis. Lactate dehydrogenase (LDH) levels may be elevated. Survival rates are greater than 90% for stage 1 tumours.

Microscopically, it consists of masses of large, clear, epithelial cells with large nuclei, resembling primitive germ cells, in cords or alveoli. Fine connective tissue that has been infiltrated by lymphocytes separates the bundles of epithelial cells. The malignancy varies, but many appear to be relatively benign and do not recur. Those in children tend to be more malignant.

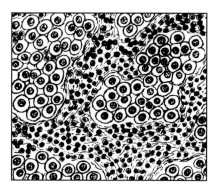

Gonadoblastoma

This is a tumour associated with dysgenetic gonads, usually streak gonads. The patient is an apparent female and may have a diminutive uterus, tubes and vagina, but usually there is a sex chromosome mosaicism such as 45X/46XY.

The tumour is composed of two types of cells: (a) a large primitive germ cell and (b) small cells of the granulosa type. Call-Exner bodies (small rosettes) may be seen in the latter. These two types of cells form epithelial islands in a stroma which may contain Leydig-like cells. Sometimes, the germ cells may undergo rapid proliferation and give rise to a dysgerminoma. Some of the dysgerminomata in children probably arise in this way. Choriocarcinoma may also originate in a gonadoblastoma.

About 60% of women show some signs of virilisation and 17-ketosteroid excretion may be raised.

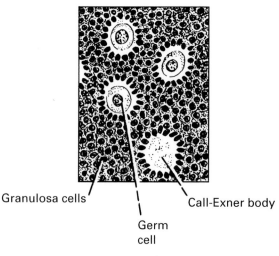

Granulosa cells   Germ cell   Call-Exner body

GERM CELL OVARIAN TUMOURS

TERATOMATA

These are broadly divided into mature and immature forms.

Mature Cystic Teratoma or Dermoid

This is one of the commonest ovarian tumours and is usually diagnosed during the child-bearing period, but may be found at any age and may be bilateral in 10% of cases.

It is often ovoid. The wall consists of dense fibrous tissue lined by stratified squamous epithelium. The cyst may contain sebaceous glands, teeth, hair, nervous tissues, cartilage, bone, respiratory and intestinal epithelium and thyroid gland tissue.

Thick yellow sebaceous material fills the cyst and if it ruptures o a severe granulomatous reaction can occur.

They are particularly liable to have a long pedicle and easily undergo torsion in up to 15% in some series. Malignant transformation is rare and an ovarian cystectomy is adequate for most cases.

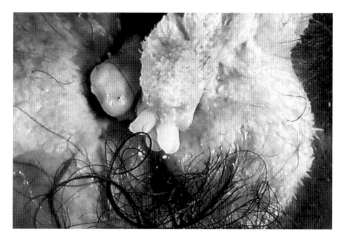

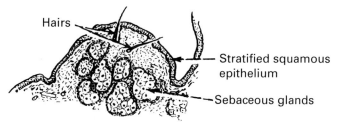

Hairs
Stratified squamous epithelium
Sebaceous glands

Immature Teratoma

These occur at an earlier age than dermoids, often in childhood. They are solid and may contain any tissue from the three germinal layers, mixed in a completely disorderly fashion. They are particularly liable to undergo malignant change, with the malignancy arising in any one of the tissues present.

GERM CELL OVARIAN TUMOURS

Yolk Sac Tumour

This is a rare tumour found in children and young adults. It has a variable histological structure and is highly malignant. The main interest lies in the fact that it produces alpha-fetoprotein and therefore its blood levels can be used as a diagnostic test and as a means of monitoring response to treatment.

Choriocarcinoma is mentioned in the succeeding part that deals with hormone-producing tumours.

OTHER OVARIAN TUMOURS
Krukenberg Tumour

This is a secondary carcinoma of the ovary. It is remarkable for its characteristic histological appearance and the fact that the primary growth, which is usually seen in the stomach and less commonly in the large intestine, is often clinically silent. The ovarian tumours are frequently bilateral, of equal size, smooth and lobulated. They remain freely mobile with no adhesions. Being firm and fibrous in appearance they are frequently mistaken for fibromata, but these are usually unilateral.

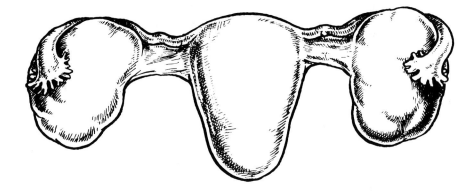

Histologically, they have a well-defined appearance. There is a very cellular stroma, resembling a sarcoma, in which there are large epithelial cells lying singly or in alveoli. These epithelial cells have a clear cytoplasm with a crescentic nucleus that has been pushed to one side, giving a signet-ring appearance that is typical. The cytoplasm is full of mucin.

The majority of patients with this tumour have a poor prognosis.

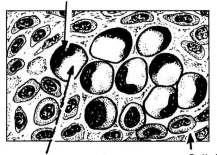

Nucleus of 'signet-ring' cell

Clear mucin-filled cytoplasm

Cellular stroma

HORMONE-PRODUCING TUMOURS

Brenner Tumour

A benign tumour, mainly solid and most common in the 6th decade, it is composed of fibrous and epithelial elements in varying proportions. It forms 2% of all solid ovarian neoplasms.

It is usually solid and resembles a fibroma. Occasionally, there may be microcysts or even an associated large mucinous cyst. Microscopically, it is mainly composed of fibrous tissue with small islands of clear epithelial cells of squamous appearance. Sometimes the islands become cystic and the epithelial cells become mucinous.

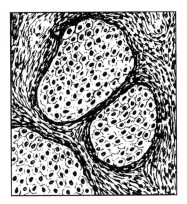

HORMONE-PRODUCING TUMOURS

The most common tumours of this kind are steroid-producing, particularly sex steroids. Both androgenic and oestrogenic effects have been described with every histological variety as some tumours have a mixed steroid cell composition, but certain tumours of well-defined histological structures are commonly associated with the production of only one type of steroid.

OESTROGEN-PRODUCING TUMOURS

These belong to the granulosa-theca cell group and are found in all ages. They account for 3% of all solid tumours of the ovary.

Oestrogen excess can cause hyperplasia of:

1. Myometrium → enlarged uterus.
2. Endometrium → Irregular and/or postmenopausal bleeding.
3. Breast tissue → enlargement, tenderness of breasts.

In childhood there is accelerated skeletal growth and appearance of sex hair.

> 5% of these occur in children → precocious puberty.
> 60% occur in child-bearing years → irregular menstruation.
> 30% occur in postmenopausal women → postmenopausal bleeding.

Diagnosis

Granulosa cell tumour in childhood may be found as the cause of female precocity with a pelvic mass being demonstrated on imaging. Following puberty, and even into postmenopausal years, diagnosis on clinical grounds is difficult owing to the multiplicity of factors that can cause irregular vaginal bleeding. Often, the diagnosis is made following the removal of an abnormal cyst or ovary.

Pathology

These tumours vary very much in function. Large tumours may be virtually functionless. In childhood and early adult life, the tumours are composed mainly of granulosa cells. In later life they are usually thecomata. The granulosa-cell type of growth should be considered as a carcinoma. Recurrence may occur many years after removal of the primary growth. It is not possible to accurately correlate malignancy with histological appearances. In 14% of the cases endometrial hyperplasia becomes atypical and an endometrial carcinoma develops.

FIBROMA

This is composed of fibrous tissue and resembles the fibromata found elsewhere. It is most common in the elderly and accounts for 4–5% of all ovarian neoplasms.

The fibroma is believed by many to be a thecoma which has undergone fibrous transformation. It is sometimes associated with Meig's syndrome where a pleural effusion is also noted.

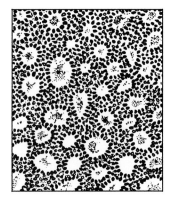

HORMONE-PRODUCING TUMOURS

ANDROGEN-PRODUCING TUMOURS

Three distinct types of masculinising ovarian tumour are recognised: (a) Sertoli-Leydig cell tumour (arrhenoblastoma), (b) Hilar cell tumour, (c) Lipoid cell tumour. All the three can cause amenorrhoea.

Sertoli-leydig Cell Tumour

This is a rare tumour and accounts for much less than 1% of all ovarian tumours. It occurs in young adult females. Clinically two stages are recognised:

1. **Period of defeminisation**
2. **Period of masculinisation**

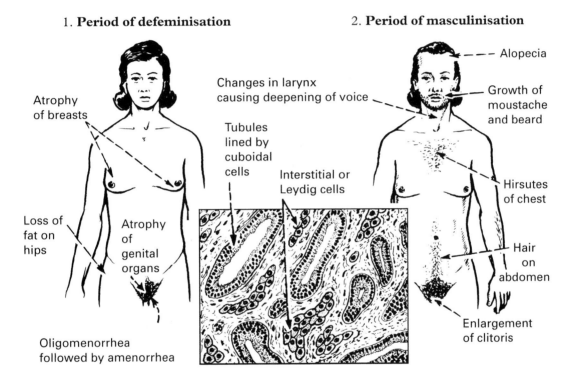

Pathology

It usually appears as a small white or yellowish tumour within the ovarian substance. Cystic degeneration may occur. These tumours are usually only of a low-grade malignancy.

Histologically it consists of primitive tubules surrounded by Leydig cells which contain crystalloids of Reinke. These are rod-shaped structures in the cytoplasm of Leydig cells and are said to be diagnostic of these cells.

Crystalloids of Reinke

273

HORMONE-PRODUCING TUMOURS

ANDROGEN-PRODUCING TUMOURS—(cont'd)

Biochemistry

The symptoms are due to the secretion of testosterone. The quantities of 17-ketosteroids are within the normal range, unlike in adrenal virilising tumours where their levels may be elevated. Direct estimations of blood testosterone can be made. Some of these tumours secrete oestrogens. Removal of the tumour results in regression of symptoms in the same order as their appearance. Menstruation returns within a month or two. Voice changes tend to be permanent.

Hilar Cell Tumour

This is a very rare tumour found in postmenopausal women. Defeminisation occurs but signs of virilism are usually mild, consisting of hirsutes, alopecia and an enlargement of the clitoris.

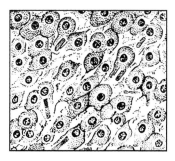

Pathology

Hilar cell tumours are small, brown, simple tumours of the ovarian hilum consisting of polyhedral Leydig cells. Crystalloids of Reinke are occasionally present. 17-ketosteroids are usually within the normal postmenopausal range. Small quantities of androgen are produced.

Lipoid Cell Tumour (Ovoblastoma, Masculinovoblastoma, Adrenal-like Tumour)

This is also a rare tumour that causes masculinisation and produces symptoms and signs of Cushing's syndrome such as skin striae, obesity, polycythaemia, impaired glucose tolerance and hypertension.

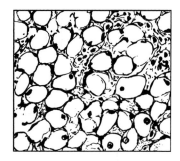

Pathology

The tumour consists of cells with high lipid content and are commonly large and yellowish.

Unlike other virilising tumours, the 17-ketosteroid output is greatly increased and the excretion of 17-hydroxycorticosteroids is also raised. ACTH or chorionic gonadotrophin will cause a further increase, but dexamethasone does not diminish the output, thus helping to differentiate the condition from virilising adrenal tumours.

OTHER HORMONE-PRODUCING TUMOURS

CARCINOID (Serotonin-Producing Tumour)

This tumour arises in association with a cystic teratoma of the ovary from cells related to the respiratory or intestinal epithelium that are sometimes found in these cysts.

It may give rise to a typical carcinoid syndrome with patchy cyanosis, flushing, diarrhoea, intestinal colic, oedema and cardiac failure due to a tricuspid valve lesion. Usually the syndrome does not appear until the tumour has metastasised to the liver.

STRUMA OVARII (Thyroid Type Tumour)

Small foci of thyroid tissue are common in ovarian teratomata, but large amounts are rare and functioning thyroid tissue is even rarer. When the thyroid tissue actually proliferates and forms a tumour, 5–10% of these become malignant.

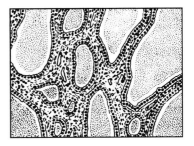

CHORIOCARCINOMA OF THE OVARY

This is an extremely rare tumour of the ovary. It is also known as a non-gestational choriocarcinoma, in that it does not arise as a consequence of conception. Most commonly, it is associated with a dysgerminoma and both, in turn, may be derived from germinal cells in a dysgenetic gonad. A syncytiotrophoblast is always present, but sometimes a cytotrophoblast is also formed. The principal hormone produced is β-human chorionic gonadotrophin (βHCG). This can prove to be useful in the diagnosis and follow-up of these tumours. Metastases may occur, as in any choriocarcinoma.

HORMONE PRODUCTION BY NON-FUNCTIONING TUMOURS

Occasionally, the presence of tumour growth in the ovary induces a thecal transformation of the ovarian stroma which in turn produces steroids, sometimes androgenic, but more commonly oestrogenic. This has been reported in association with benign and malignant cysts, Brenner tumours, fibroma and secondary carcinoma of ovary. The secretion of steroids can result in menstrual disorders, and in the case of androgens, virilisation.

SURGICAL TREATMENT OF OVARIAN TUMOURS

Benign ovarian tumours that are greater than 10 cm in diameter must be removed, but clinically and ultrasonically diagnosed cysts below 10 cm in women under 35 years of age may be reviewed in a few months if there is no suspicion of a malignancy. A follicular or luteal cyst may resolve spontaneously.

Cystectomy: It involves enucleation of the tumour from its capsule of ovarian tissue, which is then rolled into a little bundle and held together with sutures, thus preserving ovarian function.

Indications:
A tumour that is apparently benign.

This operation would not be feasible in the case of a very large tumour, or where there had been previous inflammation.

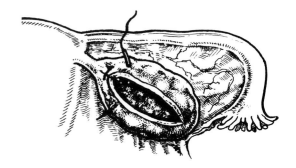

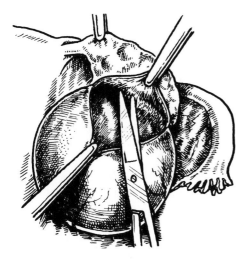

Ovariotomy: Removal of an ovary containing a tumour. (Removal of an ovary not containing a tumour is called oöphorectomy.)

Indications:
(a) Malignancy. (The uterus and other ovary are also removed.)
(b) The patient declines a hysterectomy and the other ovary is normal.

Laparoscopy: This may be diagnostic and/ or therapeutic – small benign cysts may be removed. Where a malignancy is not suspected on the basis of preoperative investigations, some larger simple cystic lesions can be placed in a laparoscopic bag for removal and then aspirated to reduce their size before removal.

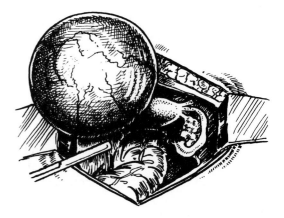

TREATMENT OF OVARIAN CANCER

Epithelial ovarian cancer is now the most frequent cause of death from gynaecological malignancy. The principles of treatment are:

1. Surgical staging.
Ovarian carcinoma is staged surgically, so laparotomy is an essential part of its management in most patients.

2. Surgical debulking of tumour volume.
Surgical removal of as much malignant tissue as possible, even if this should call for resection of structures outside the normal field of the gynaecologist.

3. Adjuvant chemotherapy.
This is followed-up with intensive chemotherapy. Currently, the most commonly used regimen is taxanes (paclitaxel) combined with the platinum compound, carboplatin.

Surgery remains an important aspect of management and referral to a specialised gynaecological oncology surgeon at the initial laparotomy has been shown to provide the best outcomes. Co-operation with a colorectal surgeon may be necessary. Increasingly, some centres offer chemotherapy prior to surgery, with an operation after three of the six planned chemotherapy treatments so as to reduce the incidence of surgical morbidity.

The diagnosis of ovarian cancer is often delayed due to the non-specific nature of the symptoms. Accordingly, as many as 66% of patients will be at an advanced stage, at the time of presentation.

SPREAD OF OVARIAN CANCER
It is important to know the direction of spread of ovarian cancers, so that the true extent of the disease and the symptoms that it may induce can be recognised and managed.

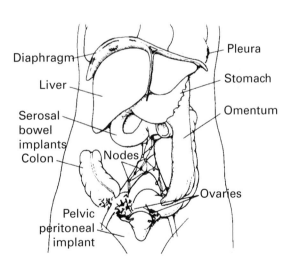

1. *Direct*
Spread directly into neighbouring structures – uterus, bladder or bowel.

2. *Transcoelomic*
Cancer cells are carried across the peritoneum and achieve widespread seeding. This results in tumour deposits in the peritoneum, bowel mesentery, visceral surfaces and the omentum. The tumour marker CA125 is usually raised in advanced ovarian cancer and is used to assess the response to chemotherapy.

3. *Lymphatics*
Ovarian drainage is to the para-aortic glands, but sometimes also to the pelvic and even the inguinal groups. Cells seeded on to the peritoneum are drained via the lymphatic channels on the underside of the diaphragm into the subpleural glands and thence to the pleura.

4. *Blood stream*
Blood spread is usually late and is to the liver and the lungs.

TREATMENT OF OVARIAN CANCER

All patients with an elevated risk of malignancy should be discussed at a preoperative multi-disciplinary meeting. The management of all patients remains as a combined surgical and chemotherapeutic regimen – primary surgery followed by adjuvant chemotherapy. Surgery may be delayed until three cycles of chemotherapy have been administered in selected cases – 'delayed primary surgery'.

The objectives are:

1. To classify the growth according to its extent of spread (staging) as accurately as possible.
2. To remove as much cancerous tissue as possible ('surgical debulking'; 'cyto-reductive treatment').

Chemotherapy is recommended for all stages of ovarian tumour greater than Stage 1B grade 2.

INCISION
A vertical incision, which can be extended, is essential to allow a full inspection. Reduction of a cyst by tapping and extraction through a suprapubic incision is not an acceptable practice. Surgical rupture of a cyst will increase its staging to a 1C tumour from what may have been a Stage 1A tumour. This has important implications for patient management.

INSPECTION
The entire peritoneal cavity must be palpated, including the liver, subdiaphragm, bowel and mesenteries, omentum and nodal areas. Suspicious areas are to be biopsied or removed.

ORGANS REMOVED
These must always include the uterus, tubes, ovaries, appendix and the omentum. Partial resection of bladder and bowel may also be required, but an epithelial cancer tends to spread over invaded tissue rather than penetrate it, and a plane of cleavage can often be found. The best patient outcomes are associated with either a complete or an optimal cytoreduction. The definition of optimal can vary but at least to a size of <2 cm largest tumour deposit or, preferably <1 cm largest tumour deposit.

CYTOLOGY
Before handling the tumour, specimens of ascitic fluid or peritoneal saline washings for cytological examination must be taken.

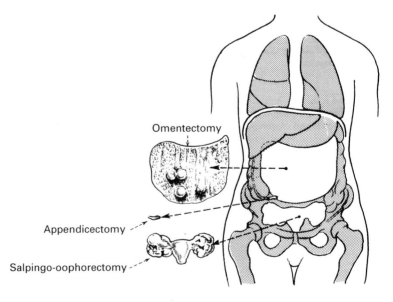

Omentectomy

Appendicectomy

Salpingo-oophorectomy

STAGING OF OVARIAN CANCER

STAGE I Growth limited to ovaries.

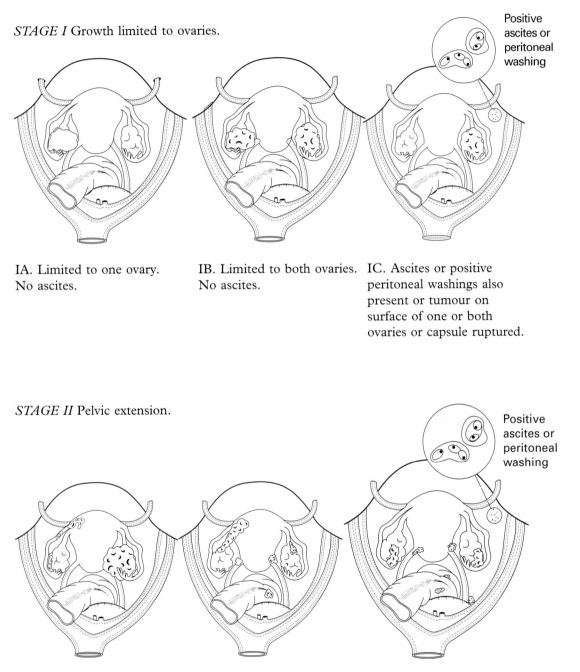

IA. Limited to one ovary.
No ascites.

IB. Limited to both ovaries.
No ascites.

IC. Ascites or positive
peritoneal washings also
present or tumour on
surface of one or both
ovaries or capsule ruptured.

STAGE II Pelvic extension.

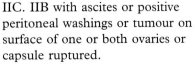

IIA. Spread to uterus/tubes.

IIB. Spread to other pelvic
tissues.

IIC. IIB with ascites or positive
peritoneal washings or tumour on
surface of one or both ovaries or
capsule ruptured.

STAGING OF OVARIAN CANCER

Stage III Extrapelvic, intraperitoneal spread and/or retroperitoneal or inguinal positive nodes, or superficial liver metastases.

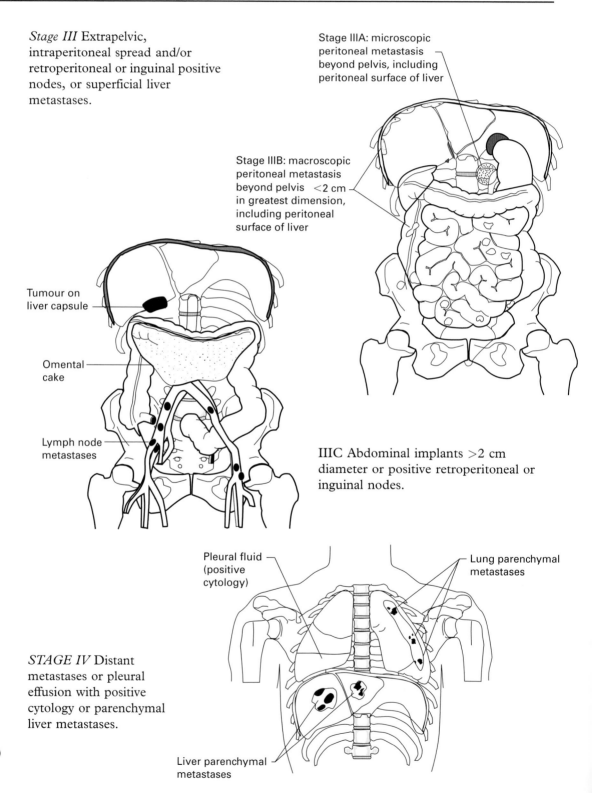

Stage IIIA: microscopic peritoneal metastasis beyond pelvis, including peritoneal surface of liver

Stage IIIB: macroscopic peritoneal metastasis beyond pelvis <2 cm in greatest dimension, including peritoneal surface of liver

Tumour on liver capsule

Omental cake

Lymph node metastases

IIIC Abdominal implants >2 cm diameter or positive retroperitoneal or inguinal nodes.

Pleural fluid (positive cytology)

Lung parenchymal metastases

STAGE IV Distant metastases or pleural effusion with positive cytology or parenchymal liver metastases.

Liver parenchymal metastases

PRINCIPLES OF CHEMOTHERAPY

MALIGNANT TUMOUR GROWTH

Tumour growth is a result of the failure of normal cell cycle control and a failure of apoptosis (the natural mechanism for removal of abnormal cells). Tumour cells multiply at the same rate or more slowly than normal cells, but have more actively dividing cells that are not subjected to the same physiological control, so that a cancer gradually develops.

MODE OF CHEMOTHERAPEUTIC ACTION

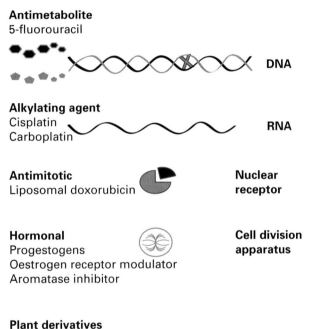

Antimetabolite
5-fluorouracil

DNA

Alkylating agent
Cisplatin
Carboplatin

RNA

Antimitotic
Liposomal doxorubicin

Nuclear receptor

Hormonal
Progestogens
Oestrogen receptor modulator
Aromatase inhibitor

Cell division apparatus

Plant derivatives
Taxane derivatives (Pacific yew tree)
Paclitaxel

CHEMOTHERAPEUTIC AGENTS IN OVARIAN CANCER

The current first line agents used in ovarian cancer treatment are carboplatin and paclitaxel. Carboplatin is an alkylating type agent that forms DNA cross links that prevent cell replication, ultimately leading to cell death. Paclitaxel similarly prevents cell replication by acting on another aspect of the cell, namely interfering with cell microtubule formation.

The antimetabolites inhibit DNA synthesis by disrupting essential metabolic events in nucleic acid synthesis. Another currently used treatment is liposomal doxorubicin which is an anti-mitotic agent with a complex mechanism of action that includes prevention of RNA synthesis, where the agent is delivered in liposomes to enhance its mechanism of action.

Hormonal therapies are employed to either directly bind to nuclear steroid receptors or influence the production of steroids that can bind to the nuclear steroid receptors. By binding to such receptors they can influence steroid gene regulation to bring about an antitumour effect. Response rates have been noted in ovarian cancer treatment and they are well-tolerated therapies.

Targeted anticancer therapies are currently being investigated as new therapies to increase the efficacy and decrease the toxicity of traditional chemotherapy. They target different pathways that are important for cancer growth and metastasis such as angiogenesis, cell cycle and the apoptotic pathways.

Chemotherapy trials are leading to evolutions of standard therapies. It has been noted that patients involved in chemotherapy trials have better outcomes than those not involved in these trials.

CHEMOTHERAPY TOXICITY
Common adverse effects of chemotherapy include nausea, vomiting and fatigue. Such side effects can be controlled well with antiemetics. Other side effects are related to the individual drugs. *Carboplatin* is well tolerated in general but is often myelosuppressive, necessitating blood transfusions or delayed treatments. *Paclitaxel* will lead to alopecia and it can also cause neuropathy, arthropathy and myalgia. *Liposomal doxorubicin* has a particular side effect called palmar/plantar erythema and it can also be cardiotoxic.

PRESENT PROGNOSIS FOR INVASIVE EPITHELIAL OVARIAN CANCER

Stage	5-year survival (%)
I	76
II	37
III	27
IV	15

Borderline epithelial tumours have excellent 5-year survival rates of 90–95% and a 15-year survival rate of 70–85%.

BROAD LIGAMENT CYSTS

BROAD LIGAMENT CYSTS (Parovarian Cysts)

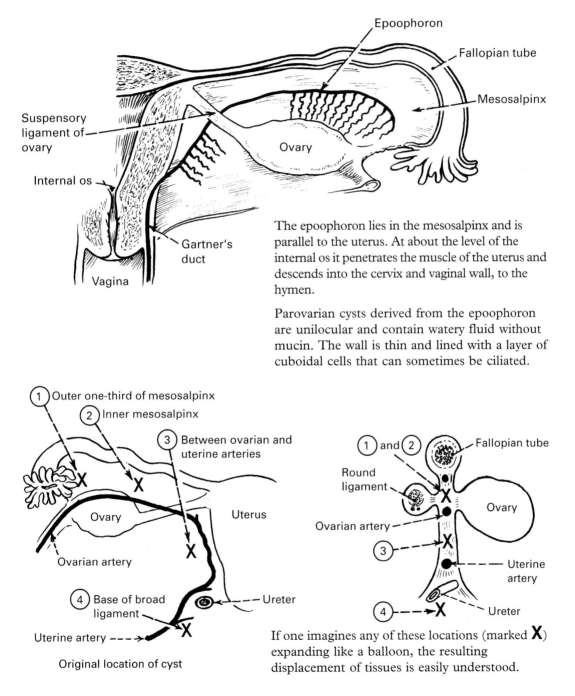

The epoophoron lies in the mesosalpinx and is parallel to the uterus. At about the level of the internal os it penetrates the muscle of the uterus and descends into the cervix and vaginal wall, to the hymen.

Parovarian cysts derived from the epoophoron are unilocular and contain watery fluid without mucin. The wall is thin and lined with a layer of cuboidal cells that can sometimes be ciliated.

If one imagines any of these locations (marked **X**) expanding like a balloon, the resulting displacement of tissues is easily understood.

BROAD LIGAMENT CYSTS

DIAGNOSIS

On palpation, the cyst, which is not mobile, may displace the uterus and may be closely related to it. An ovarian cyst with adhesions may feel very similar and it is seldom possible to distinguish between the two before a laparotomy.

OPERATION

Great care must be taken while identifying tissues, as the location of the original site of the cyst determines its displacement and its characteristics.

In the outer third of the broad ligament, the cyst tends to develop a pedicle.

In the middle of the broad ligament, the tumour is sessile but relatively fixed.

The ovarian vessels are displaced and may be stretched leading to interference with the ovarian blood supply.

It is possible for the ureter and uterine artery to be displaced outwards, but usually they are below and medial to the cyst.

The tumour may increase in size and strip the peritoneum off the pelvic walls and spread laterally and posteriorly, obliterating the Pouch of Douglas.

The broad ligament is incised anteriorly where the blood vessels are few, and the cyst is enucleated digitally. The oozing area is now exposed and should be obliterated. Care is necessary to avoid damage to the blood vessels, ureter and bladder. Redundant broad ligament may have to be excised.

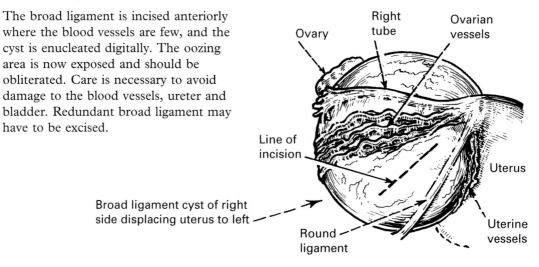

CYSTS OF KOBELT'S TUBULES, HYDATIDS OF MORGAGNI, FIMBRIAL CYSTS

These are names given to small cysts found in the mesosalpinx and around the terminal portion of the fallopian tubes. They are of indeterminate embryonic origin and are of no clinical significance.

CARCINOMA OF FALLOPIAN TUBES

The fallopian tubes are often involved in an ovarian carcinoma but an isolated fallopian tube carcinoma is very rare. There is, however, some evidence to suggest that ovarian carcinomas in BRCA gene mutation patients may actually arise from the distal fallopian tube.

PATHOLOGY

The growth is usually an adenocarcinoma of the tubal epithelium which grows inwards and secretes a copious amount of serosanguinous fluid which discharges *per vaginam,* if the proximal tube remains patent. This classical sign of a tubal carcinoma is rare.

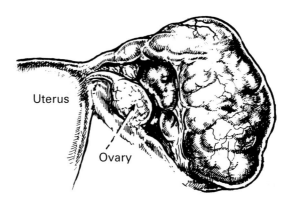

CLINICAL FEATURES

The patient is usually in her fifties and often nulliparous or of low parity. She may complain of postmenopausal bleeding, pain, and sometimes, a watery vaginal discharge. In the absence of definite symptoms the diagnosis is often made rather late. Pelvic signs suggestive of infection in a postmenopausal woman should always be investigated. The differential diagnosis includes carcinoma of the uterus or the ovary.

Aetiology is unknown, but increasing evidence suggests that some are BRCA linked.

CLINICAL STAGING

Stage I   confined to one or both tubes
Stage II   pelvic extension
Stage III spread to other structures (omentum, bowel, etc.), positive retroperitoneal or inguinal nodes or superficial liver metastases
Stage IV   distant metastases (including bladder), pleural effusion with positive cytology or parenchymal liver metastases

TREATMENT

Total hysterectomy and bilateral salpingo-oöphorectomy should be done as a minimum, followed by chemotherapy, as for an ovarian carcinoma.

CHAPTER 14

COMPLICATIONS OF GYNAECOLOGICAL SURGERY

Urinary Tract Injuries	288
Injury to the Ureter	289
Management of Ureteric Injury	290
Bowel Injury	*291*
Fistula Formation	292
Urinary Fistula	*292*
Adhesions	*293*
Lymphoedema and Lymphocyst	294
Infectious Morbidity	*294*
Hernia	*294*
Venous Thrombosis	295
Pathology	*296*
Sites of Thrombus Formation	*297*
Clinical Features of Deep Venous Thrombosis	298
Investigations for Deep Venous Thrombosis	299
Fibrin D-Dimer Assay	*299*
Ultrasound	*299*
Methods of Thromboprophylaxis	300
General Measures	*300*
Mechanical Methods	*300*
Unfractionated and Low Molecular Weight	
Heparins	*301*
Treatment of DVT	*301*
Pulmonary Embolism	302
Peripheral Pulmonary Embolism	*302*
Central Pulmonary Embolism	*302*
Pulmonary Embolism Management	*303*
Investigations	*303*
Treatment of Pulmonary Embolus	305
Mortality	306

URINARY TRACT INJURIES

Gynaecological surgery, in common with other surgical specialties, can be associated with complications. Most complications are minor, self limiting and have no long-term consequence for the patient, but they must still be avoided where possible, and actively managed where necessary, to make sure they do not become major complications.

Gynaecological surgery involves close dissection to viscera including the bladder, rectum, ureters as well as the great vessels of the pelvis. Complications can occur during difficult surgical dissections, especially when the anatomy is distorted (e.g. malignancy, endometriosis or infection).

Other complications, such as pulmonary embolus, myocardial infarction, pneumonia, or fluid or electrolyte imbalance are common to all surgery. For the purposes of this chapter, the most common complications related only to gynaecological surgery will be discussed.

URINARY TRACT INJURIES

Bladder Injuries

If a bladder injury is suspected intraoperatively, it can be localised by intravenous injection of indigo carmine, retrograde instillation of methylene blue through the urethral catheter or by opening the dome of the bladder and inspecting the mucosa. Subtle injuries can also be diagnosed using cystoscopy. Early involvement of an urologist is advised.

Primary closure of a cystotomy can be performed using a simple one or two-layered running closure with absorbable suture.

In general, it takes approximately 3–4 days for the bladder to re-epithelialise and about 3 weeks to regain its normal strength. A catheter can be left *in situ* for about 7 days with a cystogram performed just prior to its removal, to confirm healing.

In circumstances where a primary closure is difficult (e.g. vaginal surgery, unstable patient, history of pelvic irradiation) and there is a small injury (3 cm or less) in the bladder dome, a suprapubic catheter can be placed. A Foley catheter is placed through the cystotomy, with the bulb remaining in the bladder and the catheter exiting through a stab wound in the lower abdomen.

Women who have received prior lower pelvic radiation or have severe bladder injury require a stronger repair. A carefully dissected omentum, from the hepatic flexure to the splenic flexure, can be used over the two-layer closure to provide neovascularity.

After any repair to the bladder, it must be ensured that the ureteral orifices near the trigone are not compromised. This can be done by passing a stent, retrograde from the bladder toward the kidney or by dissection and visual identification of the distal ureter.

INJURY TO THE URETER

The ureter will occasionally be damaged no matter how much skill and care are exercised. It is essential to directly visualise the ureters at surgery to check for peristalsis, gross dilation (obstruction) or urine leakage, in order to prevent ureteral damage.

The operating surgeon must have a thorough knowledge of the location of the ureter and where it is most susceptible to trauma. The three most common sites of ureteral injury, in the order of frequency of occurence are:

1. While dividing the infundibulopelvic ligament
2. During division of the uterine artery
3. When mobilising the bladder.

The ureter's course is to some extent variable, and when under pressure, it will gradually change its position in the pelvis. A large tumour filling the pelvis will displace it laterally. A tumour in the broad ligament may displace the ureter outwards and upwards. Duplex (double) ureters are occasionally met with.

A ureter displaced by a fibroid which has occupied the broad ligament.

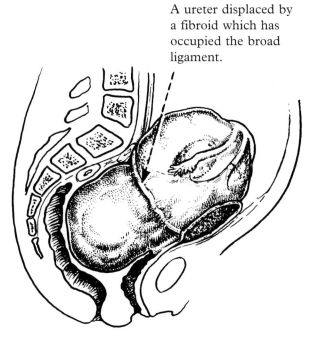

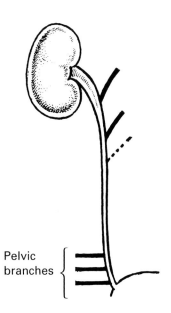

Pelvic branches

Radical surgery may destroy so much of the pelvic blood supply that the pelvic ureter becomes ischaemic, leading to fibrotic narrowing or fistula. Damage to the blood vessels may also be produced by pelvic irradiation.

MANAGEMENT OF URETERIC INJURY

Ureteric injury should be managed in consultation with a urologist, or a gynaecologist with subspecialty training in urogynaecology.

1. *Types of ureteric injury identified at operation.*
   a. Crush injury from clamp or ligature.
      The clamp or ligature should be removed, and a ureteric stent inserted.
   b. Ligation of the ureter.
      The ligation of the ureter should be treated by an end-to-end anastomosis, reimplantation of the ureter into the bladder or by uretero-ureteric anastomosis into the opposite ureter.

2. *Ureteric injury identified postoperatively.*

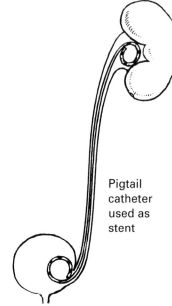

Pigtail catheter used as stent

Clinical Features

The signs and symptoms relate to the leakage of urine into the ureteric fistulae, and to ureteric obstruction, when the ureter has been ligated. If a ureteric fistula is present, urine leakage may be observed in an abdominal drain, or from the surgical incisions. The patient may develop lower abdominal pain and pyrexia. If the ureter has been ligated, the patient may develop loin pain and pyrexia.

Investigations

1. *Ultrasound.*
   If ureteric obstruction is suspected, an ultrasound may be a useful initial test to identify hydronephrosis.

2. *Computerised tomography (CT).*
   This is becoming another useful test with an increase in the widespread availability of CT scanning. It has the advantage of showing clear anatomical relationships as well as the site of any injury.

3. *Intravenous urography.*
   Intravenous urography (IVU) is useful in the investigation both of ureteric fistulae and of ureteric obstruction. The urinary tract is outlined by radio-opaque dye and the site of leakage or obstruction of urine can be identified. Small fistulae may not be identified by this approach.

MANAGEMENT OF URETERIC INJURY

4. *Percutaneous nephrostomy followed by antegrade pyelography.*

This manoeuvre is both therapeutic and diagnostic. Percutaneous nephrostomy is carried out under an ultrasound or X-ray control. Using local anaesthesia, a catheter is passed through the skin and into the renal pelvis or ureter (percutaneous nephrostomy). This allows drainage of the kidney, and prevents further renal damage. Contrast medium can then be injected through the catheter (antegrade pyelography), and this gives further information on the extent of ureteric damage.

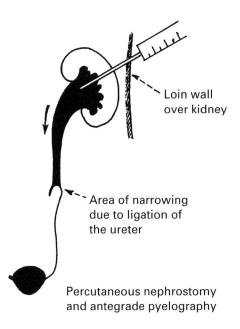

Loin wall
over kidney

Area of narrowing
due to ligation of
the ureter

Percutaneous nephrostomy
and antegrade pyelography

Treatment of Ureteric Injury

When ureteric injury is diagnosed, the principle of treatment, in the first instance, is to relieve the ureteric obstruction, thus preventing back pressure on the kidney and subsequent renal necrosis. Clearly, if both ureters have been damaged, and renal compromise/failure is already apparent, consideration should be given to renal dialysis. The following manoeuvres may be useful in the short term:

1. Percutaneous nephrostomy with or without antegrade stenting (see above).
2. Cystoscopy and retrograde insertion of ureteric stents.

In the longer term, formal repair of the ureter is necessary, and this may be achieved using one of the techniques outlined above. It should be emphasised again that these techniques are outside the areas of expertise of most gynaecologists.

BOWEL INJURY

Serosal abrasions should be assessed and repaired where appropriate, particularly when it is a diathermy injury. Injuries involving the muscularis or both the muscularis and the mucosa should also be repaired.

For colonic injury, the lack of a preoperative bowel prep is not an indication for colostomy. After the bowel is repaired, the abdomen is copiously irrigated. Occasionally, a segment of the bowel must be resected, and if reanastomosis is performed, routine care can resume. If bowel reanastomosis cannot be performed due to extensive injury or pathology (i.e. dense adhesions or inflammatory changes), a diverting colostomy may be required.

FISTULA FORMATION

URINARY FISTULA

(L. *fistula*: a pipe) It is a pathological connection between the urinary tract and an adjacent structure through which urine escapes. A fistula between the bladder base and the vagina is the condition that is most often seen.

Aetiology

1. The exposed bladder wall is torn or penetrated during a vaginal operation, or during total abdominal hysterectomy. This is the commonest cause in this country.

A tear develops during mobilisation of the bladder.

Prolonged pressure of vertex on the vagina during obstructed labour. In a few days, a slough forms. (This should not occur with modern obstetrics in developed countries.)

2. The vaginal wall and bladder are torn during an obstetric operation, or pressure necrosis develops during a prolonged and difficult labour.

3. The ureter is damaged or made ischaemic during a pelvic operation, especially during radical hysterectomy. This produces a ureterovaginal fistula.

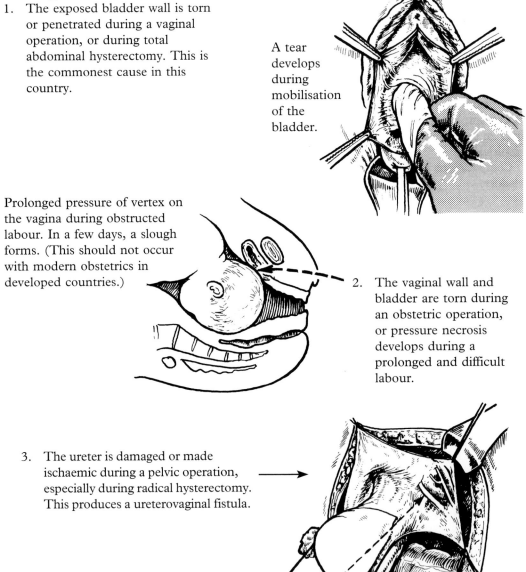

Exposing ureter in radical hysterectomy

FISTULA FORMATION

4. Radiation burns following treatment for carcinoma of the cervix. This fistula may appear several years after treatment.
5. Untreated or recurrent cancer of bladder or the genital tract. (This may also be complicated by radiation effects.)
6. Chronic tuberculosis or syphilis. Fistulae may complicate the surgical treatment of pelvic tuberculosis.
7. Congenital fistula. An accessory ectopic ureter may open into the vagina. This condition should be recognised in childhood.

Symptoms

Incontinence may immediately follow the injury, but, usually, the patient has several days of dysuria and haematuria with symptoms of urinary infection. A discharge appears followed by sloughing, and the patient finds that her vulva and perineum are constantly wet. This is soon followed by excoriation of the skin, accompanied by a strong ammoniacal smell and an incrustation of the vulva and vagina with urinary salts. The area becomes extremely tender.

Diagnosis

The fistula is localised by cystoscopy, an intravenous pyelogram and retrograde studies of the ureter. Further imaging with CT or magnetic resonance imaging (MRI), where available, can help to localise the fistulae.

Treatment

Simple vesicovaginal fistulae can be managed by prolonged bladder drainage to allow an opportunity for spontaneous healing. When healing fails to occur, surgical correction is necessary and this may be performed through a vaginal or transabdominal approach.

Simple ureterovaginal fistulae usually heal after being stented, preferably by percutaneous antegrade stents as they have higher success rates. If this fails, surgical repair will be necessary. Complex ureterovesicovaginal fistulae require stenting and drainage until inflammation and infection have resolved and surgical procedures may also be required for their resolution.

ADHESIONS

One function of the peritoneal surface of the pelvic and abdominal structures is to prevent adherence of these structures when they touch. If the peritoneum is injured as a result of surgery, the damaged areas may stick to each other and a permanent adhesion may form. This typically occurs within the first 5 days after surgery.

Postoperative adhesions occur in 60–90% of women undergoing major gynaecologic surgery. The incidence of adhesion-related intestinal obstruction after gynaecologic surgery is greater upon surgery for malignant conditions and pelvic radiation, compared to benign conditions. Symptoms may occur from weeks to several years after the procedure.

LYMPHOEDEMA AND LYMPHOCYST

Unilateral or bilateral lymphoedema of the lower extremities can occur after radical surgery, and the risk is greater when postoperative radiation is given.

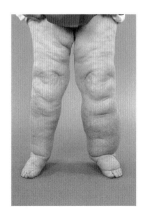

This is a chronic problem for the resolution of which a referral to a specialist clinic can help. Support hosiery and leg wraps will minimise the oedema, elevation of the extremities while sitting and elevation of the foot of the bed also help to control the problem. Women with lymphoedema should be warned to take care of their skin and pay special attention to the development of erythema or tenderness, as these may indicate infection and a need for systemic antibiotics. Diuretics do not improve lymphoedema, and may lead to electrolyte abnormalities.

Lymphocysts are uncommon after pelvic lymphadenectomy, occurring in about 1–3% of women, 11–12 days after surgery. They are seldom symptomatic and are detected when radiologic studies are performed for the purpose of surveying the woman for recurrent neoplastic disease. Symptoms consist of vague, colicky, lower abdominal pain. Symptomatic lymphocysts and those causing hydronephrosis can be drained percutaneously. Recurrent lymphocysts should be re-drained by tetracycline instillation to sclerose the cavity.

INFECTIOUS MORBIDITY

Fever within the first 48 h of surgery is almost always cytokine related. Fever-associated cytokines are released due to tissue trauma and do not necessarily signal infection. Fever due to the trauma of surgery usually resolves within 2–3 days.

Chest radiography, urinalysis, and blood and urine cultures are NOT indicated for all postoperative patients with fever. The need for laboratory testing should be determined from the findings of a careful history and physical examination. The febrile postoperative patient should be evaluated systematically, taking into account the timing of the onset of fever and its many possible causes.

Significant febrile morbidity after gynaecological surgery is usually attributable to infection of the urinary tract, wounds (including the vaginal cuff and necrotising fasciitis), or pelvic cellulitis and abscess. After the first two postoperative days, a thorough inspection of the wound and a good rectovaginal examination are the most important components of the fever work-up. Empiric broad spectrum antibiotics may then be started.

It may be appropriate to arrange further investigations to determine any septic source.

HERNIA

Incisional hernia can occur in areas of weakness in incompletely healed surgical wounds. An approach to their prevention is the closure of the incision by incorporating a permanent suture of a length that is at least four times the length of the incision. Symptomatic or cosmetically unacceptable hernias are repaired surgically.

VENOUS THROMBOSIS

Deep vein thrombosis (DVT) of the lower limbs is a common disease and is often asymptomatic. Complications include pulmonary thromboembolism (PE) and post thrombotic leg syndrome (PLS).

Patients undergoing major general or gynaecological surgery, who are aged 40 years or more, or who have other risk factors (see below) have a significant risk of venous thrombosis. In many of these patients DVT remains asymptomatic, but, in others, it can cause serious morbidity and, potentially, mortality.

There is evidence that routine prophylaxis reduces morbidity, mortality and costs in hospitalised patients at risk of DVT and PE, as highlighted in national and international guidelines. In contrast, screening for asymptomatic DVT and its treatment, are expensive, insensitive and not cost-effective compared to routine prophylaxis in at-risk patients.

Risk factors for venous thrombosis
(SIGN Guidelines October 2002)

Age	Exponential increase in risk with age. In the general population: <40 years annual risk 1/10,000 60–69 years annual risk 1/1000 >80 years annual risk 1/100 May reflect immobility and coagulation activation
Obesity	3 × risk if obese (BMI ≥ 30 kg/m^2) May reflect immobility and coagulation activation
Varicose veins	1.5 × risk after major general/orthopaedic surgery But low risk after varicose vein surgery
Previous VTE	Recurrence rate 5%/year, increased by surgery
Thrombophilias	Low coagulation inhibitors (antithrombin, protein C or S) Activated protein C resistance (e.g. Factor V Leidin) High coagulation factors (I, II, VIII, IX, XI) Antiphospholipid syndrome High homocysteine
Other thrombotic states	Malignancy 7 × risk Heart failure Recent myocardial infarction/stroke Severe infection Inflammatory bowel disease, nephrotic syndrome Polycythaemia, paraproteinaemia Bechet's disease, paroxysmal nocturnal haemoglobinuria
Hormone therapy	Oral combined contraceptives, HRT, raloxifene, tamoxifen 3 × risk High dose progestogens 6× risk
Pregnancy, puerperium	10 × risk
Immobility	Bedrest >3 days 10× risk (increases with duration)
Hospitalisation	Acute trauma, acute illness, surgery, 10× risk
Anaesthesia	2× general vs. spinal/epidural

VENOUS THROMBOSIS

PATHOLOGY

Virchow's triad encompasses the three broad categories of factors that are thought to contribute to the formation of venous thrombosis:

1. *Changes in the vessel wall*

   Injury or trauma to the vascular endothelium encourages the platelets to adhere to the exposed collagen tissue and these then release substances which further facilitate platelet aggregation. Fibrin and leucocytes then adhere to the platelets. Recent work suggests that a balance is maintained between different groups of prostaglandins.

2. *Changes in the pattern of blood flow (flow volume)*

   Venous flow in the legs is much reduced in the postoperative period and is a result of inactivity and poor muscle tone.

3. *Changes in the constituents of blood (hypercoagulability)*

   Increased procoagulant activity, including elevated platelet count, platelet 'stickiness' and fibrinogen levels, contribute to hypercoagulability. Fortunately, there is also a compensating increase in fibrinolytic activity so that nearly all thrombi are naturally broken down.

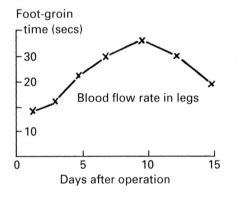

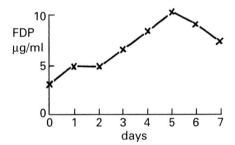

Post-operative increase in fibrin degradation products (FDP) as a result of thrombus destruction.

VENOUS THROMBOSIS

SITES OF THROMBUS FORMATION

Common sites of thrombus formation include:

(1) The calf veins extending to the popliteal
(2) The long and short saphenous veins, especially those lateral to the knee
(3) The ilio-femoral segment extending to the vena cava
(4) Superficial thrombosis in the distal leg veins.

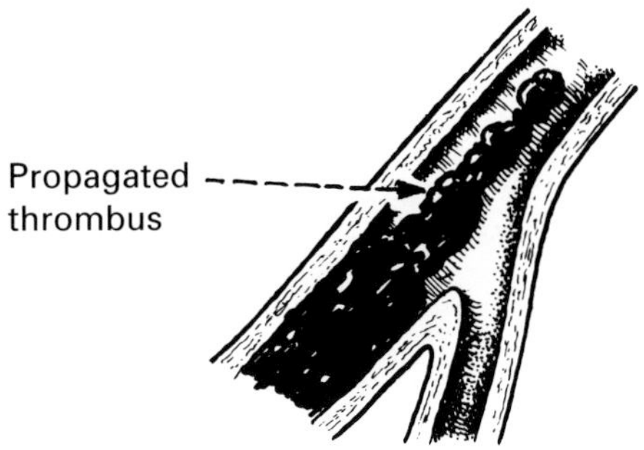

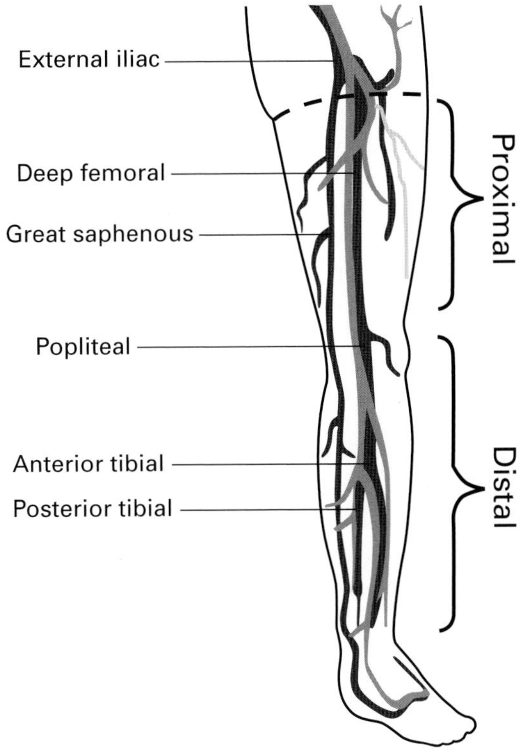

External iliac

Deep femoral

Great saphenous

Popliteal

Anterior tibial

Posterior tibial

Proximal

Distal

Propagated thrombus

CLINICAL FEATURES OF DEEP VENOUS THROMBOSIS

In many cases deep venous thrombosis (DVT) is asymptomatic. It is, therefore, imperative to carefully look for clinical features, particularly in the presence of any risk factors (see Risk Factors for Venous Thrombosis). The classical symptoms of DVT include swelling, pain and discoloration in the affected extremity. Physical examination may reveal the palpable cord of a thrombosed vein, unilateral oedema, warmth and superficial venous dilation. Other signs include the Homan's test of dorsiflexion of the foot for eliciting pain in posterior calf (it should be noted that it is of little diagnostic value and is theoretically dangerous because of the possibility of dislodgement of a loose clot) and Pratt's sign – the ability to elicit pain by squeezing the posterior calf.

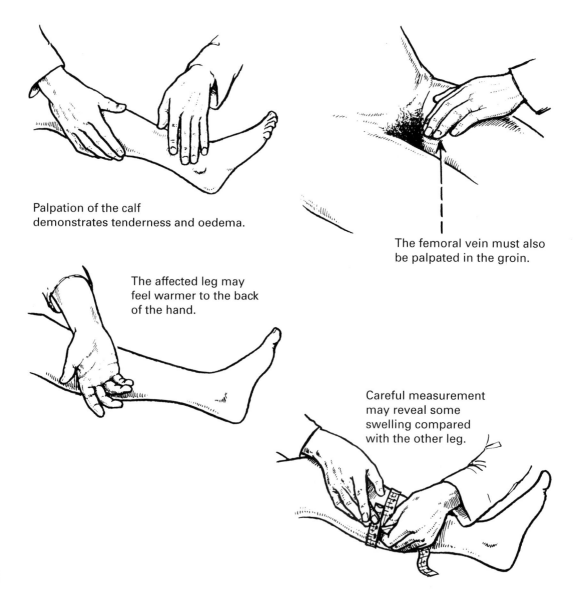

Palpation of the calf demonstrates tenderness and oedema.

The femoral vein must also be palpated in the groin.

The affected leg may feel warmer to the back of the hand.

Careful measurement may reveal some swelling compared with the other leg.

INVESTIGATIONS FOR DEEP VENOUS THROMBOSIS

Diagnostic imaging (venography, ultrasound) should be performed expeditiously (within 24 h if possible) in patients with suspected DVT. In all patients with clinically suspected DVT, the diagnosis should be confirmed or excluded by diagnostic imaging, either by non-invasive testing by ultrasound (compression or Duplex scanning) followed by contrast venography, if negative (to detect calf and non-occlusive proximal DVT) or contrast venography (to detect both calf and proximal DVT). It may be necessary to carry out serial (repeat after 7 days) ultrasound examinations to detect a proximal extension of a calf DVT. A single negative ultrasound may be sufficient to exclude DVT in patients with low clinical pre-test probability and/or a normal fibrin D-dimer assay.

FIBRIN D-DIMER ASSAY

Plasma D-dimers are specific cross-linked derivatives of fibrin that are produced when fibrin is degraded by plasmin, so its concentration is raised in patients with venous thromboembolism. Although sensitive for venous thromboembolism, high concentrations of D-dimers are insufficiently specific for making a positive diagnosis because they occur in other disorders such as a malignancy, pregnancy and after operations. Nevertheless, D-dimer tests generally have a high negative predictive value and are useful rule-out tests that reduce the need for imaging when used in conjunction with clinical probability, plethysmography and the ultrasound.

ULTRASOUND

This is the best non-invasive technique for diagnosing venous thrombosis. It has a better sensitivity and specificity (97%) in diagnosing of proximal DVT compared to the distal calf vein thrombosis (approximately 75% sensitivity).

Colour flow duplex ultrasonography evaluates blood flow characteristics within the vessel using a pulsed Doppler signal.

METHODS OF THROMBOPROPHYLAXIS

GENERAL MEASURES

(1) *Early ambulation* – immobility increases the risk of DVT by about 10 fold and, hence, early mobilisation and leg exercises should be encouraged in postoperative patients.

(2) *Postoperative physiotherapy* – the physiotherapist encourages the patient to perform deep breathing and exercises to restore muscle tone.

(3) *Hydration* – haemoconcentration increases blood viscosity and reduces blood flow, especially in the deep veins of the leg in immobile patients; hence adequate hydration should be ensured in immobilised patients.

MECHANICAL METHODS

Mechanical thromboprophylactic methods have been shown to increase mean blood flow velocity in the leg veins and to reduce venous stasis. Unlike pharmacological methods, they do not increase the risk of bleeding. Mechanical methods are contraindicated in patients at risk of ischemic skin necrosis, for example those with critical limb ischemia or severe peripheral neuropathy. Mechanical methods include:

(1) *Graduated elastic compression stockings* (*GECS*) – these reduce the pooling of blood in the leg veins. Graduated static compression stockings exert a greater pressure at the ankle than at the thigh.

(2) *Pneumatic stockings* – inflatable lower leg stocking device that applies intermittent pneumatic pressure to the legs during an operation.

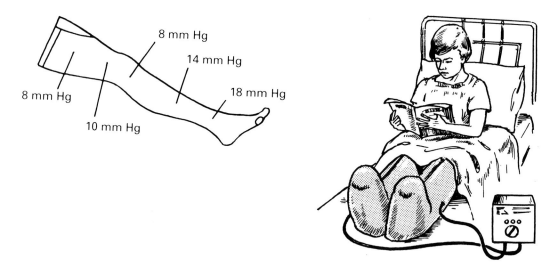

METHODS OF THROMBOPROPHYLAXIS

UNFRACTIONATED AND LOW MOLECULAR WEIGHT HEPARINS
Unfractionated heparin (UFH) and low molecular weight heparins (LMWHs – dalteparin, enoxparin, reviparin and tinzaparin) are effective in the prophylaxis of VTE in both surgical and medical patients.

The risk of wound haematomas can be minimised by avoiding injection sites close to wounds.

TREATMENT OF DVT
The goals of treatment for DVT are to stop clot propagation and to prevent clot recurrence, pulmonary embolism (PE), and pulmonary hypertension (a potential complication of multiple recurrent PEs). These goals are usually achieved with anticoagulation therapy using heparin followed by warfarin, according to local protocols.

COMPLICATIONS OF GYNAECOLOGICAL SURGERY

PULMONARY EMBOLISM

An embolism arises from a thrombus which was non-occlusive in the vessel in which it was formed and it is therefore symptomless. This then travels to the lung, causing occlusion of the pulmonary vessels.

PERIPHERAL PULMONARY EMBOLISM
Small emboli are lysed rapidly and are symptomless unless an infarction occurs. They often precede a major embolism, unless treatment is given.

Symptoms	Signs
Fever	Pyrexia
Tachypnoea	Pleural rub
Pleural pain	Crepitations
Haemoptysis (40%)	Perhaps opacity on lung X-ray

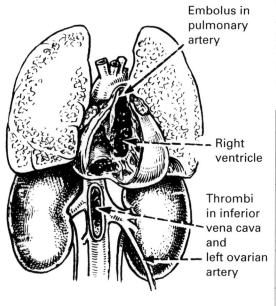

Embolus in pulmonary artery

Right ventricle

Thrombi in inferior vena cava and left ovarian artery

CENTRAL PULMONARY EMBOLISM
A large embolus impacting the main pulmonary artery will be immediately fatal, but if it is a little more peripheral, circulatory obstruction will be incomplete and there is a chance of survival.

Symptoms	Signs
1. Collapse	1. Shock – vasoconstriction – hypotension
2. Faintness	2. RV failure – distended neck veins – Gallop rhythm
3. Respiratory distress	3. Cyanosis
4. Pain	

The cardiac output drops at once and there is intense reflex vasoconstriction leading to tachycardia, hypotension and syncope if the patient is sat up. The respiratory distress is very severe and pulmonary cyanosis may be aggravated by a right-to-left shunt through a patent foramen ovale which exists in 25% of the individuals.

PULMONARY EMBOLISM

PULMONARY EMBOLISM MANAGEMENT

1. Remember the risk factors for thromboembolism.
2. Suspect PE in all women presenting with a sudden onset of shortness of breath, chest pain, unexplained tachycardia or cardiovascular collapse.
3. Involve senior medical staff.
4. Assess and ensure adequate airway, breathing and circulation. Commence cardiopulmonary resuscitation if the patient is in cardiac arrest.
5. Transfer the patient to the high-dependency area when appropriate and commence monitoring: non-invasive blood pressure, pulse oximetry, ECG, urine output.
6. Send samples for a full blood count, clotting studies, urea and electrolytes, liver function tests and thrombophilia screen.
7. Request ECG, arterial blood gas and chest X-ray.

INVESTIGATIONS

ECG
ECG is non-specific for the diagnosis of a PE. Right axis deviation and right ventricular strain pattern may be present with a large PE. S waves in lead 1, Q wave in lead 3 and inverted T waves in lead 3 (s1Q3T3) patterns are very rare.

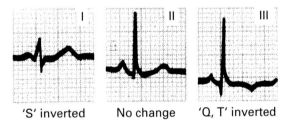

'S' inverted   No change   'Q, T' inverted

Chest X-Ray
This will help to exclude a pneumothorax and pneumonia. The non-specific radiological changes in PE include segmental collapse, a raised hemi diaphragm, consolidation and unilateral pleural effusion. A wedge-shaped infarction is a rare finding.

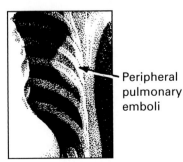

Peripheral pulmonary emboli

Arterial Blood Gases
With massive PE, PaO_2 may be reduced with and a normal or low $PaCO_2$.

PULMONARY EMBOLISM

Ventilation/Perfusion (V/Q) Scans

V/Q scanning is the most useful initial test in patients with suspected PE. They are interpreted using standardised criteria and, based on the extent of ventilation-perfusion mismatches, the scan is interpreted as normal, low probability, intermediate probability or high probability for a PE. A normal scan reliably excludes PE and a high-probability V/Q scan is considered as sufficient evidence for the diagnosis of a PE in a patient with a high clinical suspicion. Perfusion scan alone can be performed with a ventilation scan being performed only if the perfusion scan is abnormal.

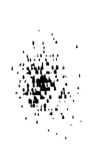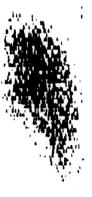

Right lung perfusion much reduced.

Duplex Doppler Leg Ultrasound

Bilateral Doppler ultrasound leg studies should be performed in all cases of suspected PE.

CT Pulmonary Angiography

CT, after contrast injection, permits excellent visualisation of the pulmonary arteries and a direct visualisation of pulmonary arterial clots in larger vessels – all during a single breath hold.

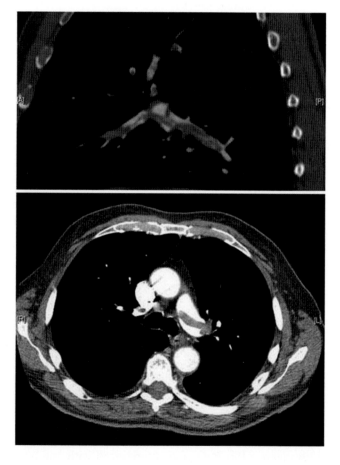

TREATMENT OF PULMONARY EMBOLUS

In most cases, anticoagulant therapy is the mainstay of the treatment. Heparin or LMWHs (such as enoxaparin and dalteparin) are administered initially, while warfarin therapy is commenced.

Massive PE causing haemodynamic instability is an indication for thrombolysis, the enzymatic destruction of the clot with medication. The aim of this therapy is to dissolve the clot, but there is an attendant risk of bleeding or stroke.

Surgical management of acute PE (pulmonary thrombectomy) is uncommon and has largely been abandoned because of poor long-term outcomes.

Chronic PE leading to pulmonary hypertension (known as *chronic thromboembolic hypertension*) is treated by a surgical procedure known as a pulmonary thromboendarterectomy.

If anticoagulant therapy is contraindicated and/or ineffective, or to prevent new emboli from entering the pulmonary artery and combining with an existing blockage, an inferior vena cava filter may be implanted.

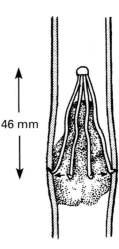

46 mm

MORTALITY

A retrospective study of 1.45 million gynaecology inpatients in England reported a mortality rate of 0.2% within 30 days of admission and 0.5% within 90 days.
The 30-day death rate in patients with cancer was higher than for patients without cancer (5.1% vs. 0.1%).

CHAPTER 15

EARLY PREGNANCY

Miscarriage 308
Threatened Miscarriage 308
Inevitable Miscarriage 308
Complete Miscarriage 308
Incomplete Miscarriage 309
Missed Miscarriage 309
Other Terms 309
Management 310
Early Pregnancy Loss (≤12 Weeks' Gestation) 310
Late Pregnancy Loss (>12 Weeks' Gestation) 313
Recurrent Miscarriage 314
Introduction and Definitions 314
Causes of Recurrent Miscarriage 314
Investigation and Treatment of Recurrent Miscarriage 316
Termination of Pregnancy 317
First Trimester Termination of Pregnancy 317
Second Trimester Termination of Pregnancy 319

Complications of Termination of Pregnancy 319
Ectopic Pregnancy 320
Aetiology 320
Diagnosis of Tubal Pregnancy 321
Symptoms 321
Signs 321
Diagnosis of Tubal Pregnancy 321
Sites of Implantation 323
Rupture of the Tube 323
Rupture into Lumen of Tube 323
Treatment of Tubal Pregnancy 324
Methotrexate 324
Salpingectomy 324
Salpingostomy 324
Conservative 324
Gestational Trophoblastic Disease 325
Pathology 326
Presentation and Genetics 327
Treatment 328
Gestational Trophoblastic Neoplasia 328
Chemotherapy for Choriocarcinoma 330

MISCARRIAGE

Miscarriage occurs in 10–20% of clinical pregnancies, and in the UK it is defined as a pregnancy loss before the 24th week of gestation. In Australia, miscarriage is a pregnancy that spontaneously ends before 20 weeks. After the 20th week of pregnancy, the loss of a fetus is called a stillbirth.

THREATENED MISCARRIAGE
Technically this refers only to bleeding from the placental site, which is not yet severe enough to terminate the pregnancy. Usually the bleeding is slight and the cervix remains closed. The pregnancy is likely to remain viable.

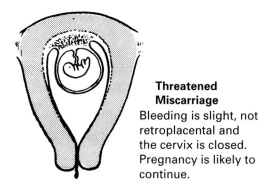

Threatened Miscarriage
Bleeding is slight, not retroplacental and the cervix is closed. Pregnancy is likely to continue.

INEVITABLE MISCARRIAGE
Clinically, the amount of bleeding is variable but the cervix is open. On ultrasound examination, the bleeding is retroplacental and often, fetal heart activity is absent.

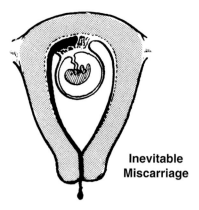

Inevitable Miscarriage

COMPLETE MISCARRIAGE
A miscarriage in which the fetus, membranes and chorionic tissue are completely expelled from the uterus is termed a complete miscarriage.

MISCARRIAGE

INCOMPLETE MISCARRIAGE

A miscarriage in which the fetus or membranes or chorionic tissue are incompletely expelled from the uterus. An ultrasound will show debris (retained products of conception) within the uterine cavity.

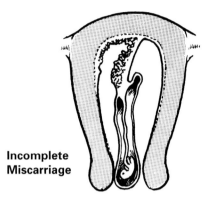

**Incomplete
Miscarriage**

MISSED MISCARRIAGE

It is defined as the retention of a non-viable fetus for several weeks without any clinical symptoms.

OTHER TERMS

The term *early fetal demise* is now used to describe what used to be known as an *anembryonic pregnancy* or a *blighted ovum* and denotes pregnancies in which a gestational sac is present without the development of a fetal pole.

MANAGEMENT

The method of management of miscarriage depends upon the gestation of miscarriage and clinical facilities available. Apart from expectant management, these methods are identical to those performed during an elective termination of pregnancy.

EARLY PREGNANCY LOSS ($\leq$12 Weeks' Gestation)

Surgical

Clinical indications for surgical evacuation include: persistent excessive bleeding, haemodynamic instability, evidence of infected retained tissue, suspected gestational trophoblastic disease and patient choice. Surgical uterine evacuation for a miscarriage should be performed using a suction curettage. Where infection is suspected, delaying surgical intervention for 12 h is recommended to allow intravenous antibiotic administration.

Preoperative cervical preparation essentially softens the cervix making it easier to dilate and, in doing so, minimises force of dilatation required, haemorrhage and uterine/cervical trauma. The cervix can be prepared using:

- gemeprost (prostaglandin E_1) given as a vaginal pessary 3 h before surgery
- misoprostol (a prostaglandin analogue) given vaginally 3 h before surgery
- mifepristone (an antiprogesterone) given orally at least 12 h before surgery
- laminaria tents inserted into the external cervical os.

Surgical Evacuation of the Products of Conception

Curettage

The patient is anaesthetised and the cervix is dilated. Once dilatation is sufficient, vacuum aspiration of the uterine contents is carried out.

A plastic suction curette is commonly used and is less likely to damage the uterus than metal instruments. Plastic curettes are available in diameters from 4 to 12 mm. The cervix is conventionally dilated to a diameter that is 2 mm less than the gestation age in weeks.

MANAGEMENT

Surgical Evacuation of Products of Conception—(cont'd)

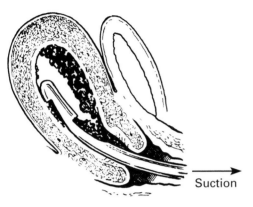

Suction

Complications

1. Incomplete uterine evacuation.
2. Uterine perforation and/or damage to abdominal viscera.
3. Sepsis. Broad spectrum antibiotics have been shown to minimise the risk of post-abortal infection.
4. Haemorrhage. Blood loss can be minimised by the use of prostaglandins for preoperative cervical ripening. Bleeding during or after the procedure can be reduced by oxytocic agents such as ergometrine or Syntocinon.
5. Rhesus isoimmunisation. Anti-D should be administered to all rhesus negative women.

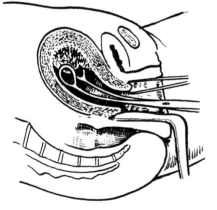

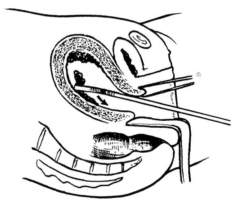

Further tissue can be removed with a sponge forcep or a curette. The concave side of the curette loop is pressed against the uterine wall and pulled down. A 'clean' uterine wall gives a characteristic sensation to the operating hand.

Reported serious complications of surgery include perforation of the uterus, cervical tears, intra-abdominal trauma, intrauterine adhesions and haemorrhage.

MANAGEMENT

EARLY PREGNANCY LOSS (≤12 Weeks' Gestation)—(cont'd)

Medical
Medical methods are an effective alternative in the management of a confirmed first-trimester miscarriage. Various medical methods have been described which use prostaglandin analogues (gemeprost or misoprostol) with or without antiprogesterone priming (mifepristone).
Protocols should be developed locally with appropriate selection criteria, therapeutic regimens and arrangements for follow-up. To avoid unnecessary anxiety, women should be informed that bleeding may continue for up to 3 weeks after medical uterine evacuation.

Expectant
Expectant management is a method that can be offered in cases of confirmed first trimester miscarriage. Patient counselling is particularly important for those women with an intact sac who wish to adopt an expectant approach. They should be aware that complete resolution may take several weeks. Expectant management for incomplete miscarriage is highly effective. Occasionally, the passage of tissue may be associated with heavy bleeding.

Medical and expectant management should only be offered in units where women have access to 24-h telephone advice and emergency admission, if required.

Anti-D Immunoglobulin
Non-sensitised rhesus (Rh) negative women should receive anti-D immunoglobulin in the following situations: ectopic pregnancy, all miscarriages over 12 weeks of gestation (including threatened) and all miscarriages where the uterus has been evacuated (whether medially or surgically).

Anti-D immunoglobulin is not required threatened miscarriages under 12 weeks of gestation unless the bleeding is heavy or is associated with significant pain. It is not required in cases of complete miscarriage under 12 weeks' gestation and when there has been no formal intervention to evacuate the uterus.

MANAGEMENT

LATE PREGNANCY LOSS (>12 Weeks' Gestation)

Surgical

Surgical uterine evacuation remains an option for some women. Dilatation and suction curettage is commonly performed up to 14 weeks' gestation. Beyond this point, dilatation and evacuation (D & E) can be carried out which involves cervical dilatation to a maximum diameter and the removal of intrauterine contents, usually following a destructive procedure. This procedure is not commonly performed in the UK.

Medical

Again, medical methods are effective in the management of a second trimester miscarriage. As in the case of first trimester loss, there are various medical regimens that have been described using prostaglandin analogues (gemeprost or misoprostol) with or without antiprogesterone priming (mifepristone). Again, local protocols should be developed appropriately with selection criteria, therapeutic regimens and arrangements for follow-up.

In cases where antiprogesterones and vaginal prostaglandins are not available, PGE2 can be very slowly instilled into the cervix through a Foley catheter to facilitate cervical ripening.

RECURRENT MISCARRIAGE

INTRODUCTION AND DEFINITIONS

Recurrent miscarriage, defined as the loss of three or more pregnancies, is a distressing problem that affects up to 1% of women. Recurrent miscarriage is a heterogeneous condition that has many possible causes; more than one contributory factor may underlie the recurrent pregnancy losses.

CAUSES OF RECURRENT MISCARRIAGE

Maternal Age

This is an independent risk factor. Advanced maternal age adversely affects ovarian function, giving rise to a decline in the number of good quality oocytes and resulting in chromosomally abnormal conceptions that rarely develop further.

Previous Number of Miscarriages

This is an independent risk factor in so far as the more miscarriages an individual has had, the more likely she is to have another one.

Genetic Factors

In approximately 3–5% of couples with recurrent miscarriage, one of the partners carries a balanced structural chromosomal anomaly. These are most commonly balanced reciprocal or Robertsonian translocations.

Abnormalities in the Embryo

Recurrent pregnancy loss may be owing to an abnormal embryo which is incompatible with life. As the number of miscarriages increases, the presence of a chromosomal abnormality decreases and the chance of a recurring maternal cause increases.

Uterine Abnormalities

It is difficult to assess the exact contribution that congenital uterine anomalies make to recurrent miscarriage. The estimates of the number of women with recurrent miscarriage, who also have uterine abnormalities, range from 2% to 37%. Women who have serious anatomical abnormalities and have not had treatment for them seem to be more likely to miscarry or give birth early. Minor variations in the structure of the womb generally do *not* cause miscarriage

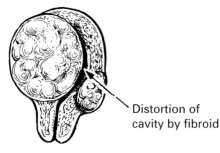

Distortion of cavity by fibroid

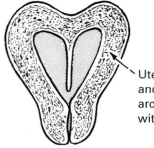

Uterine anomaly — arcuate uterus with septum

Cervical Weakness

The diagnosis of cervical weakness (previously known as incompetence) is usually based on a history of late miscarriage, preceded by spontaneous rupture of membranes or a painless cervical dilatation. This is often over diagnosed as there is currently no satisfactory, objective test that can identify women with cervical weakness in the non-pregnant state.

RECURRENT MISCARRIAGE

CAUSES OF RECURRENT MISCARRIAGE—(cont'd)

Endocrine Factors

Maternal diabetes and thyroid disease
Systemic endocrine disorders have been associated with miscarriage. However, they do not cause recurrent miscarriages as long as they are treated and well controlled.

Hyperprolactinaemia
There is insufficient evidence to assess the effect of hyperprolactinaemia as a risk factor for recurrent miscarriage.

Polycystic ovarian syndrome (PCOS)
The characteristic features of this condition are polycystic ovaries associated with an imbalance of hormones. Approximately 50% of women with recurrent early miscarriages have polycystic ovaries (almost double the number of women in the general population). The link between PCOS and recurrent miscarriage is not clear. Many women with PCOS and recurrent miscarriage have elevated levels of luteinising hormone (LH) in their blood. However, reducing the level of LH prior to pregnancy has not been shown to improve the chances of a successful birth.

Thrombophilias

Inherited thrombophilic defects including activated protein C resistance (most commonly owing to factor V Leidin gene mutation), deficiencies of protein C and S and antithrombin III, hyperhomocysteinaemia and prothrombin gene mutations are established causes of systemic thrombosis. Studies have established an association between inherited thrombophilias and fetal loss and late pregnancy complications, with the presumed mechanism being thrombosis of the uteroplacental circulation. Women with recurrent miscarriage who carry the factor V Leidin (FVL) mutation are at a significantly increased risk of miscarriage compared to those with a normal factor V genotype. However, carriage of the FVL mutation did not preclude an uncomplicated pregnancy that could be delivered at term. There is currently no test that can reliably discriminate those women with recurrent miscarriage and the FVL mutation who are destined to miscarry from those who are destined to have a successful pregnancy.

Autoimmune Factors

Approximately 15% of women who have recurrent miscarriages have the antiphospholipid syndrome. This syndrome is characterised by some or all of the following: recurrent miscarriage, thrombosis, thrombocytopenia, poor obstetric history. Anticardiolipin antibodies and lupus anticoagulant levels are also often abnormal.

Infections

Any serious systemic infection can potentially lead to a miscarriage. The presence of bacterial vaginosis in the first trimester of pregnancy has been reported as a risk factor for second trimester miscarriage and preterm delivery but the evidence for its association with first trimester miscarriage is inconsistent.

Environmental Factors

Smoking and alcohol may play a role.

RECURRENT MISCARRIAGE

INVESTIGATION AND TREATMENT OF RECURRENT MISCARRIAGE

Even after careful investigation, the majority of women have no obvious cause for recurrent miscarriage. Notwithstanding, the prognosis is generally good, with a mean probability of a live birth in the next pregnancy being around 70%.

1. *Genetic factors*
   Essentially no treatment is available.
2. *Uterine abnormalities*
   All women with recurrent miscarriage should have a pelvic ultrasound to assess uterine anatomy and morphology. Uterine surgery may correct the abnormality, but may not necessarily improve the prognosis. Ironically, these procedures may cause intrauterine adhesions and, thus, reduce fertility.
3. *Cervical weakness*
   The diagnosis is based on a history of mid-trimester miscarriage preceded by a spontaneous rupture of the membranes or a painless cervical dilatation. A transvaginal ultrasound assessment of the cervix during pregnancy may be useful in predicting preterm birth in some cases of suspected cervical weakness. Cervical cerclage is associated with potential hazards that are related to the surgery and the risk of stimulating uterine contractions and, hence, should only be considered in women who are likely to benefit.

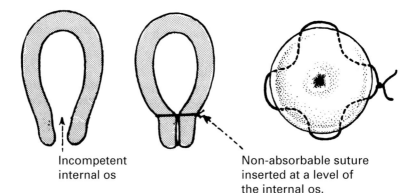

Incompetent
internal os

Non-absorbable suture
inserted at a level of
the internal os.

4. *Endocrine problems*
   The aim is to obtain optimal control of the condition.
5. *Immunological factors*
   In women with the anticardiolipin antibody syndrome, treatment with low dose aspirin and heparin has been shown to improve the outcome of future pregnancies.
6. *Thrombophilias*
   If protein C and protein S deficiency are found, thromboprophylaxis should be considered. A few well-conducted trials exist for the treatment of these conditions, although there is a rationale for low dose aspirin therapy.
7. *Environmental factors*
   All women wishing to become pregnant should be advised to stop smoking and to minimise their alcohol intake.

TERMINATION OF PREGNANCY

Some people elect to terminate their pregnancy for various reasons which must fall within the Indications for Therapeutic Abortion under the Abortion Act (1967, UK) which was amended 1992. These include:

1. ...the continuance of the pregnancy would involve risk to the life of the pregnant woman greater than if the pregnancy were terminated.

2. ...the termination is necessary to prevent grave permanent injury to the physical or mental health of the pregnant woman.

3. ...the pregnancy has NOT exceeded its 24th week and the continuance of the pregnancy would involve risk, greater than if the pregnancy were terminated, of injury to the physical or mental health of the pregnant woman.

4. ...the pregnancy has NOT exceeded its 24th week and the continuance of the pregnancy would involve risk, greater than if the pregnancy were terminated, of injury to the physical or mental health of the existing child(ren) of the family of the pregnant woman.

5. ...there is substantial risk that if the child were born it would suffer from such physical or mental abnormalities as to be seriously handicapped.

To facilitate this process, a certificate of opinion is given by two medical practitioners prior to commencement of the termination process to which it refers.

A single practitioner may give an emergency certificate before termination or, where not reasonably practical, within 24 h of termination, and terminate a pregnancy if it is necessary to save the life of the pregnant woman or to prevent grave permanent injury to her physical or mental health.

FIRST TRIMESTER TERMINATION OF PREGNANCY

In the first trimester of pregnancy termination can be carried out by surgical or medical methods.

1. *Surgical termination of pregnancy (Stop)*
    This is usually performed up to 14 weeks' gestation. It involves preoperative cervical ripening with prostaglandin agents preceded by the administration of an antiprogesterone, and (mifepristone) followed by dilatation of the cervix and suction curettage of the products of conception. The methods are almost identical to those already described for the surgical management of a miscarriage.

TERMINATION OF PREGNANCY

2. *Medical termination of pregnancy*

    Mifepristone is an antiprogestogen which offers a medical alternative to vacuum aspiration of an early pregnancy and can be used up to 63 days from the first day of the LMP or as dated by an ultrasound. The use of mifepristone is strictly controlled to approved NHS hospitals and premises that have been approved under the Abortion Act. Mifepristone is contraindicated in a suspected ectopic pregnancy, in smokers over 35 years of age, in chronic adrenal failure, porphyria, corticosteroid therapy, coagulation disorders and in women on anticoagulant therapy.

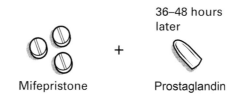

Mifepristone   +   Prostaglandin

36–48 hours later

200 mg mifepristone is taken orally and the patient is admitted 36–48 h later for a vaginal administration of prostaglandins (in certain situations prostaglandins can be also given orally). Over 95% of pregnancies are completely aborted. In a small number of cases, surgical evacuation of uterus may be required for any retained products of conception. Side effects include abdominal pain with up to 20% of the patients requiring opiate analgesia following prostaglandin administration. Blood loss is similar to that following surgical termination of pregnancy at the same gestation.

TERMINATION OF PREGNANCY

SECOND TRIMESTER TERMINATION OF PREGNANCY

1. *Surgical termination – dilatation and evacuation (D&E)*
   Dilatation and evacuation (D & E) involves cervical dilatation to a maximum diameter of 20 mm and removal of the intrauterine contents. This is not commonly performed in the UK.

2. *Medical termination*
   Again mifepristone and prostaglandins are used to facilitate the process, in accordance with the local protocols. The use of mifepristone significantly reduces the interval from induction (prostaglandin administration) to abortion, and so, the vast majority of patients abort within 24 h. Curettage for retained products of conception may be required in up to 30% of patients undergoing a second trimester abortion using medical methods.

3. *Extra-amniotic termination*
   This method may be used if the mifepristone and prostaglandin pessaries are unavailable.

   PGE2 is very slowly instilled into the cervix through a Foley catheter.

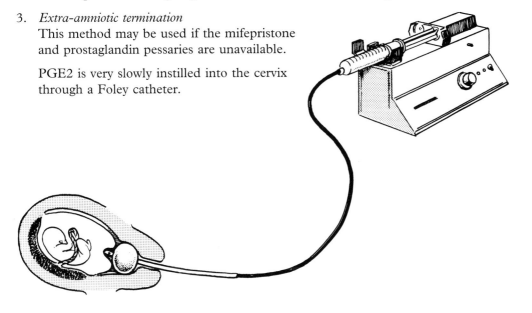

COMPLICATIONS OF TERMINATION OF PREGNANCY

Immediate
Major complications occur in approximately 2% of the cases and include haemorrhage, thromboembolism, operative trauma and infection. Minor complications (10%) include lower abdominal pain, bleeding and pelvic infection.

Late
Infertility can occur if a termination is complicated by infection as this increases the risk of tubal occlusion. In general, if women are screened and treated for genital tract pathogens prior to an evacuation procedure, the risk of postoperative infection is significantly reduced. However in the absence of infection, results from several well-designed studies have shown no adverse effects on a future pregnancy from a single uterine evacuation procedure.

Rhesus isoimmunisation can be minimised by administering anti-D to rhesus negative women.

ECTOPIC PREGNANCY

The term 'ectopic' comes from the Greek 'ektopis' meaning 'displacement' ('ek', out of + 'topos', place = out of place). An ectopic pregnancy is an extrauterine pregnancy. This occurs with an incidence of approximately 11.1 per 1000 pregnancies. It is still a cause of maternal death with 10 deaths being reported in the UK between 2002 and 2005.

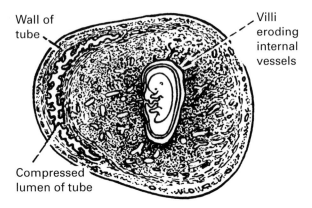

An ectopic pregnancy is usually caused by various conditions that block or slow the movement of a fertilised egg through the fallopian tube to the uterus.

The trophoblast can successfully implant on any tissue that has an adequate blood supply. The most common site for an ectopic pregnancy is within the fallopian tube. Other less common sites include the cervix, ovary, liver, spleen, stomach and the intestine.

AETIOLOGY

Often unknown, but there are a number of associated factors:

Pelvic Inflammatory Disease

About half the patients will have signs of salpingitis or a history of infection, including gonorrhoea or chlamydia or tuberculosis. This may affect tubal ciliary activity.

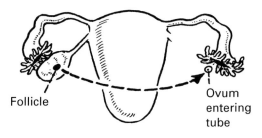

Intrauterine Devices (IUDs)

The IUD may introduce infection. As the aim of the IUD is to prevent implantation in the uterine cavity, a relative increase in ectopic pregnancy is to be expected.

Tubal Damage

Previous tubal damage such as an ectopic pregnancy treated conservatively, previous pelvic surgery leading to adhesion formation, endometriosis or reversal of sterilisation may also be causes.

Assisted Conception

This is associated with an increased incidence of ectopic pregnancies.

DIAGNOSIS OF TUBAL PREGNANCY

Tubal pregnancy can present in many ways and misdiagnosis can occur. Many patients now present with mild symptoms as methods of investigation that detect early pregnancy problems such as ectopics, can do so earlier than previously. However, acute ruptures with significant patient compromise still occur.

SYMPTOMS

Pain
Pain in the lower abdomen is always present in the acute presentation. Described as either stabbing or cramp-like, it may be referred to the shoulder if blood tracks to the diaphragm and stimulates the phrenic nerve, and may be so severe as to cause fainting.

Vaginal Bleeding
In about 75% of the cases, a tubal pregnancy presents with vaginal bleeding.

Fainting/Collapse
These pregnancies will cause pain and fainting, leading to anaemia.

If haemorrhage is severe the usual signs of collapse and shock will appear.

SIGNS

Abdominal Tenderness
Tenderness may be elicited on the left, right or across the lower abdomen.

Pelvic Tenderness
Care should be taken when examining the patient to make sure that an ectopic pregnancy is not ruptured during the process.

Adnexal Mass
Gentle bimanual palpation may reveal a pelvic adnexal mass.

DIAGNOSIS OF TUBAL PREGNANCY

1. **Serum hCG tracking** can aid in its diagnosis. An ongoing intrauterine pregnancy should have a doubling (minimum of 2/3) of serum beta hCG in 48 h. A non-continuing pregnancy will usually show a fall in beta hCG. An ectopic pregnancy will show a suboptimal rise, static value or a decline.

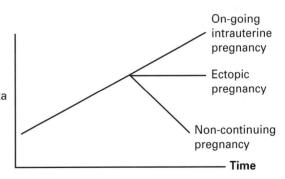

2. **Ultrasound Features** of ectopic pregnancy include:
    – absence of a gestation sac within the uterine cavity
    – presence of a gestation sac outside the uterus (usually in the adnexal regions)
    – demonstration of a live embryo with fetal heart activity outside the uterus.
    – free fluid or blood in the adjacent parts of the pelvis.

DIAGNOSIS OF TUBAL PREGNANCY

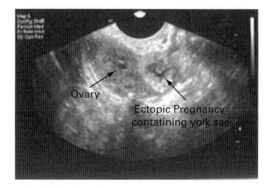

A transvaginal ultrasound is the diagnostic modality used. In general, ultrasound findings in association with serum beta hCG tracking can help establish the diagnosis of an ectopic pregnancy. In general, there is a serum hCG level at which it is assumed that all viable intrauterine pregnancies will be visualised by a transvaginal ultrasound. This is referred to as the discriminatory zone. When serum hCG levels are below the discriminatory zone (<1000 iu) and there is no pregnancy (intra- or extrauterine) visible on transvaginal ultrasound scan, the pregnancy can be described as being of unknown location.

SITES OF IMPLANTATION

Sites of Implantation

The tubal ampulla is the commonest location followed by the isthmus, but the developing ovum can implant anywhere inside or outside the uterus.

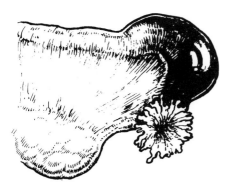

Ampullary implantation: note the thinning of the tube wall.

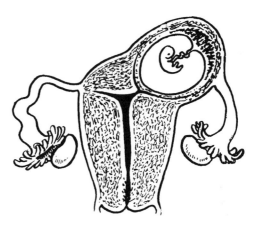

Cornual implantation is not common but is very dangerous because its rupture is accompanied by bleeding from uterine arteries.

RUPTURE OF THE TUBE

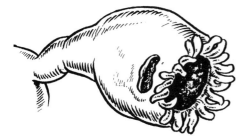

The muscle wall of the tube does not have the capacity of uterine muscle for hypertrophy and its distension and a tubal pregnancy nearly always end in its rupture and the death of the ovum.

RUPTURE INTO LUMEN OF TUBE

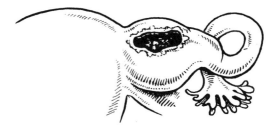

Tubal Abortion

This is usual in an ampullary pregnancy at about 8 weeks. The conceptus is extruded, complete or incomplete, towards the fimbriated end of the tube.

Rupture into the Peritoneal Cavity

This usually occurs spontaneously, and often from the narrow isthmus before 8 weeks, or from the interstitial portion at 12 weeks. Haemorrhage is likely to be severe.

TREATMENT OF TUBAL PREGNANCY

Patients presenting with collapse and shock with a positive pregnancy test must be assessed and managed like any other critically ill patient. Intravenous access with appropriate blood tests including a full blood count, a coagulation screen and an emergency blood cross match should be established. Fluid resuscitation and an emergency theatre should be organised to deal with the bleeding. In such cases, all procedures are performed as traditional open operations.

If the patient is stable, then management can be medical (using methotrexate intramuscular injection) or surgical.

METHOTREXATE
Most ectopics follow a chronic course and are confidently diagnosed with ultrasound and βHCG. To avoid surgical intervention, women can be offered this treatment if the βHCG is <3000 and there are no symptoms of rupture. If βHCG levels do not fall, then, 14% may need a further injection and only <10%, in this group, will eventually need surgery if the treatment fails or if the ectopic shows signs of rupture during treatment. The dose is usually 50 mg/m^2 body surface area.

SALPINGECTOMY
This can be performed following the diagnosis at surgery. Before removing the tube, the other fallopian tube should be examined, because if it is abnormal, then a more conservative surgical approach may have to be adopted. Laparoscopic salpingectomy is the preferred method.

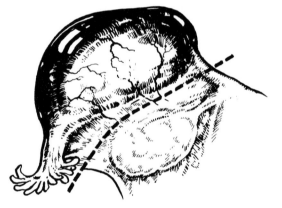

SALPINGOSTOMY
This is a conservative approach to the surgical management of ectopics. An incision is made over the antimesenteric border of the tube, the ectopic is removed and the tube left to heal once haemostasis is achieved. There is a risk of a persistent trophoblast that may need to be treated, so follow up βHCG values should be checked. There is also an increased risk of a recurrent ectopic pregnancy.

CONSERVATIVE
If there is a raised βHCG of <1000 with no further increase in the βHCG levels and no intra-uterine pregnancy on an ultrasound scan, then the pregnancy can be described as being of unknown location. Such cases can be treated conservatively as up to 70% will resolve by themselves. Surgery or medical therapy will be required in some cases.

GESTATIONAL TROPHOBLASTIC DISEASE

Hydatidiform Mole

The incidence of molar pregnancies in Europe and North America is approximately 0.2–1.5 per 1000 live births but there may be a higher incidence in Africa and Asia.

Complete and **partial** are two distinct forms of a molar pregnancy. The gross specimen from a complete molar pregnancy shows diffuse hydropic placental villi. On scanning, this gives a multicystic appearance to the uterine contents. A partial molar pregnancy can have a similar appearance but the findings can be variable and subtle.

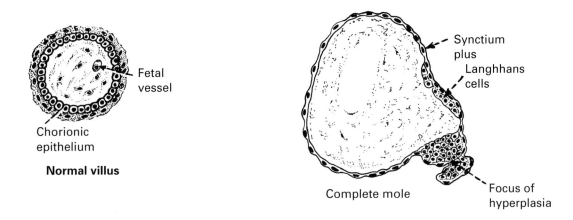

Normal villus

Fetal vessel

Chorionic epithelium

Synctium plus Langhhans cells

Complete mole

Focus of hyperplasia

Table 15.1 Features of Partial and Complete Hydatidiform Moles (From DISAIA Clinical Gynecologic Oncology 7E Mosby 2007)

Feature	Partial mole	Complete mole
Karyotype	Most commonly 69, XXX or –, XXY	Most commonly 46, XX or –, XY
Pathology Fetus Amnion, fetal RBC Villous edema Trophoblastic proliferation	Often present Usually present Variable, focal Focal, slight–moderate	Absent Absent Diffuse Diffuse, slight–severe
Clinical presentation Diagnosis Uterine size Theca lutein cysts Medical complications Post-molar GTN	Missed miscarriage Small for dates Rare Rare 2.5–7.5%	Molar gestation 50% large for dates 25–30% 10–25% 6.8–20%

RBC, red blood cells; GTN, gestational trophoblastic neoplasia.

GESTATIONAL TROPHOBLASTIC DISEASE

GESTATIONAL TROPHOBLASTIC DISEASE – PATHOLOGY

Premalignant
Complete Hydatidiform Mole

In a complete hydatidiform mole, the villi are grossly swollen and are likened to 'bunches of grapes'. There is no embryo. Microscopically, the villi are enormously distended. Hyperplasia of both the syncytio-trophoblast and the cytotrophoblast can be observed.

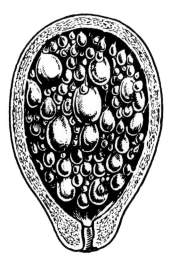

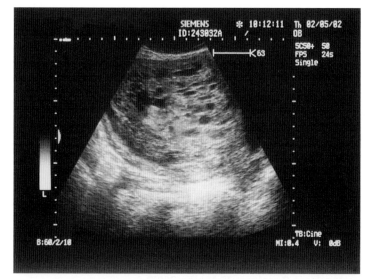

Partial Mole

In this case, there are two populations of villi. Some are of normal size and configuration, and contain fetal vessels, while others show the typical grape-like appearance of hydatidiform change. Frequently, an embryo or embryonic tissue is present. Trophoblast hyperplasia is very focal and is usually confined to the syncytio-trophoblast.

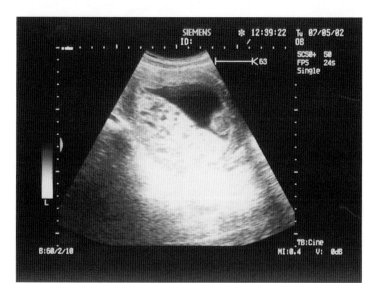

GESTATIONAL TROPHOBLASTIC DISEASE

GESTATIONAL TROPHOBLASTIC DISEASE – PRESENTATION AND GENETICS

Presentation

Early pregnancy bleeding
The degree of bleeding is variable but can be significant.

Excessive nausea and vomiting in early pregnancy
This is related to high levels of serum βHCG.

Symptoms of hyperthyroidism
βHCG is a thyrotropic molecule and when in excess, they bind to the TSH receptor

Larger than expected uterine size for gestation

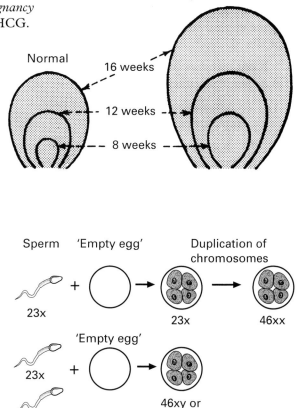

Cytogenetics

Genetics of hydatidiform mole

1. **Complete Mole**
   The karyotype of a complete mole is 46XX in 95% and 46XY in 5%, but all of the chromosomes are of **paternal** origin. The pronucleus of the ovum is absent. The empty egg is fertilised by a haploid 23X sperm which duplicates its chromosomes without cell division (less commonly) or by two different sperm. Why the ovum should fail to contribute to the process is not known. As complete moles are more likely to become malignant, the karyotype of every mole should be determined.

2. **Partial Mole**
   In a partial mole, fetal tissue of some type is present and the karyotype is entirely different. It is usually triploid – 69XXX or 69XXY with both **maternal** and **paternal** DNA. This is due to fertilisation of the egg by two sperm. Partial moles are less likely to undergo malignant change.

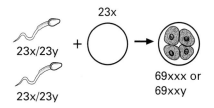

327

GESTATIONAL TROPHOBLASTIC DISEASE

GESTATIONAL TROPHOBLASTIC DISEASE – TREATMENT

The diagnosis is made using an ultrasound (see p. 326) and βHCG levels. Partial moles may appear as a missed miscarriage and may not detected until the pathology is available. If a molar pregnancy is suspected, then uterine evacuation should be performed.

Prior to Evacuation

A full blood count, clotting studies and crossmatching for blood type should be performed.
Renal and liver function analysis.
βHCG levels.
Chest X-ray.

Evacuation

No cervical ripening agents to be used, for example misoprostol.
There is increased incidence of post-evacuation neoplasia.
Suction evacuation using a large suction cannula should be performed.

Post Evacuation

Registration with a gestational trophoblastic disease centre should be done.
Serial βHCG estimation should be performed.
Advise use of reliable contraceptive during follow-up.
Advise not to attempt pregnancy for at least 6 months following treatment.
βHCG levels to be checked after any subsequent pregnancy.

Post-Molar Gestational Trophoblastic Neoplasia

7.5–20% incidence following complete molar pregnancy
2.5–7.5% incidence following partial molar pregnancy.
Chemotherapy is indicated where there is persistent post-molar disease.

GESTATIONAL TROPHOBLASTIC NEOPLASIA

Malignant

Invasive mole

This is a condition in which the molar tissue invades through the decidua and into the myometrium and its associated blood vessels. It almost always results from a complete, rather than a partial, mole. Perforation of the uterus may occur, resulting in invasion of the parametrium.

Spontaneous resolution can occur, but to prevent morbidity and mortality these lesions are treated with surgery where fertility is of no concern and with chemotherapy if fertility sparing is required.

GESTATIONAL TROPHOBLASTIC DISEASE

Gestational Choriocarcinoma

This occurs most commonly after a complete molar pregnancy but can also occur after any pregnancy. This is a rare condition and a non-gestational variant can arise directly in the ovary. Only about 2% of moles give rise to a choriocarcinoma but the risk is 1000 times greater than the risk after normal delivery.

These tumours metastasise, with the lung being the commonest site.

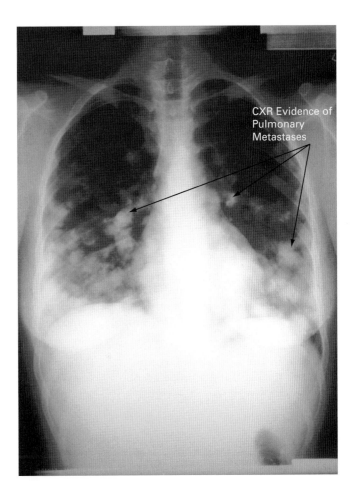

CXR Evidence of Pulmonary Metastases

Placental Site Trophoblast Tumour

This is a rare lesion in which a few villi are formed. The bulk of the tissue consists of the chorionic epithelium, much of which has not properly differentiated into the usual two types. These can occur at variable lengths of time after pregnancy.

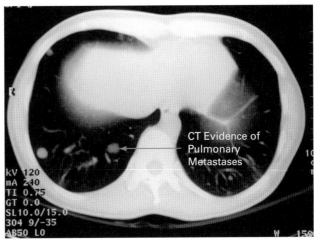

CT Evidence of Pulmonary Metastases

329

GESTATIONAL TROPHOBLASTIC DISEASE

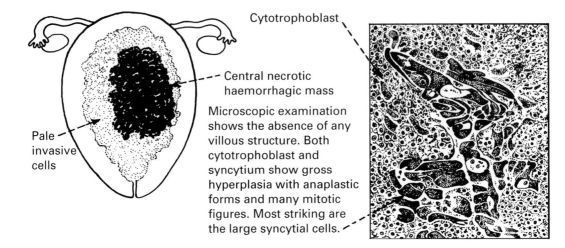

Cytotrophoblast

Central necrotic haemorrhagic mass

Microscopic examination shows the absence of any villous structure. Both cytotrophoblast and syncytium show gross hyperplasia with anaplastic forms and many mitotic figures. Most striking are the large syncytial cells.

Pale invasive cells

CHEMOTHERAPY FOR CHORIOCARCINOMA

A choriocarcinoma is very chemosensitive and its rates of cure can be high. Prognostic variables which help determine a suitable chemotherapeutic regimen are calculated following patient referral to a specialist centre.

Patients in the Low Risk Group
They are treated using a single agent chemotherapy regimen.

Recurrence rates <5%

Patients in High Risk Group
They are treated with multiagent chemotherapy regimen.

CHAPTER 16

SEXUALITY AND CONTRACEPTION

Physiology of Coitus	332
Excitement Phase	*332*
Plateau Phase	*332*
Orgasm	*333*
Postcoital Phase or Resolution	
Phase	*333*
Sexual Problems	*333*
Loss of Libido	*333*
Failure to Achieve Orgasm	*333*
Dyspareunia	334
Dyspareunia (Painful Coitus)	*334*
Sexual Problems Affecting the	
Male	335
Premature Ejaculation	*335*
Erectile Dysfunction	*335*
Treatment Options for Erectile	
Dysfunction	336
Organic Causes	*336*
Psychosexual Counselling	*336*
Sildenafil (Viagra)	*336*
Sex Hormones	*336*
Papaverine	*336*
Ejaculatory Failure	*336*
Medico-Legal Problems	337
Rape	*337*
Methods of Contraception	338
Failure Rates in Contraception	*339*
Patient Suitability for	
Contraception	*339*
Hormonal Contraception	340
Combined Oral Contraception	*340*
Minor Side Effects of OCs	342
Failure of the Pill	*342*
Oral Contraception: Risks	343

Vascular Disease	*343*
Hypertension	*343*
Oral Contraceptives and	
Neoplasia	*344*
Endometrium and Ovary	*344*
Progestogen-Only Pill (POP)	*344*
Other Routes	*344*
Vaginal Rings	*344*
Injectable Progestogens	*344*
Progestogen-Only Implants	*345*
Intrauterine Devices (IUDs)	346
Mode of Action	*346*
Principle of Insertion of IUDs	*347*
Complications of Intrauterine	
Devices	348
Diaphragms and Caps	349
Condoms	350
The Sponge	*350*
Contraception Based on Time	
of Ovulation	351
The Rhythm Method	
('Safe Period')	*351*
The Ovulation Method	
(The Billings' Method)	*351*
Postcoital Contraception	352
Postcoital Contraception	
('Morning After'	
Contraception)	*352*
Irreversible Methods	353
Sterilisation	*353*
Laparoscopic Sterilisation	355
Vasectomy	356

PHYSIOLOGY OF COITUS

It is important to understand the physiology of sexual function as sexual dysfunction cannot only be the primary reason for a referral to gynaecology, but often may be a secondary issue that is related to other complaints, for example pain and fertility. Sexual history should be taken sensitively and the patients should be able to express their concerns in a non-judgmental environment.

The response to sexual stimulation is primarily an autonomic nervous reflex which can be reinforced or inhibited by psychological, hormonal and social factors. These factors are infinitely variable and understanding the social and psychological influences that are affecting an individual cannot be easily covered during a single consultation. Referral to a specialist psychosexual counselling service should also be considered.

The normal sexual response has been categorised into a series of phases by researchers Masters and Johnson in the 1960s. These are excitement, plateau, orgasm and refractory. The initial interest in sex, also known as libido, is probably harder to define, but as a generalisation, it may be said that the female responds to the consciousness of being desired as a whole person, while satisfaction in the male depends to a greater extent on visceral sensation.

EXCITEMENT PHASE

Female	Male
Vasodilatation and vasocongestion of all erectile tissue. Breasts enlarge, the vaginal ostium opens and secretion from the vestibular glands and vaginal exudations cause 'moistening'	Penile erection occurs and may be transient and recur if this stage is prolonged. Scrotal skin and dartos muscle contract and draw testes towards the perineum

PLATEAU PHASE

In both, the male and the female, the pulse rate, blood pressure and respiratory rate increase. Both partners make involuntary thrusting movements of the pelvis towards each other.

Female	Male
Vasocongestion increases, and contraction of the uterine ligaments (which contain muscle) lift the uterus and move it more into alignment with the axis of the pelvis. The cervix dilates. There is engorgement of the lower third of the vagina and ballooning of the upper two thirds	The intensity of penile erection increases and the testes are enlarged by congestion. Seminal fluid arrives at the urethra as a result of sympathetic nervous stimulation of the vas deferens, seminal vesicles and the prostate. There is some pre-ejaculatory penile discharge which may contain sperm

PHYSIOLOGY OF COITUS

ORGASM

Pulse and respiration rate are at double their resting rate, and blood pressure may reach 180/110. Pelvic and genital sensations are completely dominating, and there is a noticeable reduction in the sensory awareness in other parts of the body. The pelvic floor contracts involuntarily, with rhythmic contraction of the vagina, urethra and the anal sphincter.

Female	Male
Climactic sensations appear to be caused by spasmodic contractions of vaginal muscles and uterus. The female is potentially capable of repeated orgasm	Strong contractions pass along the penis causing ejaculation of seminal fluid. The greater the volume of ejaculate (after several days' abstinence) the more intense the sensations of orgasm

POSTCOITAL PHASE OR RESOLUTION PHASE

Pulse, respiratory rate and blood pressure rapidly return to normal and there is marked sweating. Vasocongestion recedes over about 5 min and there is complete relaxation of all muscles and a detumescence of erectile tissue. In the male, but less so in the female, there occurs a refractory period, which varies with individuals, from a few minutes to several hours during which there is no response to further stimuli.

SEXUAL PROBLEMS

Normal sexual activity and behaviour change with a number of factors including age, social circumstances, background and values, but it can also be affected by illness or medication and adverse psychological experiences.

LOSS OF LIBIDO

As previously discussed, interest in sex is a more complex process for women and it can be adversely affected by a number of common social factors, for example having a baby, stress at work, bereavement, etc. There is some evidence that it is influenced by hormonal factors; in particular, it has been shown that women who have had their ovaries removed have lower levels of androgens and these women may benefit from testosterone supplementation. For some postmenopausal women standard hormone replacement therapy may be of benefit.

FAILURE TO ACHIEVE ORGASM

The failure to achieve an orgasm is a common problem in women, although relatively few women seek medical advice. As with the loss of libido, there may be a number of causative factors. However, many women do not experience orgasm during penetrative intercourse and require stimulation of the clitoris or other erogenous zones. Psychosexual counselling should be offered.

DYSPAREUNIA

DYSPAREUNIA (PAINFUL COITUS)

Superficial Dyspareunia

It is vaginal pain during sexual intercourse.

Causes include:

1. Vulvovaginitis (especially infection by trichomonas or candida).
2. Vaginal cysts. Small ones are usually symptomless.
3. Infection of the Bartholin's gland.
4. Postmenopausal atrophy.
5. Rarely, there is a congenital narrowing of the ostium or a thick hymen.
6. Painful perineal scar.
   This may be due to an inflamed or fibrous scar following childbirth, or to an imperfectly repaired episiotomy or tear.

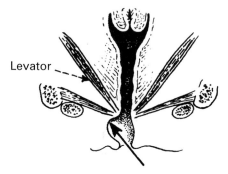

Levator

Deep Dyspareunia

Pain is due to pressure on an area of tenderness near the vaginal vault. The cause is often difficult to identify and there may be no obvious disease but a number of pelvic pathologies should be considered.

Examples include:

Pelvic infection.
Endometriosis.
Pelvic masses including an ectopic pregnancy.
Scarring of the vaginal vault following hysterectomy.

Vaginismus

It is a partly voluntary contraction of the pelvic muscles that takes place when the introduction of the penis is attempted, making coitus impossible. It can also occur with insertion of tampons or during a vaginal examination.

Causes are as those for the other forms of sexual dysfunction.

Treatment

Referral to psychosexual counselling can often be helpful in treating vaginismus and should be a key element of any treatments offered.

Vaginal dilators of graduated sizes are useful. The purpose is not to dilate a narrow vagina but to give the patient control over her vaginal muscle and the confidence that sexual intercourse will not be painful.

Mild vaginismus usually responds well to these simple measures, but in severe cases the results are poor.

Botox therapy is a new technique which may be beneficial in severe cases. The pelvic floor muscles are temporarily paralysed and for many women normal sexual function continues after muscle function has resumed.

SEXUAL PROBLEMS AFFECTING THE MALE

The gynaecologist is not normally called upon to deal directly with the male, but it can be useful to be aware of their sexual problems and know something of their management.

PREMATURE EJACULATION

The male ejaculates with minimal sexual stimulation or before he wishes it to occur.

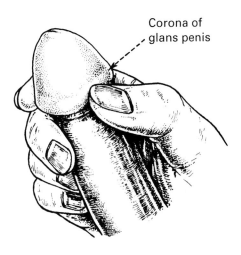

Corona of glans penis

There are a number of behavioural techniques that can prolong the sexual episode, such as stopping repeatedly or the squeeze technique where intermittent pressure is applied to the penis by the partner.

There are also some medications that may be beneficial, including some antidepressants, but referral should be made to a specialist with an interest in male sexual disorders.

ERECTILE DYSFUNCTION

This is also known as impotence, is the inability to achieve or sustain an erection. Erectile dysfunction becomes more common with age and may have either a physical or psychological basis. Social, domestic and relationship pressures can have significant effects, but it has been increasingly recognised that organic causes are common.

These include:

- Diabetes mellitus
- Vascular disease and hypertension
- Neurological conditions such as multiple sclerosis, spinal injury
- Radical surgery: extended prostatectomy or abdomino-perineal resection
- Drugs: antihypertensives, antidepressants
- Endocrine causes: prolactinoma, testosterone deficiency
- Urological conditions such as Peyronie's disease.

TREATMENT OPTIONS FOR ERECTILE DYSFUNCTION

ORGANIC CAUSES
These may be reversible, as in endocrine lesions and drugs, and, where possible, treatment of the underlying condition may be of benefit.

PSYCHOSEXUAL COUNSELLING
This is most useful when social and psychological factors predominate and is often used in conjunction with drug treatment.

SILDENAFIL (VIAGRA)
An oral therapy for erectile difficulties, this does not produce an erection without sexual stimulation. Side effects have been reported in men with cardiovascular problems who are on cardiovascular medication.

SEX HORMONES
Simple prescription of a male sex hormone is seldom successful and its part in the physiology of erection and ejaculation is not yet known. It has been shown that testosterone levels do decline with age, but there does not appear to be a male equivalent of the female menopause, and the role of testosterone replacement therapy remains unclear.

PAPAVERINE
This is a smooth muscle relaxant. Intracavernosal injection is an effective treatment for impotence.

EJACULATORY FAILURE
It is the inability to ejaculate although there is no loss of erotic drive, erection and intromission are normal.

The ejaculatory reflex requires intact pathways in both the autonomic and somatic systems. Somatic nerves receive the sensory stimuli of coitus and pass these impulses to the sympathetic nerves which then stimulate the delivery of seminal fluid to the urethra by the vasa deferentia, seminal vesicles and prostate, and prevent retrograde ejaculation into the bladder by causing contractions of the internal urinary sphincters.

Sympathectomy from T12 to L3 will abolish ejaculation without affecting erectile ability or the sensations of an orgasm, producing a phenomenon known as 'dry sex'.

MEDICO-LEGAL PROBLEMS

RAPE

The doctor may on occasion be asked to examine a victim of alleged rape. This crime has heavy penalties and the examination must be thorough and careful. Ideally, the examination should be performed by a clinician with requisite specialist training and experience. The victim is likely to have experienced significant trauma and an appropriate supportive environment and staff trained in counselling techniques, should be available. Major police forces have specially trained rape investigation teams whose expertise is invaluable.

The following preliminary notes should be made:

1. Authority for examination.
2. Consent for examination.
3. General appearance of person and clothing.
4. History of the circumstances of crime.

Rape is defined as unlawful sexual intercourse with a woman by force and against her will.

Sexual intercourse is described as the slightest degree of penetration of the vulva by the penis and entry of the hymen is therefore not necessary. (Use of vaginal tampons by virgins may confuse the issue.)

The vulva should be inspected for signs of bruising, scratching or tearing. The hymen may be torn and bleeding.

When the orifice is small or the hymen is vestigial, bruising may be present because of the force needed for penetration against the resistance of the victim. The presence of seminal fluid in the vagina and cervix may, sometimes, be the only sign. This fluid is removed and examined microscopically.

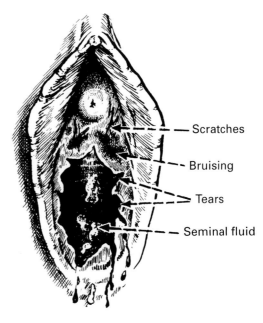

Scratches

Bruising

Tears

Seminal fluid

General examination of the patient may show injuries and bruising, confirming a story of resistance that has been overcome by violence.

Skin should be swabbed for blood, semen or saliva, if there is evidence of these fluids, using a swab moistened with sterile water, for DNA analysis. Finger nail clippings should be taken if there is blood or debris under them.

Comb the head and pubic hair for hairs from the assailant and cut 10 hairs from each site of the victim for comparison. Blood and urine samples should be taken. These may require to be tested for drugs.

Careful record keeping is essential. Collection, storage and transport of specimens must comply with legal requirements so that their source cannot be challenged.

METHODS OF CONTRACEPTION

Natural methods	Rhythm or Billings Breastfeeding (while baby is totally breast fed)	
Barrier methods	Diaphragm Cervical cap Condoms male and female	
Spermicides (usually used in conjunction with barrier methods)	Creams, films, foams, jellies, pessaries, sponges	(These are mainly Nonoxynol based)
Hormonal methods	Oral contraceptive Depot progestogens Vaginal	Combined oestrogen/progestogen Progestogen only Injections Subcutaneous silicone implants Silicone rings releasing oestrogen and progestogen
Intrauterine devices	Inert Copper bearing Progestogen releasing (Mirena).	
Surgical methods	Laparoscopic sterilisation Hysteroscopic tubal occlusion (Essure) Intrauterine quinacrine producing tubal fibrosis, in developing countries Vasectomy	

The ideal contraceptive would have a 100% success rate, have no side effects, and be completely reversible and totally convenient. Clearly, none of the above fulfil all of these conditions. Many people are often ill-informed about contraception, and fears about possible side effects, together with problems experienced by friends and relatives, may play a greater role in influencing choice than medical advice and statistics. Some medical professionals have limited knowledge of the details of contraceptive choices and are therefore unable to give appropriate advice. An informed choice should provide information and counselling, and written details should, ideally, be supplied along verbal details. Within the UK, specialist family planning services offer free contraception and advice.

METHODS OF CONTRACEPTION

FAILURE RATES IN CONTRACEPTION

There are four factors that affect the failure rate of any method of contraception:

1. *Inherent weakness of the method*
    For example, the rhythm method, which depends on the accurate determination of the time of ovulation, can never be as reliable as an oral contraceptive (OC).

2. *Age*
    With all methods, the failure rate declines as age increases and fertility and frequency of intercourse also decrease.

3. *Motivation*
    Every method depends on the determination of the woman to use it correctly. Thus pills may be forgotten, diaphragm users 'take a chance', even with intrauterine devices (IUDs), a suspicion that the device is out of place may be ignored.

4. *Duration of use*
    The failure rate, especially with occlusive methods, declines as duration of use and therefore habit, increase.

PATIENT SUITABILITY FOR CONTRACEPTION

Many factors need to be taken into consideration when choosing an appropriate contraceptive method. These include age, parity, recent pregnancy, smoking, body mass index, medical history and concomitant medication. The Faculty of Sexual and Reproductive Healthcare provides evidence-based guidance on its website www.fsrh.org.uk

Potential contraindications are categorised as below

UKMEC categories	Definition
UKMEC 1	A condition for which there is no restriction for the use of the contraceptive method
UKMEC 2	A condition for which the advantages of using the method generally outweigh the theoretical or proven risk
UKMEC 3	A condition where the theoretical or proven risks usually outweigh the advantages of using the method. The provision of a method required expert clinical judgement and/or referral to a specialist contraceptive provider since the use of this method is not generally recommended, unless other more appropriate methods are not available or are unacceptable
UKMEC 4	A condition which represents an unacceptable health risk if the contraceptive method is used

HORMONAL CONTRACEPTION

COMBINED ORAL CONTRACEPTION

The pill is a mixture of oestrogen and progestogen, the combined oral contraceptive pill (COCP)

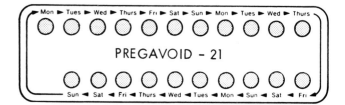

Mode of Action

The high oestrogen and progestogen levels reduce the negative feedback effect so that follicle stimulating hormone (FSH) secretion is depressed and the luteinising hormone (LH) peak is abolished. The combined pill, therefore, reliably prevents ovulation.

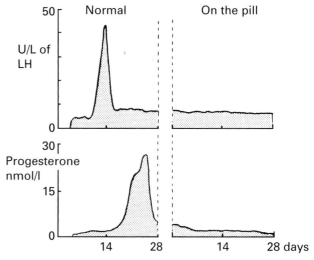

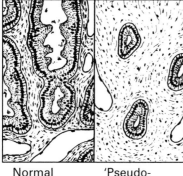

Normal endometrium   'Pseudo-atrophy'

The absence of a corpus luteum inhibits the preparation of an endometrium that is suitable for implantation, and a 'pseudo-atrophy' develops.

Changes in cervical mucus make sperm penetration less likely.

All these effects are the result of a synergistic action between oestrogen and progestogen.

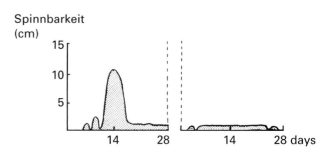

HORMONAL CONTRACEPTION

Constituents

Oestrogens (O)	Progestogens (P)
Ethinyloestradiol Mestranol (ethinyloestradiol-3-methyl-ether)	Levonorgestrel Norethisterone Ethynodiol diacetate Desogestrel Gestodene Norgestimate Drospirenone

Choice of Pill

There are over 30 brands available, using different drugs in different proportions.

Low dose preparations contain 20 µg of ethinyloestradiol and are particularly suitable for women with risk factors for circulatory disease.

Standard strength preparations contain 30–35 µg of ethinyloestradiol; however, the risk of venous thromboembolism varies with the progestogen used.

There are a range of different progestogens, and may have a variety of effects, depending on their derivation. Side effects such as acne are more likely to be associated with progestogens that have an androgenic derivation. Drospirenone, a new progestogen, is derived from spironolactone and has antiandrogenic and anti-mineralocorticoid activity. It is been found to be useful in women who have fluid retention and is useful in women with the premenstrual syndrome.

Women should however be offered levonorgestrel- and norethisterone-containing pills as a first line and alternatives considered only if side effects are problematic.

Risk of venous thromboembolic disease	
Non-pregnant, not on the pill	5–10 women per 100,000 per year
Levonorgestrel-and norethisterone-containing pills	15 women per 100,000 per year
Desogestrel and gestodene	25 women per 100,000 per year
Pregnancy	60 women per 100,000 per year

MINOR SIDE-EFFECTS OF OCs

Oestrogen	Oestrogen and progestogen	Progestogen
Breakthrough bleeding Nausea Painful breasts Headache	Weight gain Post-pill amenorrhoea	Acne Depression Dry vagina Loss of libido

Higher doses of 50–60 µg (taking two pills) can be used by women who are on enzyme inducing drugs that affect hepatic metabolism. However, this not an ideal long-term option and it may be best for the woman to consider an alternative approach of contraception that is not affected by hepatic metabolism.

In the combined pill, the oestrogen and progestogen component is usually given as a uniform dose for 21 days. This is followed by a 7-day pill-free interval. This break is usually associated with a withdrawal bleed. Some women opt to exclude the pill-free interval to avoid a withdrawal bleed. This works well but may be associated with breakthrough bleeding if used for long periods and it may be best to 'tricycle' the COCP, meaning that they run three packets together at a time followed by a 7-day break to allow a withdrawal bleed.

FAILURE OF THE PILL

The failure rate of the combined pill is very small, between 0% and 1%, and there is often an avoidable factor.

1. The patient may forget to take the pill. Packing by the pharmaceutical firms is ingenious but not foolproof. If one pill is missed, two are taken the next day and additional precautions should be undertaken.
2. Gastroenteritis may impair absorption.
3. Certain groups of drugs such as anticonvulsants, usually phenytoin and phenobarbitone, and the antibiotic rifampicin are known to increase the metabolic activity of hepatic enzymes and increase the rate of excretion of contraceptive steroids.
4. Several antibiotics, including ampicillin, are associated with an increase in breakthrough bleeding, and pregnancy has been reported. Oral contraceptives are conjugated in the liver, excreted in the bile, and partly reabsorbed. If gut bacteria are inhibited by antibiotics, reabsorption may not occur, leading to increased bowel excretion but lower circulating levels of steroids.

ORAL CONTRACEPTION: RISKS

Conditions where COCP is contraindicated or special precaution is required:

History of cardiovascular disease	Collagen diseases
Hypertension	Otosclerosis
Smoking	Diabetes mellitus
Obesity	Sickle cell anaemia
Chronic hepatitis	Severe varicose veins
Depression	Migraine
Acute porphyria	Arterial or venous thrombosis

A great deal of clinical and laboratory research and epidemiological analysis are available to support an association between COCPs and thromboembolism and stroke, and there is a increase in the risk of ischaemic heart disease in women with underlying risk factors. Women on the COCP, who are over 35 and smoke, have a significant increase in the risk of stroke. Women with migraine on the COCP are more at risk of stroke.

VASCULAR DISEASE

The risk of vascular disease, either venous or arterial, depends on the dose of oestrogen and also on the type of progestogen (see above). The risk remains low, but traditional risk factors increase the risk during pill use. These include thrombophilic tendencies, hypertension and obesity.

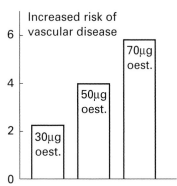

HYPERTENSION

OCs gradually raise the blood pressure, sometimes to the hypertensive range. The blood volume is increased by fluid retention, and the secretion of angiotensin is increased.

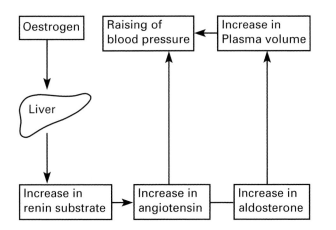

ORAL CONTRACEPTION: RISKS

ORAL CONTRACEPTIVES AND NEOPLASIA

No causal link has yet been established between OCs and any kind of neoplasia, but there is evidence of a small increase in risk of cervical and breast cancer. There has been much epidemiological debate about the possible mechanisms. It may be that pill users are less likely to use barrier contraception and, as such, have a higher risk of human papilloma virus infection.

ENDOMETRIUM AND OVARY

Prolonged OC use depresses mitotic activity in the endometrium and follicular maturation in the ovary, and these effects significantly reduce the risk of both cancers.

There is also a lower risk of benign conditions such as fibroids. Dysmenorrhoea, premenstrual syndrome and menstrual loss are also reduced.

PROGESTOGEN-ONLY PILL (POP)

Some 50% of women, on progestogen-only oral contraceptives, ovulate and menstruate, and the main contraceptive effect is a change in the cervical mucus. Some women bleed irregularly and around 15% of women are amenorrhoeic with no follicular development. The POP should be taken at the same time every day for maximum efficacy. Cerazette, a new POP containing desogestrel, has a 12-h missed pill window similar to COCP, and its contraceptive efficacy is over 99%.

OTHER ROUTES

VAGINAL RINGS

Silastic ring pessaries have been developed which release either a progestogen alone or both oestrogen and a progestogen, which are absorbed vaginally, thereby avoiding the first pass through the liver that results in a subsequent reduction in dosage.

INJECTABLE PROGESTOGENS

The most widely used injectable progestogen is medroxyprogesterone acetate (Depo-Provera), an intramuscular injection.

Three-monthly injections offer an effective method for contraception for women. The higher dose of progesterone inhibits ovulation and many women will be rendered amenorrhoeic. Irregular bleeding is common in the first months of use and some weight gain may also occur.

Long-term use is associated with some loss of bone mineral density and careful consideration should be given to the risks and benefits. Particular caution should apply in adolescents as skeletal development is ongoing.

ORAL CONTRACEPTION: RISKS

PROGESTOGEN-ONLY IMPLANTS

Implanon is available in the UK. It consists of a single rod for subdermal insertion in the inner aspect of the upper arm and releases etonogestrel. The mode of action involves inhibition of ovulation but irregular bleeding is common and it may sometimes be persistent. Insertion and removal should always be performed by someone trained in the procedure.

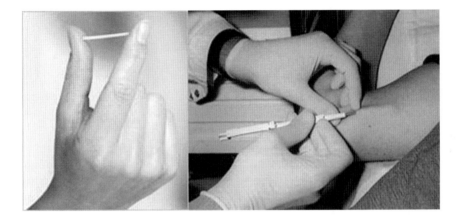

INTRAUTERINE DEVICES (IUDs)

Intrauterine devices (IUDs) have been made from a number of different materials. Inert coils simply contain plastic but the common devices also contain a copper or progestogen implant (Mirena). Most devices have threads that hang through the cervix to enable easy removal of the device.

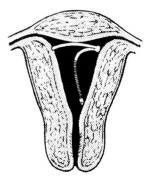

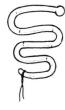

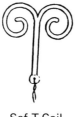

| Lippes Loop | Saf-T-Coil | Copper-7 IUD in place |

MODE OF ACTION

Intrauterine devices prevent fertilisation and implantation. Copper is toxic to both the ova and the sperm and an inflammatory reaction is induced in the endometrium. Progestogen releasing intrauterine systems deliver the progestogen directly to the endometrium, rendering it unreceptive to implantation, and cervical mucus is thickened.

There is an increased risk of pelvic infection. It is thought that lower genital tract organisms enter the uterus either during insertion of the device or via the threads. The risk of pelvic infection is much lower with Mirena as it thickens the cervical mucus which in turn helps prevent lower genital tract organisms from entering the uterus.

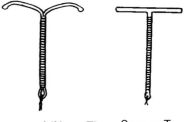

Novagard (Nova-T)   Copper-T

These devices can also be colonised by actinomyces. This does not merit a removal of the coil, but occasionally, pelvic actinomycosis can occur. This is a chronic, granulomatous infection which should be treated aggressively with antibiotics and, possibly, surgery.

The length of time that an IUD can last for depends on the type of device.

The Mirena

This levonorgestrel releasing (20 μg/24 h) intra-uterine system is licensed for 5 years. It is said to be as effective as female sterilisation, but the effects are immediately reversible upon removal.

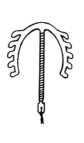

IUDs commonly cause heavy painful periods but the Mirena reduces menstrual loss and dysmenorrhoea due to the local effect of the progestin on the endometrium and its muscle relaxant effect on the myometrium.

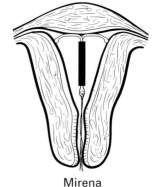

Multiload   Mirena

INTRAUTERINE DEVICES (IUDs)

PRINCIPLE OF INSERTION OF IUDs

Insertion Technique

Insertion of an IUD is always easier when a woman has had a previous vaginal delivery. Coil insertion can also be achieved in nulliparous women. The woman should be examined vaginally to assess of the size and direction of the uterus, to reduce the risk of uterine perforation.

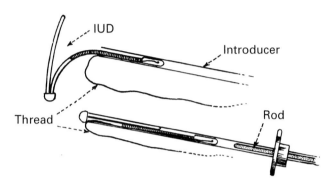

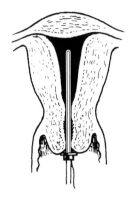

1. The IUD is first of all folded and pulled into a plastic tube called the introducer.

2. The introducer is then inserted into the uterus until it reaches the fundus.

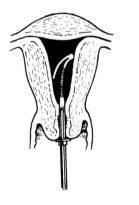

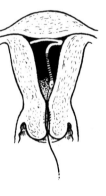

3. The surrounding introducer is drawn back holding the rod in place so that the device has now opened out in the uterine cavity.

4. The rod and introducer is now removed carefully and the threads are trimmed to about 4 cm.

A local anaesthetic and a tenaculum forceps can be useful. The Mirena has a specific introducer that makes insertion simpler, although it is very slightly thicker than most copper coils, at 4 mm.

Occasionally some sedation or even a general anaesthetic may be required to insert a coil.

COMPLICATIONS OF INTRAUTERINE DEVICES

1. *Increased menstrual loss*
   The cause may be due to the increased fibrinolytic activity that occurs around the IUD. It can be minimised by the use of antifibrinolytic agents such as tranexamic acid. Antiprostaglandin agents, such as mefenamic acid or diclofenac, are also effective. Progestogen releasing devices *decrease* loss.

2. *Infection*
   There is an increase in the risk of pelvic inflammatory disease, especially during the first months after insertion. Inert IUDs can be associated with actinomycosis infection if retained for long periods. Women with active pelvic infection should not have a coil fitted. Women with an existing coil in place may be given antibiotic treatment with the coil left in place, but with severe or persistent infection, consideration should be given to coil removal.

   Progestogen releasing systems *reduce* the incidence of infection as the cervical mucus is thickened due to the effect of progestin.

3. *Pregnancy*
   The chances of pregnancy are about 1–1.5 per 100 woman years and it is most likely to occur in the first 2 years. It is lower with copper-bearing coils and may be as low as 0.1 per 100 with the Mirena.[†] The risk of ectopic pregnancy is lower in IUD users as the risk of pregnancy is very low, but in those women who become pregnant with a coil *in situ*, the risk of ectopic pregnancy is higher.

4. *Expulsion*
   There is a 5–10% incidence, usually in the first 6 months. It is recommended that a speculum examination be performed at 6 weeks after coil insertion to check that the threads are visible. If the threads are not visible, an ultrasound scan should be performed to check for the presence of an intrauterine coil.

5. *Translocation*
   The IUD passes through the uterine wall into the peritoneal cavity or the broad ligament. It is thought that this begins at the time of a faulty insertion.

   An intrauterine coil is usually identified on scan but an extrauterine coil can be very difficult to visualise using the ultrasound. If an intrauterine location has not been confirmed, an abdominal/pelvic X-ray should be performed. If the coil is outside the uterus, a laparoscopy, and possible laparotomy, may be needed to locate it.

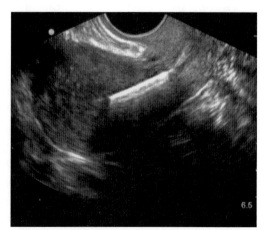

[†]Sivin I, et al. *Contraception* (1991) 44:473.

DIAPHRAGMS AND CAPS

The diaphragm is inserted into the vagina prior to intercourse. It is used in conjunction with a spermicidal cream and it acts by preventing sperm cells from reaching the cervical canal. It has a higher failure rate compared to oral contraceptives or IUDs but it has few side effects.

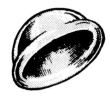

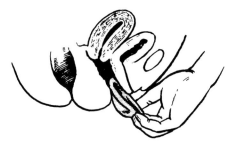

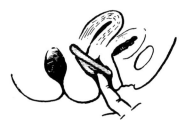

1. The diaphragm is smeared with spermicidal cream round the edges and on both sides, and guided into the posterior fornix.

2. The front end is tucked up behind the symphysis pubis.

The diaphragm must not be removed until 6 h after intercourse, and if intercourse is repeated in that period more cream must first be injected using an applicator.

Caps act in a similar way but are designed to fit over the cervix.

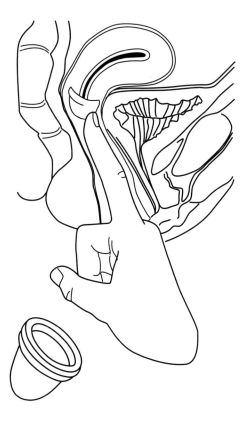

CONDOMS

A thin rubber sheath fits over the penis. Condoms can interfere with sensation; however, they reduce the risk of sexually transmitted infections and may be used in addition to other contraceptive methods. Condoms can split and they are liable to come off as the penis is withdrawn after the act. The failure rate is higher than for oral contraceptives. Lubricants, such as 'baby oil', can weaken condoms.

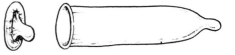

THE SPONGE
A disposable plastic sponge, impregnated with spermicide, is inserted into the vagina and can be left *in situ* for at least 24 h. Sponges need no fitting and are comfortable; however, they have a higher pregnancy risk than the diaphragm.

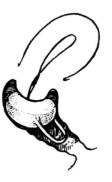

CONTRACEPTION BASED ON TIME OF OVULATION

THE RHYTHM METHOD ('Safe Period')

The woman must take her temperature every morning and watch out for the sustained rise which indicates ovulation. Women with regular periods can often usually identify the peri-ovulatory time with a fair degree of accuracy. However, an episode of hormonal irregularity may occur without warning and this can put the woman at risk of pregnancy.

However, assuming the cycle is regular and lasts for 28 days, ovulation usually occurs between the 12th and 14th days of the cycle. 24 h are allowed for ovum survival and 3 days should be allowed as survival time of the sperms in the genital tract, although sperm have been shown to survive for up to a week.

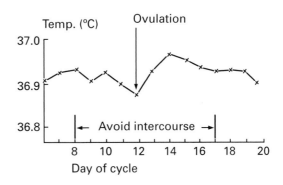

This means that intercourse must be avoided from the 9th to the 15th day and a 24 h safety margin at either end increases the avoidance period from the 8th to the 17th day, both inclusive.

THE OVULATION METHOD (The Billings' Method)

The woman is taught to identify the peri-ovulatory phase by noting the changes in cervical mucus.

This method provides the same opportunities for coitus as the rhythm method. In practice, many women will use these methods concurrently. The failure rate depends very much on the motivation of the couple and on an understanding of the method. It may be more useful to help women understand and know if they are fertile when they wish to conceive.

Say 5 days	Menstruation	
2–3 days	'Early safe days'	Sensation of vaginal dryness
4–5 days	Moist days – not safe	Increasing amounts of sticky mucus
2 days	Ovulation peak – not safe	Copious, clear 'slippery' mucus
3 days	Post-ovulation Peak – not safe	Gradual decrease in secretion
11 days	'Late safe days'	Minimal secretion

Breastfeeding

For many women, particularly in the developing world, lactational amenorrhoea is an effective method of contraception. It is most effective where an infant is exclusively breast fed, and ovulation is more likely to occur when the frequency of feeding is reduced. This is usually due to supplementary milk feeds or weaning of the infant (introduction of solid foods).

POSTCOITAL CONTRACEPTION

POSTCOITAL CONTRACEPTION ('Morning After' Contraception)

Effective postcoital contraception has been sought for many years, usually in the form of douching with various liquids, but these have been unsuccessful because of the rapidity with which the sperm leave the vagina and enter the cervical canal and uterus. Modern methods are extremely effective, if started early enough.

Hormonal Methods

Levonorgestrel is given as a once-only dose, as soon as possible after unprotected intercourse (up to 72 h). This is available over the counter, in the UK, to maximise accessibility.

Method of Action

The preparation of the endometrium for implantation is prevented.

Insertion of IUD

This method is highly effective and can be used for up to 5 days after coitus or 5 days after the estimated date of ovulation. The IUD can be used for continued contraception, if desired.

IRREVERSIBLE METHODS

STERILISATION

For Women

The reasons for seeking sterilisation as a contraceptive method are numerous, but many women seek a method by which they no longer need to be concerned with, for example, remembering to take pills, etc., and can essentially forget about.

Careful counselling is required as this method should be considered as irreversible and the woman needs to be sure that her family is complete. It is useful to explore how long she has felt that this is the case, and it is best to avoid making such a decision at a time of particular stress, such as the early postnatal period. Possible future change in circumstances should be considered in a sensitive manner. Careful consideration should be given before patients under 30, and those who have no children, are sterilised. Reversal operations have a success rate of around 50% but are now only funded, under exceptional circumstances, by the NHS.

Many women come with the expectation that female sterilisation is 100% successful. This is not the case and this procedure has a failure rate of 1 in 200. The failure rates for long-acting reversible contraceptives (LARCs) are similar. LARCs include Mirena and Implanon in the UK. Only a vasectomy is more successful, with 1 in 2000 women becoming pregnant after their partner has been sterilised.

Alternative contraceptive options should also be discussed. Experience of previous contraceptive methods should be considered. Clearly, if a woman has conceived or has had side effects with another method, she may well be unwilling to use it again.

The method of sterilisation should be explained to them, including the need for anaesthesia, recovery period and risks associated with the procedure. In most women, this will be performed as a day-case under laparoscopic guidance, but, occasionally, laparotomy may be the only feasible procedure, for example in extensive adhesions. There is a small risk of visceral injury as with any laparoscopic procedure, and laparotomy can occasionally be required as an emergency procedure.

Some women request sterilisation during a caesarean delivery. There is a higher failure rate and, possibly, a higher incidence of regret. This should be carefully discussed in the antenatal period. The Royal College of Obstetricians and Gynaecologists recommend that consent for sterilisation, at the time of a caesarean section, should be taken at least 1 week prior to the procedure.

If a woman does become pregnant after sterilisation, it is more likely to be a tubal pregnancy and she should be counselled to seek medical advice.

The woman should be made aware that her periods are likely to be unchanged by sterilisation, unless she has been on hormonal contraception which may make them lighter. This is not unusual, and, in women who expect this to be the case, it may be best to opt for the Mirena.

IRREVERSIBLE METHODS

It is important to remind the woman to continue with her current contraceptive method until the next menstrual period, after the procedure is performed.

All of this information should be clearly documented and written information should be given to the patient.

<table>
<tr><td colspan="2">CLINICAL/COUNSELLING NOTES
FOR FEMALE STERILISATION</td><td>ADDRESSOGRAPH
LABEL</td></tr>
</table>

DATE:

AGE:	PARITY:		LMP:		BMI:

REASONS FOR WANTING STERILISATION:

CURRENT CONTRACEPTIVE METHOD: PREVIOUS CONTRACEPTION:

ALTERNATIVE CONTRACEPTION DISCUSSED:	DISCUSSED	INTERESTED
Vasectomy – *failure rate 1/2000, can be done under local anaesthetic, complications less*	☐	☐► urology
Mirena - *>99% effective, lasts for 5 years, periods less heavy, may cause initial menstrual upset*	☐	☐► FPC
Implanon - *>99% effective, lasts for 3 years, local anaesthetic, initial menstrual upset, weight gain*	☐	☐► FPC
Depo-provera – *('The Jag') >99% effective, lasts for 12 weeks, periods may be irregular or stop, weight gain*	☐	☐► GP/FPC
IUCD - *99% effective, lasts 3 to 10 years depending on type, periods may be heavier & more painful*	☐	☐► GP/FPC
Oral contraception (COCP/POP) – *COCP >99% effective, periods less heavy; POP 99% effective; compliance issues*	☐	☐► GP/FPC

FEMALE STERILISATION	DISCUSSED	
GENERAL ANAESTHETIC, usually undertaken laparoscopically with clips as day surgery	☐	
LAPAROTOMY may be required if surgical complications are encountered	☐	ACTION
IRREVERSIBLE – difficult to reverse and NHS may not fund reversal	☐ →	
FAILURE RATE 1/200; if subsequent pregnancy, risk of ECTOPIC is approx. 5%	☐	
SURGICAL RISKS greater in high risk women (BMI, abdominal scars, medical disorders)	☐	
CONTINUE current contraception until after the procedure	☐	
PERIODS will be unchanged (unless on hormonal method pre-op, or an IUCD is removed)	☐	

MEDICAL/SURGICAL HISTORY:	DRUG HISTORY: ALLERGIES:
EXAMINATION: ABDOMINAL	VAGINAL CERVICAL SMEAR NEEDED: YES / NO

PREVIOUS ABDOMINAL SURGERY

CONSENT FORM SIGNED	LEAFLET GIVEN		

COMMENTS/PLAN:

SIGNATURE/PRINT NAME & GRADE:	Patient signature:

Instillation of chemical substances. In developing countries with limited facilities and budgets, insertion of a pellet of quinacrine into the uterine cavity through the cervical canal on two occasions, 4 weeks apart, has proved to be effective.

Hysteroscopic insertion of implants within the fallopian tubes has recently been used to achieve permanent contraception.

LAPAROSCOPIC STERILISATION

The tubes can be occluded by the application of clips or rings under laparoscopic vision. (Two clips are applied to each tube by some operators.)

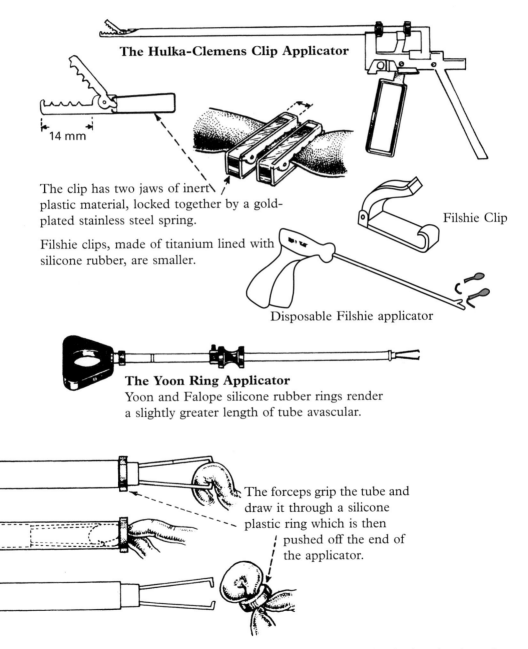

The Hulka-Clemens Clip Applicator

14 mm

The clip has two jaws of inert plastic material, locked together by a gold-plated stainless steel spring.

Filshie clips, made of titanium lined with silicone rubber, are smaller.

Filshie Clip

Disposable Filshie applicator

The Yoon Ring Applicator
Yoon and Falope silicone rubber rings render a slightly greater length of tube avascular.

The forceps grip the tube and draw it through a silicone plastic ring which is then pushed off the end of the applicator.

These applicators, whether for clips or rings, are passed into the abdominal cavity through a trocar, after the passage of a laparoscope. The clips should be placed about 1 cm from the cornu, and the rings as near to that point as possible. Thick and vascular tubes are more difficult to occlude by these methods.

VASECTOMY

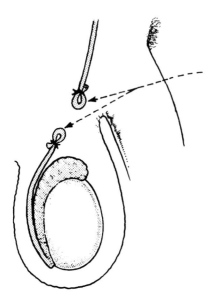

The same principles apply when counselling for male or female sterilisation (see above). The major difference is that vasectomy can be performed by a simple operation that can be done under local anaesthesia and the success rate is significantly better. Only 1 in 2000 women become pregnant after their partner has had a vasectomy.

It takes several months for the storage system to become clear of sperm, and a few non-motile ones may persist whose significance is uncertain. It may take a year before the ejaculate is completely sperm free. About 5% of patients demonstrate minor complications, including vaso-vagal reactions, haematoma and mild infection. There are occasional reports of severe infection. Possible long-term complications include the development of sperm autoantibodies. This can lower the success rate of reversal of the procedure.

CHAPTER 17

INFERTILITY

Infertility   358
  Causes of Female Factor Infertility   359
  Causes of Male Factor Infertility   359
Investigations   360
  Investigations in the Primary
    Setting   360
  Investigations in the Secondary
    Setting   360
Evidence of Ovulation   361
  Features Suggestive of Ovulation   361
  Tests that Confirm the Occurrence
    of Ovulation   362
Seminal Analysis   364
  Tests which Confirm Normal Sperm
    Production   364
Sperm Production Tests   365
Abnormalities in Sperm
    Production   366
Sperm Function Tests   367
  Postcoital Test   367
  Measurement of Antisperm
    Antibodies   367
  In Vitro Assessment of Fertilisation
    Ability of Sperm   367
  Abnormal Sperm Function   367
Tests of Tubal Patency   368
  Requirements for the Assessment
    of Tubal Patency   369

Contraindications to the Assessment
    of Tubal Patency   369
Assisted Conception   370
  Assisted Reproduction Techniques   370
Fertility Drugs   371
Tubal Surgery   373
  Efficacy   373
  Side Effects   373
Assisted Conception Techniques   374
  In Vitro Fertilisation   374
  Risks of IVF Treatment   376
  Intrauterine Insemination
    (IUI)   378
  Intracytoplasmic Sperm Injection
    (ICSI)   378
  Donor Conception   378
  Gamete Intrafallopian Transfer
    (GIFT)   378
  In Vitro Maturation (IVM)   379
  Reproductive Immunology   379
  Pre-Implantation Genetic Diagnosis
    (PIGD)   379
Assisted Conception   380
  HFEA   380
  Counselling   380

INFERTILITY

Approximately one in seven couples has difficulties in conceiving. In general, 80% of the couples who have regular sexual intercourse and do not use contraception will get pregnant within a year. The majority of the remaining 20% achieve a pregnancy within 2 years of trying.

Percentage of couples pregnant after varying time periods of unprotected intercourse (Gutmacher 1965)

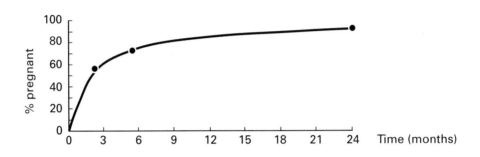

Definitions

Primary infertility is a condition where a couple, who have had no previous pregnancies, are unable to conceive.

Secondary infertility is a condition where a couple, who have had at least one previous pregnancy that may have ended in a livebirth, stillbirth, miscarriage, ectopic pregnancy or induced abortion, are unable to conceive.

Aetiology of Infertility

Lifestyle factors such as heavy smoking or being significantly over- or underweight and stress can adversely affect both male and female fertility.

INFERTILITY

CAUSES OF FEMALE FACTOR INFERTILITY

With increasing age, women become less fertile.

There are many causes of infertility (see below). Sometimes, failure to conceive can be due to a combination of factors. However, in approximately 30% of cases, a clear cause is never established.

Unexplained infertility	28%
Male factor infertility	21%
Ovulatory disorders	18%
Tubal disease	14%
Endometriosis	6%
Coital problems	5%
Cervical factors	3%

Other factors that may play a part include chronic medical conditions such as diabetes, epilepsy and thyroid and bowel diseases.

CAUSES OF MALE FACTOR INFERTILITY

Infertility is often thought of as a female issue, but in around 30% of cases, it is because of a problem in the male partner. As in women, male fertility is also thought to decline with age, although to what extent is unclear. Possible causes of male infertility include:

- problems with the tubes carrying sperm
- erectile dysfunction
- ejaculatory problems
- previous orchitis
- a past bacterial infection that caused scarring and blocked tubes within the epididymis as it joins the vas
- past medical treatment such as drug treatment, radiotherapy or surgery – for example, to correct a hernia, undescended testes or twisted testicles
- genetic problems
- chronic diseases such as diabetes
- drugs.

INVESTIGATIONS

INVESTIGATIONS IN THE PRIMARY SETTING

When a couple presents to their general practitioner with the issue of infertility, these initial investigations should be carried out.

Female partner	Cervical smear test.
	Urine test for *Chlamydia* (this can cause blockages of the fallopian tube).
	Serum progesterone level to check ovulation. This is taken 1 week prior to menstruation, hence day 21 for a 28-day cycle or day 28 for a 35-day cycle (see below).
	Rubella immunity – if rubella is contracted during the first 3 months of pregnancy it can seriously harm the developing fetus Women who are not immune to rubella should be vaccinated, and advised to avoid pregnancy for 3 months.
	Measuring serum FSH (follicle stimulating hormone), LH (luteinising hormone) and oestradiol to identify hormone imbalances or possible early menopause.
Male partner	Semenalysis to check for abnormalities of the sperm such as number, motility, and morphology (see below).
	Urine test for *Chlamydia*, which, in addition to being a known cause of infertility in women, can also affect sperm function and male fertility.

INVESTIGATIONS IN THE SECONDARY SETTING

These are done in the context of a tertiary fertility clinic and after the primary investigations have been carried out. Some or all of the following tests will be done:

Female partner	Measuring serum FSH, LH and oestradiol to identify hormone imbalances or possible early menopause.
	Serum progesterone level to check ovulation. This is taken 1 week prior to menstruation, hence day 21 for a 28-day cycle or day 28 for a 35-day cycle.
	A pelvic ultrasound scan to look at uterine and ovarian anatomy.
	Serial ultrasound tracking of the ovaries for looking at developing follicles (see below).
	Checking of tubal patency – either by hysterosalpingogram, hysteron-contrast sonography or laparoscopic hydrotubation.
	Diagnostic laparoscopy – to check for problems with tubal and uterine anatomy.
	Hysteroscopy – to check for uterine conditions such as fibroids or polyps
	Endometrial biopsy (in rare cases) see below.
Male partner	Semenalysis to check for abnormalities of the sperm such as number, motility and morphology (see below).
	Sperm antibody test to check for protein molecules that may prevent sperm from fertilising an egg.

EVIDENCE OF OVULATION

FEATURES SUGGESTIVE OF OVULATION

1. *Clinical symptoms and signs*

    Regular menstruation is usually associated with ovulation, however, no clinical symptoms or signs are sufficiently reliable to confirm ovulation. Supportive laboratory tests are always required.

2. *Changes in basal body temperature*

    The secretion of progesterone by the corpus luteum induces a rise of around 0.5 °C in basal body temperature (BBT). If BBT is recorded throughout the menstrual cycle, a fall in temperature is often observed at the time of the LH surge. Charts typical of those generated by A) a woman with a normal ovulatory cycle, and B) a woman with an anovulatory cycle, are shown below. The differences in BBT between ovulatory and anovulatory women are not sufficiently consistent for a diagnosis of ovulation to be made without further tests.

A. Normal BBT chart from an ovulating woman $\longrightarrow$

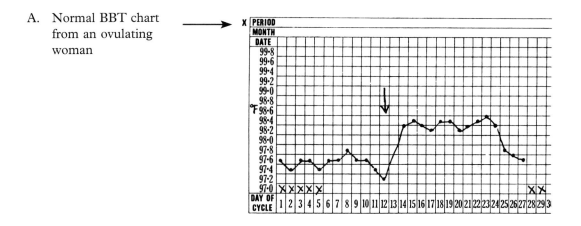

B. Abnormal BBT chart from a woman who is not ovulating $\longrightarrow$

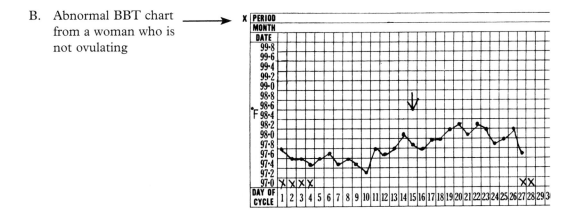

EVIDENCE OF OVULATION

TESTS THAT CONFIRM THE OCCURRENCE OF OVULATION

1. *Serum progesterone levels*

    Estimation of serum progesterone is a simple method for confirming ovulation. Progesterone is produced by the corpus luteum and its levels reach a peak in the mid-luteal phase (i.e. 7 days prior to menstruation). If the measured serum progesterone levels are low, this may indicate either that the patient is not ovulating, or that the blood sample was withdrawn at an inappropriate time in the cycle. Information about the time of the subsequent menstrual period is required to accurately interpret the relevance of serum progesterone levels.

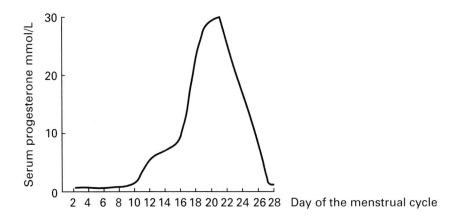

2. *Endometrial biopsy*

    The presence of a secretory endometrium confirms that ovulation has taken place. Under the influence of progesterone, the endometrial glands dilate, and secretory vacuoles may be observed within the glandular cells. If an endometrial biopsy is taken in the luteal phase and examined histologically, secretory changes can be observed. A biopsy of the endometrium is a relatively invasive process, but it gives useful information, especially if sensitive progesterone assays are unavailable.

Proliferative phase endometrium showing oestrogen stimulation. Note the narrow non-secreting glands. The epithelial and stromal cells show proliferative activity.

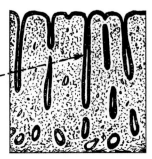

Secretory endometrium showing the effects of progesterone. Note the dilated secretory glands.

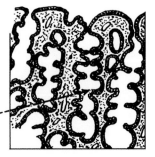

362

EVIDENCE OF OVULATION

3. *Serial ovarian ultrasound*

    Over the course of the menstrual cycle, an ovarian follicle develops, grows to 20 mm and the oöcyte is then released at ovulation. This process can be visualised by a transvaginal ultrasound examination every 2–3 days during the follicular, ovulatory and early luteal phases. This procedure is too invasive and expensive to be used in an unselected population of women complaining of infertility. However, it is often used to monitor the number and size of the developing ovarian follicles in women undergoing ovulation induction. The serial ultrasound is the only method of detecting the luteinised unruptured follicle syndrome (LUF).

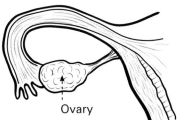

Early follicular phase (no ovarian follicle visible on ultrasound).

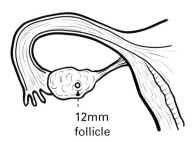

Mid-follicular phase (12 mm follicle visible on ultrasound).

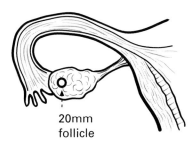

Immediate pre-ovulatory phase (ovarian follicle on 20 mm diameter).

SEMINAL ANALYSIS

TESTS WHICH CONFIRM NORMAL SPERM PRODUCTION

Semen Analysis

A basic semen analysis assesses the number, morphology and motility of spermatozoa. The patient is asked to provide a sample (usually by masturbation), which should be analysed within 2 hours of production. The sample should be kept warm (15–38 °C) during the interval from production to analysis. Abstinence from sexual activity for a period of 2–3 days is required before submitting a sample for analysis; otherwise an abnormally low count may be recorded. The patient should also be advised to keep the sample away from spermicidal agents, such as those in condoms.

The criteria for normal spermatogenesis may vary from laboratory to laboratory. The WHO criteria are shown below:

1. Volume: ≥ 2 ml
2. Concentration: ≥ 20 million/ml
3. Motility: $\geq 50\%$ with forward motility (within 60 min of ejaculation)
4. Morphology: $\geq 30\%$ normal forms
5. White blood cells: <1 million/ml

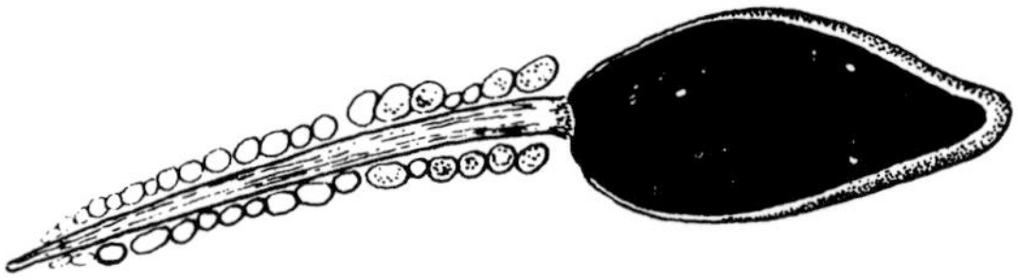

Normal human sperm (from transmission electron micrograph).

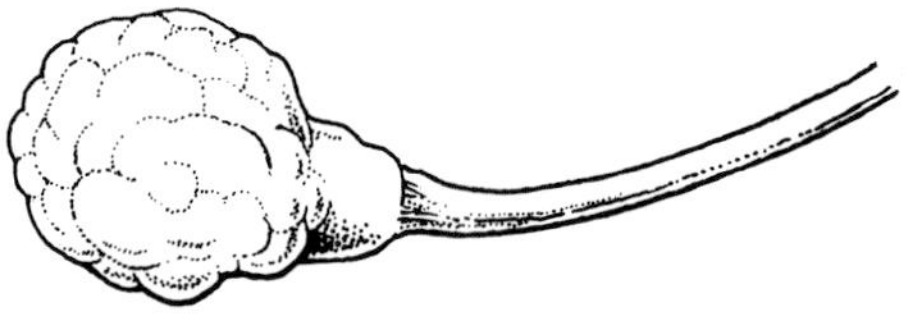

Abnormal sperm (from scanning electron micrograph).

SPERM PRODUCTION TESTS

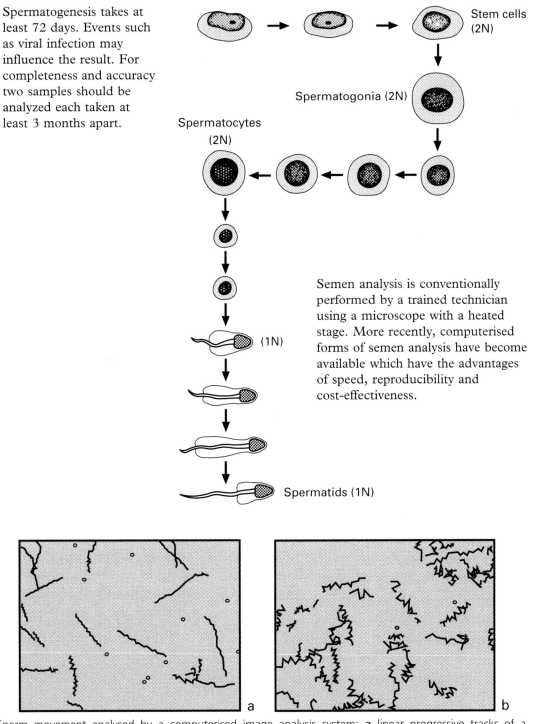

Spermatogenesis takes at least 72 days. Events such as viral infection may influence the result. For completeness and accuracy two samples should be analyzed each taken at least 3 months apart.

Stem cells (2N)

Spermatogonia (2N)

Spermatocytes (2N)

(1N)

Semen analysis is conventionally performed by a trained technician using a microscope with a heated stage. More recently, computerised forms of semen analysis have become available which have the advantages of speed, reproducibility and cost-effectiveness.

Spermatids (1N)

a

b

Sperm movement analysed by a computerised image analysis system: **a** linear progressive tracks of a non-capacitated sperm population; **b** high amplitude, non-progressive tracks of a hyperactivated, capacitated sperm population.

ABNORMALITIES IN SPERM PRODUCTION

The causes of abnormalities in sperm production include:

1. *Acute and chronic infection* of the male genital tract. Gonococcal and coliform infections respond to antibiotics but chronic prostatitis can be difficult to treat. Spermatozoa are reduced in number and tend to be malformed and non-motile.

    Chlamydial infection may be found in both partners. Sperm motility is reduced, causing infertility. Both partners should be treated and follow-up examinations of the ejaculate carried out.

    Viral infections can be important, especially mumps. Testicular atrophy may follow this infection.

2. *Immunological reactions* in the form of auto-antibodies occur in a variable number of men (3–12%). Formation of these antisperm antibodies may be stimulated by infection or by injury, but in most cases the cause is obscure. Steroids in short courses may be helpful.

3. *Environmental factors*
    These include social habits such as smoking, alcohol and drugs.

    Also included under this heading are occupational hazards such as working with heavy metals, welding processes, exposure to high temperatures, pesticides and radioactive materials.

    The list of occupations involving substances that are toxic to sperm count is remarkably long:
    Agriculture and gardening – handling pesticides, weed killers.
    Car industry, painters, battery workers, domestic decorators, smelters – all using lead products.
    Textile industry – exposure to carbon disulphide.
    Plastic manufacturing – exposure to chlorinated biphenyls.
    Grain storage – exposure to benzine hexachloride.

A large number of therapeutic agents also affect spermatogenesis.

1. Chemotherapeutic agents – these depress sperm production and cause germinal epithelial aplasia. Rising FSH levels are an indication of these changes.
2. Sulfasalazine reduces sperm motility and number. These effects are reversed if treatment is stopped.
3. Cimetidine, spironolactone and ketoconazole interfere with androgen action and may affect spermatogenesis.
4. Anabolic steroids profoundly depress spermatogenesis, but the effect is reversible when the drug is withdrawn.
5. Antihypertensive drugs, antidepressants and some sedatives cause impotence and may depress sperm count or motility.
6. Nitofurantoin, antimalarial drugs and corticosteroids depress spermatogenesis.

SPERM FUNCTION TESTS

Other tests which may be used to assess sperm function:

POSTCOITAL TEST

The postcoital test assesses the ability of sperm to penetrate the human cervical mucus. Healthy sperm are able to swim through the cervical mucus secreted at mid-cycle. To perform the test, the couple is advised to have intercourse mid-cycle, and a sample of the cervical mucus is obtained 9–24 h later. The presence of ≥ 20 motile sperm per high powered field ($400\times$ magnification) indicates a positive result.

Although the postcoital test is still widely used, the requirement for careful timing of intercourse and cervical mucus recovery means that the test can be difficult to perform. An alternative is to assess the distance travelled by sperm through a layer of 'artificial mucus', normally, a polymer of hyaluronic acid. This test is more easily quantified, and when used in combination with antisperm antibodies, gives similar information.

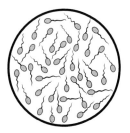

Positive postcoital test showing presence of ≥ 20 motile sperm in one high powered field.

MEASUREMENT OF ANTISPERM ANTIBODIES

Antisperm antibodies may be found in the serum, seminal fluid or the cervical mucus. Each of these may adversely affect fertility. Many tests have been devised to assess antisperm antibodies. The immunobead test (IBT) detects both IgA and IgG antibodies. In the presence of antisperm antibodies, polyacrylamide beads covered with bound antibody react with the spermatozoa. The test has good sensitivity and specificity, and this test can also be used to identify the antisperm antibody binding site – antibodies bound to the head of the sperm have the most serious effect on fertility.

IN VITRO ASSESSMENT OF FERTILISATION ABILITY OF SPERM

In practice, many couples with male factor infertility are treated with *in vitro* fertilisation (IVF). Some sperm are so abnormal that they are unable to fertilise the egg *in vitro*, and this will be detected during the course of a conventional IVF regimen. More specialised treatment, such as intracytoplasmic sperm injection (ICSI), may then be required.

ABNORMAL SPERM FUNCTION

Spermatogenesis may be adversely affected by conditions such as a viral illness; hence it is important to obtain two samples of sperm, more than 3 months, apart for complete analysis. Persistent abnormalities in spermatogenesis are rarely treated successfully without recourse to assisted reproductive technologies. Further investigation and treatment of such men is outside the scope of this book, but these should be considered before assisted reproduction technologies are embarked upon.

TESTS OF TUBAL PATENCY

1. *Laparoscopic hydrotubation*

   Tubal patency can be assessed at laparoscopy. A cannula is inserted into the cervix, and 5–20 ml of methylene blue dye is injected into the cavity of the uterus. If the fallopian tubes are patent, the dye can be seen spilling out of the end of each tube. An important advantage of laparoscopic hydrotubation is that it enables inspection of the pelvic organs during the procedure. Conditions such as pelvic adhesions and endometriosis, both of which may reduce fertility, can be noted. The major disadvantage of laparoscopy is that it is an operative procedure that requires a general anaesthetic.

2. *Hysterosalpingography*

   Hysterosalpingography is the radiological visualisation of the genital tract after the injection of a radio-opaque contrast medium through the cervix. Hysterosalpingography may be a useful supplementary test in women who have tubal blockage that is demonstrated at laparoscopy. Hysterosalpingography allows the site of tubal blockage to be determined, which is helpful if surgery is contemplated.

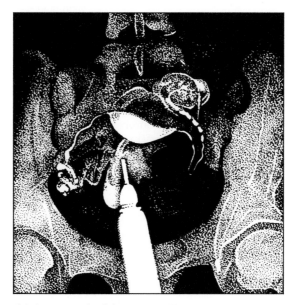

This is a normal salpingogram. Note:
1. The anteverted uterus is foreshortened.
2. The long thin tubal outline.
3. The ill-defined shadow of peritoneal spill.
4. Cervico-vaginal leakage.

TESTS OF TUBAL PATENCY

3. *Hysterosalpingo-contrast sonography.*
    Tubal patency can also be assessed by an ultrasound examination. A solution containing galactose microparticles, visible on ultrasound, is injected though the cervix. If the fallopian tubes are patent, the solution can be observed passing along the tubes and out through the fimbrial ends.

4. *Falloposcopy*
    Advances in imaging techniques have allowed the manufacture of hysteroscopes that are small enough to be passed into the fallopian tube. Internal tube morphology can be directly assessed. This procedure is only available in specialised centres, but it can be combined with operative treatments to relieve fallopian tube blockage.

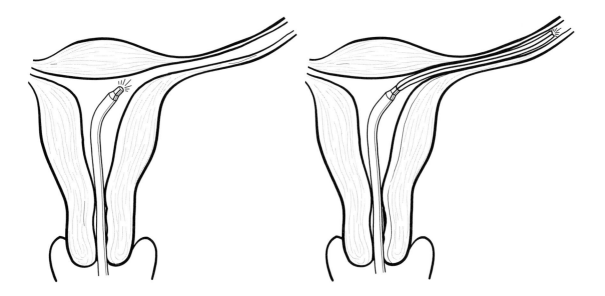

REQUIREMENTS FOR THE ASSESSMENT OF TUBAL PATENCY
1. The patient should have a clear understanding of the procedure that is going to be performed.
2. To avoid inadvertently performing the procedure when the patient is pregnant, the procedure should be done during the first half of the menstrual cycle, or may be done at any phase of a cycle if adequate contraceptive precautions have been taken.

CONTRAINDICATIONS TO THE ASSESSMENT OF TUBAL PATENCY
1. Pregnancy or possible pregnancy.
2. Active pelvic or vaginal infection.

ASSISTED CONCEPTION

Pre-Pregnancy Infection Screening
Prior to the storage of patient sperm, eggs or embryos a number of screening tests are carried out to assess the risk of contamination. These include HIV 1 and 2 (anti-HIV – 1, 2), hepatitis B (HBsAg/Anti-HBc) and hepatitis C (anti-HCV-Ab).

Folic Acid Administration
Folic acid is thought to reduce the risk of neural tube defects in the offspring of pregnant women. All women planning a pregnancy should be advised to commence folic acid.

ASSISTED REPRODUCTION TECHNIQUES
The treatment of subfertility is very much dependent on the cause. Available techniques include:

- Fertility drugs
- Surgery
- *In vitro* fertilisation (IVF) with or without pre-implantation genetic diagnosis (PIGD)
- Intrauterine insemination (IUI)
- Donor insemination (DI)
- Intracytoplasmic sperm injection (ICSI)
- Gamete intrafallopian transfer (GIFT)
- *In vitro*-maturation (IVM)
- Reproductive immunology
- Surrogacy.

FERTILITY DRUGS

FERTILITY DRUGS

These are used for inducing ovulation. Some women may become pregnant with these drugs alone, or alternatively, these may be used in combination with other treatments such as IVF or IUI. Commonly used drugs include:

1. *Clomiphene*

   Clomiphene is a non-steroidal antioestrogen. It has complex actions, including an oestrogen-agonistic activity at the endometrium. The major effect of clomiphene is at the hypothalamus, and it induces ovulation by increasing pituitary gonadotrophin production. Its side effects include hot flushes, mood swings, nausea, breast tenderness, insomnia, increased urination, heavy periods, spots and weight gain. The risk of ovarian cancer can also increase slightly if it is taken for over a year.

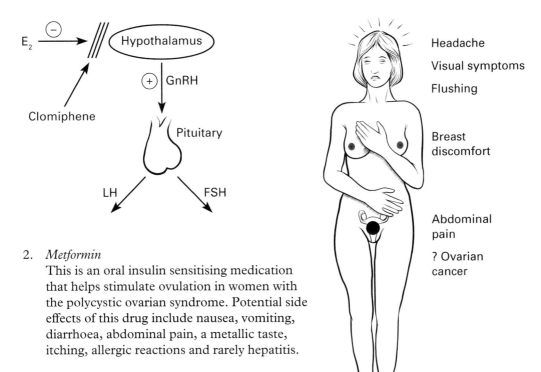

2. *Metformin*

   This is an oral insulin sensitising medication that helps stimulate ovulation in women with the polycystic ovarian syndrome. Potential side effects of this drug include nausea, vomiting, diarrhoea, abdominal pain, a metallic taste, itching, allergic reactions and rarely hepatitis.

3. *Gonadatrophin releasing hormone analogues (GnRHa)*

   This is administered by a small pump, which injects pulses of the drug into the bloodstream. It is used mainly in ovulation failure caused by a lack of GnRH. Possible side effects include abdominal pain, nausea, vomiting, heavy periods and headaches.

FERTILITY DRUGS

4. *Gonadotrophins*
   Follicle stimulating hormone (FSH), Gonal-f and Puregon

   Luteinising hormone (LH), such as Menogon, Menopur and Merional

   The use of gonadotrophins to induce ovulation should only be carried out in specialised centres. The patient should be monitored by ovarian ultrasound (to determine the number of follicles and their diameter) combined with serum or urinary oestrogen assays. These drugs are generally used before treatment cycles during assisted conception, or for polycystic ovary syndrome in which clomiphene has not been effective. They are administered as once-daily injections and act by stimulating follicle production in the ovaries. When the follicles are mature (as deemed by ovarian tracking), an injection of human chorionic gonadotrophin hormone (hCG) is given to trigger the release of an egg(s). Ovarian hyperstimulation syndrome (OHSS), risk of multiple pregnancies when used for ovulation induction, allergic reactions and skin reactions are the potential side effects.

5. *GnRH analogues/pituitary agonists (nafarelin, buserelin and goserelin)*
   These are administered via nasal sprays, daily injections, or as monthly depot injections. They downregulate the ovarian cycle which results in low levels of FSH, LH and oestradiol. They are often used before an IVF cycle is commenced. Some side effects include hot flushes, night sweats, headaches, vaginal dryness, mood swings, changes in breast size, acne and muscle aches.

6. *Gonadotrophin releasing hormone antagonists (cetrotide and orgalutran)*
   These are given daily by subcutaneous injection and simultaneously with FSH injections. These drugs act by blocking the release of LH and are administered while the ovaries are stimulated to produce eggs, in readiness for IVF treatment. Possible side effects include nausea, headache, injection site reactions, dizziness and malaise.

7. *Progesterone (Cyclogest, Gestone, Crinone, Progynova)*
   This is generally given after the hCG injection or on the day the embryos are returned to the womb. Its purpose is to prepare the endometrium for nurturing an embryo. This may help maintain the pregnancy after IVF or IUI.

8. *Bromocriptine and carbergoline*
   These tablets reduce high levels of prolactin, which can be a cause of subfertility. Side effects include nausea, headache, constipation, dry mouth, skin reactions, hair loss and a lowering of the voice.

TUBAL SURGERY

When tubal disease has been confirmed, tubal patency may be improved by surgery. The best results are obtained when surgery is performed by an operator trained in these techniques, using an operating microscope. Surgery may be performed laparoscopically, or as an open procedure. The aim of surgery is to restore tubal patency and mobility. However, the restoration of tubal patency does not guarantee pregnancy, since tubal function (e.g. the movement of cilia) may have been permanently destroyed or impaired.

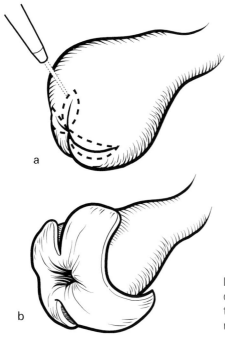

a

b

Laparoscopic salpingostomy with laser or diathermy to (a) incise the tube and scar the serosa to cause (b) eversion of the mucosa.

EFFICACY
The efficacy of tubal surgery depends on the extent of the pre-existing disease and on the particular procedure that is carried out. The best results are achieved after surgery for sterilisation reversal as pregnancy rates as high as 60%, have been reported. However, with severe disease, the cumulative pregnancy rate at 24 months after surgery is low at 10%, which is a little greater than could have been expected after no treatment.

SIDE EFFECTS
– complications of surgery
– increased risk of ectopic pregnancy during a future pregnancy.

ASSISTED CONCEPTION TECHNIQUES

IN VITRO FERTILISATION

This technique involves the fertilisation of human oöcytes '*in vitro*'. The eggs are harvested from ovarian follicles that are approximately 20 mm in diameter (i.e. immediately before ovulation). The eggs are then placed in a culture medium, in an incubator, and fertilised several hours later. Gonadotrophins are commonly employed to increase the number of pre-ovulatory oocytes available for collection. The use of a GnRH analogue allows better control of the timing of egg collection.

Indications for *in vitro* Fertilisation

1. Unexplained infertility when anatomy and function appear to be normal, and all treatable causes of infertility have been eliminated.
2. Tubal disease.
3. Lack of success with other techniques such as fertility drugs alone or IUI.
4. Minor degrees of male subfertility, for example, when the sperm count is low, but not so low that fertilisation is impossible (see ICSI).

Example of a Treatment Schedule

Suppression of the Natural Monthly Hormone Cycle
The patient is usually given a GnRH analogue, which blocks the pituitary receptors and stops the normal production of GnRH.

Boosting the Egg Supply
Once the natural cycle has been suppressed, a FSH (e.g. human menopausal gonadotrophin, hMG) is administered by daily injection.

Follicle Tracking
This is done by a transvaginal ultrasound scanning which helps monitor follicular growth. When the follicles reach 20 mm in diameter, ovulation is imminent. At this point, an injection of hCG is given to facilitate the egg maturation process.

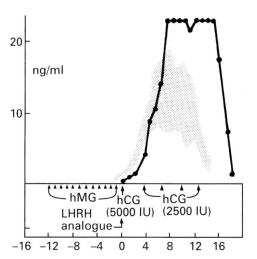

The diagram shows the sequence of hormone treatments, and the much improved luteal progesterone profile (●) compared with the normal (shaded).

ASSISTED CONCEPTION TECHNIQUES

IN VITRO FERTILISATION—(cont'd)

Collection of Eggs
Egg collection is carried out by a transvaginal ultrasound-guided aspiration of the ovarian follicles. Light sedation may be required for this process.

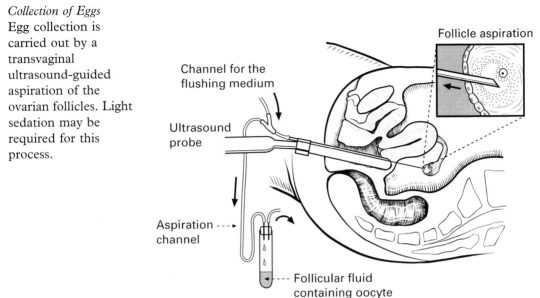

Follicle aspiration

Channel for the flushing medium

Ultrasound probe

Aspiration channel

Follicular fluid containing oocyte

Egg Fertilisation
The eggs and sperm are then cultured, *in vitro*, for 16–20 h to allow fertilisation to occur. The fertilised eggs (embryos) are then grown to the 4–8 cell stage. The best one, or two, embryos are then chosen for transfer back to the uterus.

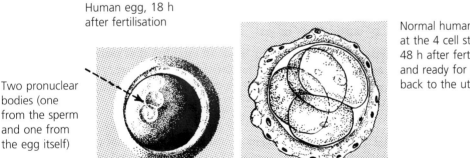

Human egg, 18 h after fertilisation

Two pronuclear bodies (one from the sperm and one from the egg itself)

Normal human embryo at the 4 cell stage 48 h after fertilisation and ready for transfer back to the uterus

After egg collection, progesterone is often given to prepare the lining of the womb for embryo transfer. This can be in the form of pessaries, an injection or a gel.

ASSISTED CONCEPTION TECHNIQUES

IN VITRO FERTILISATION—(cont'd)

Embryo Transfer

For women under 40 years of age, one or two embryos can be transferred. If the woman is over 40, however, a maximum of three embryos can be used. A restriction on the number of embryos used is to prevent multiple births and its associated risks. Any remaining embryos can be frozen for future IVF attempts, if they are suitable.

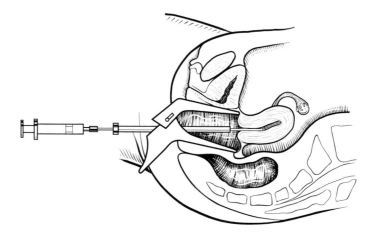

RISKS OF IVF TREATMENT

(1) *Side effects of hormonal therapy* – hot flushes, mood changes, headaches, restlessness.

(2) *Multiple births (twins, triplets or more)* – this is the single greatest health risk associated with fertility treatment. The Human Fertilisation and Embryology Authority (HFEA) has imposed restrictions on the number of embryos that can be transferred during IVF in order to reduce the number of multiple births. Multiple births carry risks for both the mother and fetuses. The babies are more likely to be premature and tend to have below-normal birth weight. The perinatal mortality rate has been shown to be four times greater in twins compared to singletons, and for triplets, the risk is seven times greater than for singletons. In addition, the risk of cerebral palsy is five times higher for twins and 18 times higher for triplets, compared to singletons.

ASSISTED CONCEPTION TECHNIQUES

IN VITRO FERTILISATION—(cont'd)

(3) *Ovarian hyperstimulation syndrome*

The ovarian hyperstimulation syndrome is a potentially dangerous overreaction to certain drugs that are used to stimulate ovarian follicle production. It is characterised by a sudden increase in vascular permeability with a massive extravascular exudate. The condition is categorised into mild, moderate and severe disease. In severe disease, there is evidence of intravascular loss, with ascites and pleural effusion. The resulting haemoconcentration can lead to hepatorenal failure and thrombosis. The condition can be fatal and should be carefully managed by fluid balance, thromboprophylaxis and, where necessary, dialysis and paracentesis. The mainstay of management is prevention, which involves careful monitoring of ovarian stimulation and a withholding of hCG in women at risk.

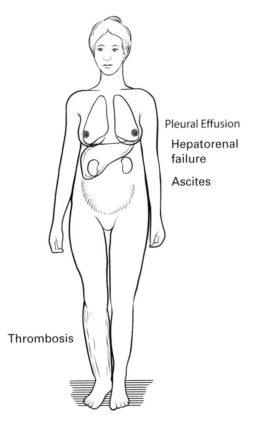

Pleural Effusion

Hepatorenal failure

Ascites

Thrombosis

(4) *Ectopic pregnancy* – there is a higher chance of this occurring after IVF (especially in the context of tubal disease) when compared to a spontaneous conception.

EFFICACY

The success of IVF is dependent on the age of the female partner, the indications for treatment, the number of embryos replaced and the skill of the IVF treatment centre. The cumulative conception rate, after three treatment cycles, varies from over 40% (in women aged 20–24) to 20% (in women aged 40–45). The live birth rate is considerably lower at around 30% (in women aged 20–24) to less than 15% (in women aged 40–45).

ASSISTED CONCEPTION TECHNIQUES

INTRAUTERINE INSEMINATION (IUI)

IUI involves a laboratory procedure that separates fast-moving sperm from more sluggish or non-moving sperm. The fast-moving sperm are then placed into the woman's womb, close to the time of ovulation, when the egg is released from the ovary in the middle of the monthly cycle. Prior to IUI, it is essential that fallopian tubes are proven to be patent. IUI can be carried out with or without the use of fertility drugs.

INTRACYTOPLASMIC SPERM INJECTION (ICSI)

ICSI involves the injection of a single sperm into an egg. This technique is used when, in the male partner, the sperm count is so low, or if the sperm function is so abnormal, that they would not normally be able to fertilise an egg, either *in vitro* or *in vivo*.

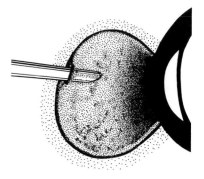

DONOR CONCEPTION

Donor conception involves using sperm, eggs or embryos from donors. DI uses sperm from a donor to achieve conception. Sperm donors are screened for sexually transmitted diseases and some genetic disorders. In DI, sperm from the donor is placed into the cervix at the time of ovulation.

Donor eggs are fertilised *in vitro*, frozen, and placed in a recipient who has been treated with oestrogens and progesterones, as described above. Such treatment may be useful in women with premature menopause.

GAMETE INTRAFALLOPIAN TRANSFER (GIFT)

GIFT involves the replacement of harvested sperm and eggs into the fallopian tube, before fertilisation occurs. The advantage of this technique is that the expertise of an embryologist is not required. Clearly, GIFT is unsuitable for women with tubal disease. Pregnancy rates are similar to those achieved by conventional IVF. However, the clinical guidelines on fertility, issued by NICE (the National Institute for Health and Clinical Excellence) state: 'There is insufficient evidence to recommend the use of GIFT . . . in preference to IVF in couples with unexplained fertility problems or male factor fertility problems.'

ASSISTED CONCEPTION TECHNIQUES

IN VITRO MATURATION (IVM)

With IVM, eggs are removed from the ovaries and collected when they are still immature. They are then matured in the laboratory, before being fertilised. The difference between IVM and conventional IVF is that the eggs are immature when they are collected. This means that the woman does not need to take as many drugs before the eggs can be collected as she might if using conventional IVF, wherein mature eggs are collected. This is a useful technique, particularly in patients who are susceptible to developing the ovarian hyperstimulation syndrome.

REPRODUCTIVE IMMUNOLOGY

Reproductive immunology (still in its infancy) is a method which offers treatments aimed at the patient's immune system, in an effort to sustain a pregnancy. The theory behind this is that the natural killer (NK) cells, found within the endometrium, may be attacking the implanting embryo, thus resulting in miscarriage. Uterine NK cells are present in large numbers in the wall of the womb at implantation and in the early months of pregnancy. They appear to facilitate the placental link between the mother and the fetus – the mechanism of this is, however, not clear.

Treatments to 'suppress NK cells', offered by some clinics, include high-dose steroids, intravenous immunoglobulin and tumour necrosis factor-a (TNF) blocking agents. These treatments are not licensed for use in reproductive medicine. As with all medical interventions, they carry risks and potential side effects.

PRE-IMPLANTATION GENETIC DIAGNOSIS (PIGD)

PIGD testing involves carrying out tests on embryos, created through IVF or ICSI, to detect certain inherited conditions or abnormalities. The embryo is grown in the laboratory for 2–3 days until the cells have divided and the embryo consists of around eight cells. An embryologist then removes one or two of the cells (blastomeres) from the embryo. The cells are tested to see if the embryo from which they were removed contains the gene that causes a genetic condition in the family. Embryos unaffected by the condition are transferred to the womb for development. Any suitable remaining unaffected embryos can be frozen for later use. Those embryos that are affected by the condition are allowed to perish. Another method, known as the trophectoderm biopsy, is also available, wherein the embryo is allowed to develop for 5–6 days such that there are 100–150 cells. At this stage, cells within an embryo have separated into two types: cells which will form the fetus (inner cell mass) and cells which will form the placenta (trophectoderm). More cells can be removed at this stage (from the trophectoderm) without compromising the viability of the embryo, possibly leading to a more accurate test.

ASSISTED CONCEPTION

HFEA (HUMAN FERTILISATION AND EMBRYOLOGY AUTHORITY)

HFEA was created by an act of the UK parliament in 1990. Its function is to license and monitor clinics that carry out ART (e.g. IVF, DI, etc.). The HFEA inspects each clinic on an annual basis. It also lays down criteria on what is considered as acceptable treatment (e.g. women under the age of 40 can have either one or two embryos transferred (if however, the woman is 40, or over, a maximum of three can be used) it requires clinics to make counselling facilities available to patients; it forbids the payment of donors, etc.). In other countries (e.g. the USA), there are no legal restraints on treatment; however, clinics have an ethical obligation to treat their patients with clinical, rather than commercial, principles in mind.

COUNSELLING

Infertility is not just a medical condition, as it also affects the couple's perceptions of themselves as individuals, their relationship and their functioning in society. The use of assisted reproductive technologies, such as IVF, has allowed many couples to bear children when they could not conceive naturally. However, these technologies may be a mixed blessing – they are stressful to undergo and are by no means completely effective.

It is important, while dealing with subfertile couples, to give them an accurate description of the cause of their infertility and their prognosis, both with and without treatment. The efficacy and the side effects of the various treatment options should be discussed. In addition to this detailed medical information, the couple should be encouraged to explore their feelings about their situation. The use of professionals with counselling skills is invaluable, and, indeed, the provision of counselling facilities is required by the HFEA, as a prerequisite for their licensing of ART providers.

CHAPTER 18

THE MENOPAUSE

The Menopause	382
Signs and Symptoms	*383*
Common Menopausal Symptoms	*383*
The Greene Climacteric Scale	384
Changes in the Genital Tract	385
Osteoporosis	386
Cardiovascular Disease and the Menopause	389
Risks and Benefits of HRT	*390*
HRT and the Breast	*390*
Hormone Replacement Therapy	391
Factors Influencing Prescription of HRT	*391*
Severity of Symptoms and Quality of Life	*391*
Duration of Therapy	*391*
Screening	*391*
Choice of Treatment	*392*
Pros and Cons of Different Routes	*392*
HRT: Miscellaneous	*393*

THE MENOPAUSE

The word menopause means the cessation of menstruation, but it is commonly also used to describe events leading up to, and following, the final menstrual period. For about 10% of women, menses cease suddenly, but for a majority of women, the final period is preceded by several years of erratic periods. This phase is known as the perimenopause.

Oestrogen levels fall over the 5 years preceding ovarian failure, which occurs usually between 45 and 55 years of age, with an average of around 50 years. The fall in oestradiol has a positive feedback effect on the pituitary, increasing the production of follicle stimulating hormone (FSH) and luteinising hormone (LH). Once menopause has occurred, the FSH level is usually above 30 iu/l. FSH levels increase in the perimenopause but levels can fluctuate. The anti-Müllerian hormone (AMH) is a better marker of ovarian reserve. The ovary eventually produces only androstenedione, also produced by the adrenals, which is converted in the peripheral fat to the weak oestrogen, oestrone.

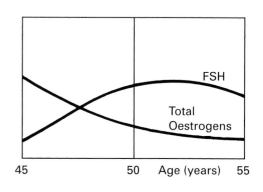

Cause of Menopause
Ovarian failure occurs when only a few thousand primordial follicles remain – an insufficient number to stimulate cyclical activity. Now that women in developed countries have a life expectancy of around 80 years, at least one-third of a woman's life is spent in the post-reproductive, 'menopausal' phase.

Premature menopause may occur due to surgical removal of the ovaries, radiotherapy or chemotherapy; however, for most women, the cause is less clear. Premature ovarian failure is associated with auto-immune conditions, but in some women there may be a genetic element.

There is a slightly higher chance that conserved ovaries may fail following a hysterectomy. Menopause occurs 6–18 months earlier in smokers.

Differential Diagnosis
Before the days of immunological pregnancy tests and effective contraception, pregnancy and menopause were easily confused. Other causes of amenorrhoea, for example, polycystic ovarian syndrome or a prolactinoma should also be considered (see Chapter 6).

		FSH (U/l)	LH (U/l)	Oestradiol (ρmol/l)
Principal changes in serum hormone levels:	Premenopausal	2–20	5–25	100–600
	Postmenopausal	40–70	50–70	60

THE MENOPAUSE

SIGNS AND SYMPTOMS

These are related to changes in circulating oestrogen levels, and the symptoms may start to occur some years before menstruation ceases.

COMMON MENOPAUSAL SYMPTOMS

Vasomotor Symptoms

Hot flushes are the classic menopausal symptom. When they occur at night, they are known as night sweats. This often affects sleep quality and this in turn can affect the quality of life. In a vast majority of women, these will settle within the first few years of menopause, but for some women there will be a long-term problem.

Psychological Symptoms

Emotional liability and mood disturbance.
Poor memory and concentration.
Loss of libido.

Urogenital Atrophy

The epithelium of the genital tract and lower part of the urethra is highly sensitive to oestrogen deprivation. Symptoms include:

Vaginal dryness and dyspareunia
Urinary urgency and frequency

Severity and Duration of Symptoms

It can be useful to attempt to quantify these symptoms, and the following questionnaire demonstrates the variety that can occur.

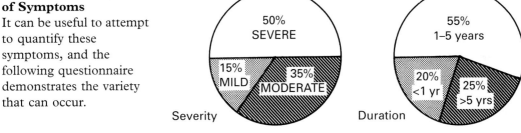

THE GREENE CLIMACTERIC SCALE

Please indicate the extent to which you are troubled at the moment by any of these symptoms by placing a tick in the appropriate box.

SYMPTOMS	Not at all	A little	Quite a bit	Extremely	Score 0–3
1. Heart beating quickly or strongly					
2. Feeling tense or nervous					
3. Difficulty in sleeping					
4. Excitable					
5. Attacks of panic					
6. Difficulty in concentrating					
7. Feeling tired or lacking in energy					
8. Loss of interest in most things					
9. Feeling unhappy or depressed					
10. Crying spells					
11. Irritability					
12. Feeling dizzy or faint					
13. Pressure or tightness in head or body					
14. Parts of body feel numb or tingling					
15. Headaches					
16. Muscle and joint pains					
17. Loss of feeling in the hands or feet					
18. Breathing difficulties					
19. Hot flushes					
20. Sweating at night					
21. Loss of interest in sex					

Psychological (1–11) = ☐ Somatic (12–18) = ☐ Vasomotor (19–20) = ☐

Anxiety (1–6) = ☐ Depression (7–11) = ☐ Sexual dysfunction (21) = ☐

[Greene, J.G. (1991), *Guide to the Greene Climacteric Scale*. University of Glasgow.]

This scale may be used to measure climacteric symptoms and their response to treatment or to compare different treatment regimes.

An Anxiety score of 10 or more indicates severe, and possibly clinical, anxiety. A Depression score of 10 or more indicates severe, and possibly clinical, depression.

CHANGES IN THE GENITAL TRACT

These changes are of atrophic type and affect the external genitalia as well as the internal organs. These changes occur over a number of years.

Not only are the main pelvic structures reduced in size but, more importantly, the fascial framework and the intrapelvic ligaments supporting the bladder and genitalia are weakened; this may lead to vaginal prolapse and urinary incontinence.

Vulva: There is flattening of the labia majora, the minor labia become more evident. Sexual hair becomes grey and sparse. The clitoris shrinks.

Uterus: The uterus becomes small with a relatively large cervix – a return to infantile proportions.

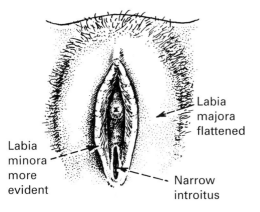

Labia majora flattened

Labia minora more evident

Narrow introitus

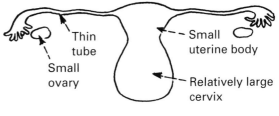

Thin tube

Small ovary

Small uterine body

Relatively large cervix

Tubes and ovaries: These show great shrinkage, the tubes becoming thin while the ovaries are reduced to small white wrinkled bodies, about 2–3 cm in length.

In addition to shrinkage of the vaginal introitus, the vagina diminishes in length and its secretions are limited, leading to vaginal dryness and dyspareunia. Changes in the vaginal epithelium are also seen. There is loss of rugosity and the epithelium becomes atrophic, with petechial haemorrhages in some cases and loss of glycogen.

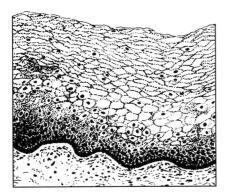

Normal premenopausal vaginal epithelium. Note the thick cornified layer.

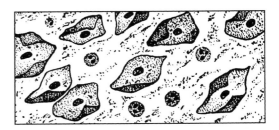

Smear of premenopausal vaginal epithelium. The cells are large with small nuclei and characteristic folded edges. Polymorphs are few in number.

385

OSTEOPOROSIS

Osteoporosis is the most common metabolic bone disease. Postmenopausal osteoporosis results from an excess of bone resorption over bone formation, and is associated with the loss of oestrogen. Women have 20% less bone than men at peak skeletal development, and hence they have less bone to lose before reaching the fragility threshold. More than 50% of Caucasian women suffer one or more osteoporotic fractures by the age of 70. Osteoporotic fractures, particularly of the neck of the femur and vertebrae, have significant impact on the lives of the affected women, and for society as a whole.

Risk factors for osteoporosis are:
1. Female sex.
2. White or oriental race.
3. Family history of osteoporosis.
4. Early menopause (natural or oophorectomy).
5. Sedentary life-style.
6. Low weight for height.
7. Tobacco and alcohol.
8. Low calcium intake.

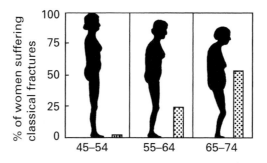

Incidence of classical osteoporotic fractures by decades of life (stipple). Note the loss of height and the development of dorsal kyphosis with age.

DEXA (dual X-ray densitometry) is currently the favoured technique for measuring the lumbar spine and femoral neck densities, even though loss of height or the radiological demonstration of vertebral crush fractures also give clear evidence of osteoporosis. Bone mineral density (BMD) above minus 1 SD below the young adult mean is normal, osteopenia lies between −1 and −2.5 SD and osteoporosis below −2.5 SD of the young adult mean.

Ultrasonic densitometry of the calcaneum is of some value, but is not at present a substitute for DEXA scanning.

OSTEOPOROSIS

BONE DENSITOMETRY

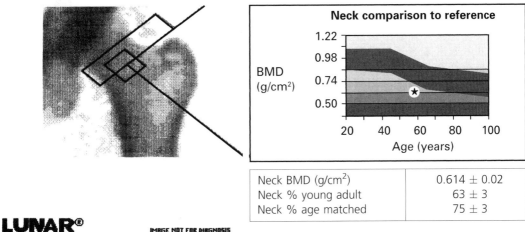

L2–L4 BMD (g/cm²)	0.809 ± 0.01
L2–L4% young adult	67 ± 3
L2–L4% age matched	79 ± 3

Region	BMD g/cm²	Young adult %	T	Age matched %	Z
L2–L4	0.809	67	−3.26	79	−1.80

At −3.26 SD of young adult, there is definite osteoporosis of lumbar spine

Neck BMD (g/cm²)	0.614 ± 0.02
Neck % young adult	63 ± 3
Neck % age matched	75 ± 3

NECK	:BMC (g) = 3.06	Area (cm²) = 4.99
WARDS	:BMC (g) = 1.50	Area (cm²) = 2.76
TROCH	:BMC (g) = 4.47	Area (cm²) = 9.45

Region	BMD g/cm²	Young adult %	T	Age matched %	Z
NECK	0.614	63	−3.05	75	−1.73
WARDS	0.542	60	−2.83	78	−1.18
TROCH	0.473	60	−2.88	67	−2.07

Osteoporosis at all three sites in this hip

OSTEOPOROSIS

Comparative cortical bone thicknesses:

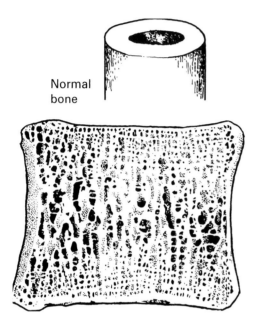

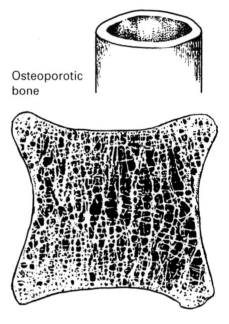

Normal
bone

Osteoporotic
bone

Normal vertebral body. Note
the thick trabeculae of bone.

Vertebrae from postmenopausal
woman showing extreme
rarefaction of the trabeculae.

Oestrogens have an antiresorptive effect on the bone, and there is good evidence that hormone replacement therapy (HRT) use is associated with a decreased risk of fractures. HRT is not recommended as a first line treatment for osteoporosis; however, HRT should be considered for women who have experienced a premature menopause, whether natural or surgical.

First line treatment for osteoporosis is the administration of bisphosphonates, a non-hormonal preparation. Other options include raloxifene, a selective oestrogen receptor modulator that has an antioestrogen effect on the breast and endometrium.

Bone loss recommences on stopping therapy, so withdrawal of HRT at age 65 results in bone density at ages 75 or 80 being no better than that of untreated women.

CARDIOVASCULAR DISEASE AND THE MENOPAUSE

In European countries, 40 to 45% of deaths are due to cardiovascular causes, with a relative increase in risk in females after the menopause. (The actual risk is greater in males even after 75 years.)

Mortality rate for selected causes per 100,000 population in Scotland, 1988.
(Source: Registrar General for Scotland.)

	Endometrial cancer	Cervical cancer	Breast cancer	Lung cancer	Fractured femur (estimated)	Ischaemic heart disease	Cerebro-vascular disease
All ages	4	7	48	52	<20	316	196
45–64	6	14	88	114	<10	170	62
65–74	12	22	130	206	<25	854	325

The risk of coronary heart disease is increased sevenfold by bilateral oophorectomy before 35 years of age and by premature menopause at 35 years. The rates of coronary heart disease are lower for women when compared to men, but there is an increase which occurs in the years after the menopause. Endogenous female hormones have a number of protective effects on the cardiovascular system and HRT has been shown to replicate some of these features.

Lipid metabolism............................. oestrogen increases high density lipoprotein (HDL) cholesterol and lowers low density lipoprotein (HDL) cholesterol.

Carbohydrate metabolism .... oestrogen reduced insulin resistance.

Blood flow... oestrogen increases arterial blood flow.

They also have multiple effects on coagulation and fibrinolysis, with evidence for activation of coagulation. This is particularly the case with oral HRT. There is also evidence of an inflammatory effect as CRP increases with oral HRT.

CARDIOVASCULAR DISEASE AND THE MENOPAUSE

RISKS AND BENEFITS OF HRT

Early observational studies had suggested a number of health benefits associated with HRT use, specifically a significantly lower risk of cardiovascular disease and osteoporosis. It had also been shown that HRT use was associated with a small increase in the risk of breast cancer and that this was higher with long-term use. It had also been shown that HRT use was associated with an increased risk of venous thromboembolic disease.

Several large randomised placebo-controlled trials were published in the late 1990s and the subsequent years. These demonstrated no evidence of HRT having a protective effect against heart disease. The largest of these studies, The Women's Health Initiative, was stopped before completion as there was an overall small increase in the risks, when compared to the benefits of HRT use. A higher risk of breast cancer, venous thromboembolic disease, heart disease and stroke, but a lower risk of osteoporosis and colon cancer, was demonstrated. There is, however, some evidence that HRT, started in the early postmenopausal years, has a cardioprotective effect, presumably before vascular disease has become established.

The results of these studies have significantly reduced HRT prescription and uptake. However, the women recruited were older than the typical HRT seeking population, for symptom control. The current recommendation is that women should be prescribed HRT for menopausal symptoms and not for health benefits such as prevention of osteoporosis. The lowest effective dose should be used for the shortest time possible. This will vary from woman to woman.

HRT AND THE BREAST

Fear of an increased risk of breast cancer is the main cause of concern about HRT, in both patients and doctors.

Breast cancer is increasing in incidence and may affect one woman out of nine in a lifetime.

Alcohol use in young women may increase the risk, and obesity, high socioeconomic status and delayed first pregnancy are other risk factors. Early menarche, late menopause and nulliparity are also risk factors. Only 20% of the subjects have a positive family history. A woman's risk of developing breast cancer is significantly increased when her mother, sister or daughter have developed the disease before the age of 50 years. A number of genetic mutations have been identified, with the commonest being the BRCA gene, and women with a strong family history of breast and ovarian cancer should be referred for genetic counselling.

Early menopause decreases breast cancer risk (70% reduction with menopause before 35 years).

Between the ages of 50 and 70 years, when most HRT is prescribed, 45 women per thousand *not taking HRT*, will develop breast cancer. Using HRT for 5 years between the ages 50 and 70 increases this by only 2 per thousand, 10 years use adds 6 per thousand and 15 years use adds 12 per thousand.

HORMONE REPLACEMENT THERAPY

Oestrogen replacement remains the most effective treatment for menopausal symptoms. The doses required are much lower than those used for oral contraception. For women with an intact uterus progesterone is also required as oestrogen alone (unopposed oestrogen) is associated with endometrial hyperplasia and an increased risk of endometrial cancer.

FACTORS INFLUENCING PRESCRIPTION OF HRT
HRT prescription should be considered carefully for any woman, but a number of factors need to be taken into account and the risks and benefits discussed on an individual basis.

SEVERITY OF SYMPTOMS AND QUALITY OF LIFE
Women who have minimal symptoms may require no treatment. Clearly, women who experience symptoms that affect their quality of life will be more likely to opt for HRT.

Contraindications	Relative contraindications
Pregnancy Uninvestigated abnormal vaginal bleeding Breast cancer or other oestrogen-dependent tumour Venous thromboembolic disease Myocardial infarction or unstable angina Severe liver disease	Cerebrovascular accident Severe migraine Thrombophilia

Route of administration: oral preparations, transdermal patches or gels, implants, local preparations.

Concurrent medication: with anticonvulsant, epileptic, or other liver enzyme inducing therapy, avoid oral HRT.

DURATION OF THERAPY
The main reason for HRT prescription is menopausal symptoms and it may be best to stop HRT at intervals and recommence if symptoms are an ongoing problem.

Women who have experienced a premature menopause should use HRT until the age of natural menopause, that is, around 50 years.

Acceptability of therapy: If side effects are problematic then a review of the regimen should be considered, as well as other treatment options. Withdrawal bleeds and hormonal effects, such as fluid retention, are common side effects and may settle with time.

SCREENING
Screening before and on HRT is similar to well-woman screening.

Women should be encouraged to take part in national breast and cervical screening programmes.

Pelvic examination should be performed only where clinically indicated.

Blood pressure should be checked every 6 months.

HORMONE REPLACEMENT THERAPY

Hormone levels can be useful in women who have had a hysterectomy with conservation of the ovaries; however, hormone levels are not required in the vast majority of women. They can even be normal in the perimenopause. HRT should only be prescribed on a clinical basis.

CHOICE OF TREATMENT
This involves the following considerations:

Routes of administration
1. Oral – tablets.
2. Transdermal – patches.
3. Percutaneous – gel.
4. Subcutaneous – implants.
5. Vaginal
   - cream
   - pessary
   - tablet
   - ring (silastic).

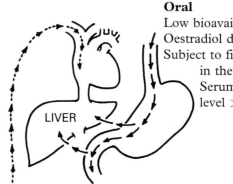

Oral
Low bioavailability.
Oestradiol dose in mg/day.
Subject to first pass metabolism
   in the liver.
Serum oestrone
level > oestradiol level.

LIVER

Parenteral
High bioavailability.
Oestradiol dose absorbed in μg/day.
No first pass metabolism in the liver.
Serum oestradiol level > oestrone level (more physiological).

PROS AND CONS OF DIFFERENT ROUTES

Oral
1. Economical.
2. Wide choice of preparations and doses.
3. Absorbed into portal system and passes through liver before reaching systemic circulation with metabolism to oestrone and liver enzyme induction. More effects on lipids and coagulation.
4. May cause nausea.

Transdermal and Percutaneous
1. More physiological, with absorption into and distribution by systemic circulation, and not the hepatic portal system.
2. Lesser effect on coagulation.
3. High patient acceptability (if no skin irritation).
4. More costly.

HORMONE REPLACEMENT THERAPY

Subcutaneous Implants (25 or 50 mg pure crystalline oestradiol)
1. Can be effective where other routes fail.
2. Risk of escalation of oestradiol levels, so strict control of dose and frequency of implants is necessary. Some women will be symptomatic even with supraphysiological oestradiol levels, this is known as tachyphylaxis.

Vaginal Preparations
Oestriol preparations and low dose oestradiol tablets (0.025 mg) do not have systemic effects, and can give local benefit in women with contraindications to systemic therapy.

Potent oestrogens given vaginally have systemic effects.

Vaginal preparations relieve atrophic vaginitis, trigonitis, vaginal dryness and dyspareunia.

Vaginal silastic ring pessaries can be low dose oestradiol for local effect, or higher dose oestradiol to get a parenteral, systemic effect, with each pessary lasting for 3 months.

Alternatives to Oestrogen
When systemic oestrogen is contraindicated, not tolerated or declined, the following may be useful:
1. Progestogens (norethisterone, megestrol acetate, medroxyprogesterone acetate). In significant doses, there is an increased risk of thrombosis.
2. Low dose vaginal oestrogen preparations for urogenital symptoms.
3. Selective serotonin reuptake inhibitors have been shown to be effective for some women.

HRT: MISCELLANEOUS

Contraception in the Climacteric
Ovulation may occur after 6 months of amenorrhoea.

Most HRT preparations are not contraceptive.

Effective contraception is recommended until 1 year after menstruation ceases, in the absence of a vasectomy or female sterilisation. After the age of 45, it is considered that intrauterine devices (IUDs) do not require to be renewed regularly and that they can be left *in situ* till there is no risk of pregnancy. Levonorgestrel releasing IUDs serve a double purpose, giving excellent contraceptive protection and also countering the effects of oestrogen on the endometrium.

Barrier contraception has a low failure rate in climacteric women.

Notes

vs. indicates a comparison or differential diagnosis

The following abbreviations have been used:

CIN - cervical intra-epithelial neoplasia

DVT - deep vein thrombosis

FSH - follicle-stimulating hormone

GnRH - gonadotrophin releasing hormone

HRT - hormone replacement therapy

IUDs - intra-uterine devices

LH - luteinizing hormone

Abdominal aorta 34, 41
Abdominal examination 75–77
  ascites 77
  hypersplenism 76
  kidney palpation 76
  liver enlargement 76
  obesity 77
  ovarian cysts 75, 77
  palpation 76
  pregnancy 75
  uterus enlargement 75
Abdominal hysterectomy
  endometrial cancer treatment 209
  total 209
  urinary fistula formation 292
Abdominal pain
  pedicle torsion 259
  tubal pregnancy 321
Abdominal ultrasound, obesity 77
Ablation, CIN treatment 180–181
Abnormal bleeding
  definition 71
  see also specific types of haemorrhage
Abortion
  tubal 323
  see also Miscarriage; Pregnancy termination
Accessory horn, uterus 65
Aciclovir, genital herpes 140

Actinomycin D, sarcoma botriodes 171
Acute pelvic inflammation, ovarian cyst accidents *vs.* 261
Acute pelvic inflammatory disease 149
Addisonian crisis, congenital adrenal hyperplasia 63
Adenocanthoma, cervical cancer 184
Adenocarcinoma
  cervical cancer 184
  Fallopian tubes carcinoma 285
Adenocarcinoma *in situ* 159
Adenomyosis 122
  microscopy 122
Adhesions, surgical complications 293
Adjuvant chemotherapy, ovarian epithelial tumours 277
Adnexal mass, tubal pregnancy 321
Adrenal-like tumours 274
Adriamycin, endometrial cancer recurrence treatment 210
Adult uterus 38
Adventitia, ureter 233
Age, contraception failure rates 339
Age-related changes 39–41
  ovary 38
  uterus 38
  vagina 38
  vulva 38
AIDS 153
  intercurrent infections 154
  lymphomas 153
  paediatric 154
  see also HIV infection
Alkylating agents, mechanism of action 281
Ambulation, DVT 300
Amenorrhoea 88
  causes 89
  history taking 102
  hyperprolactinaemia 99
  investigation 102–104
    progesterone challenge test 102
    prolactin levels 102
    TSH 102
  physical examination 102
  physiological 89
    lactation 89

menopause 89
  pregnancy 89
  primary 71
  secondary 71
  treatment 96
AMH *see* Anti-Müllerian hormone (AMH)
Ampicillin, pelvic inflammatory disease management 149
Ampule implantation, tubal pregnancy 323
Anabolic steroids, sperm production abnormalities 366
Anaemia, uterine fibroids 199
Anaesthetic, IUD insertion 347
Anal triangle 12
Anatomical perineum 12
Androgen-producing tumours
  hirsutism 105
  ovaries 273–274
Anembryonic pregnancy 309
Anorexia nervosa 101
Antegrade pyelography 291
Anterior colporrhaphy
  stress incontinence 245
  vaginal prolapse 223–224
Anterior fornix, vagina 23
Anterior vaginal prolapse 218
Anteverted uterus retroversion 214
Anti-androgens, hirsutism treatment 108
Antibiotic therapy
  broad-spectrum *see* Broad spectrum antibiotics
  Candida albicans infection 136
  combined oral contraceptive pill failure 342
Anti-cardiolipin antibody syndrome 316
Anti-coagulant therapy, pulmonary embolism 305
Anti-depressants, sperm production abnormalities 366
Anti-D immunoglobulin, miscarriage management 312
Anti-hypertensive drugs, sperm production abnormalities 366
Anti-malarial drugs, sperm production abnormalities 366

Anti-metabolites
  mechanism of action 281
  ovarian tumour treatment 282
Anti-mitotics, mechanism of action 281
Anti-Müllerian hormone (AMH)
  complete androgen insensitivity 62
  menopause 382
Anti-progesterone priming,
  miscarriage management 312, 313
Anti-retroviral drugs, HIV infection
  154
Anti-sperm antibodies 367
Appendicitis, pelvic inflammatory
  disease vs. 149
Arcuate uterus 66
Arrhenoblastoma, ovarian tumours
  263
Arterial blood gases, pulmonary
  embolism 303
Artificial urinary sphincters, stress
  incontinence treatment 244
Ascites
  abdominal examination 77
  ovarian tumours vs. 255
Asherman's syndrome 91
Assisted conception 370, 374–379
  donor conception 378
  ectopic pregnancy 320
  folic acid administration 370
  gamete intrafallopian transfer 378
  HFEA 380
  intracytoplasmic sperm injection
    378
  intrauterine insemination 378–379
  pre-implantation genetic diagnosis
    379
  pre-pregnancy infection screening
    370
  reproductive immunology 379
  in vitro fertilization see In vitro
    fertilization
  in vitro maturation 379
Asymptomatic vaginal prolapse 220
Atrophic vaginitis 139
Atypical epithelium identification,
  cervical cancer 179
Atypical hyperplasia, endometrial
  hyperplasia 201
Autoantibodies, sperm production
  abnormalities 366
Autoimmune factors, recurrent
  miscarriage 315
Autonomic nerve supply, pelvis 44
Azithromycin
  Chlamydia trachomatis infection 142
  pelvic inflammatory disease
    management 149

Backache, vaginal prolapse 220
Bacterial infections 142
  see also specific infections

Bacterial vaginosis 137
Bacteriology, pelvic inflammatory
  disease 149
Ball diathermy, CIN treatment 181
Barrier contraception methods 338
Bartholin's glands 15
  cysts 158
  ducts 14
  embryology 8
  histology 15
  infection, superficial dyspareunia
    334
  obstruction, inflammation 133
  secretions 132
  vulval examination 78
Basal body temperature changes,
  ovulation 361
Benign papilloma, genital warts vs.
  141
Benign squamous metaplasia, cervix
  174
Benign tumours
  vagina 168
  vulva 158
Bicornuate (double) uterus 65
Bilateral oophorectomy, heavy
  uterine bleeding 118
Bilateral salpingo-oophorectomy
  endometrial cancer treatment 209
  Fallopian tubes carcinoma 285
  premenstrual syndrome treatment
    130
  uterine leiomyosarcoma 212
  uterine sarcoma 212
Billings' method (ovulation method)
  351
Bimanual pelvic examination 79
  uterine retroversion 215
  vaginal discharge 135
Biopsies
  atypical epithelium identification
    179
  cervical cancer diagnosis 186
  trophectoderm 379
Bisphosphonates, osteoporosis 388
Bladder
  blood supply 39–40
  cancer, urinary fistula formation
    293
  full, ovarian tumours vs. 255
  function examination 242
  injuries, surgical complications
    288
  innervation 235
  retraining, detrusor instability
    treatment 249
Bladder neck relaxation (funnelling)
  236
Bleeding, intermenstrual
  see Intermenstrual bleeding
Blighted ovum 309

Blood flow, menopause 389
Blood loss estimation, dysfunctional
  uterine bleeding 110
Blood stream, ovarian tumour
  spread 277
Blood supply
  ovary 34
  uterus 39–40
  vagina 39–40
Blood vessel walls, venous
  thrombosis 296
BMD (bone mineral density),
  osteoporosis 386
Bone mineral density (BMD),
  osteoporosis 386
Borderline nuclear changes, cervical
  smears 177
Botox, vaginismus treatment 334
Bowel injury, surgical complications
  291
Brachytherapy, cervical cancer 189
BRCA 1, ovarian tumours 264
BRCA 2, ovarian tumours 264
Breast(s)
  examination 83–85
  hormone effects 52, 53
  HRT 390
Breast cancer, HRT 390
Breastfeeding, as contraception
  351
Brenner tumour 263, 271
Broad ligament 29, 34–37
  blood vessels 33
  cysts (parovarian cysts) 283
    diagnosis 284
    surgery 284
  cysts vs. ovarian tumours 258
  vestigial structures 33
Broad spectrum antibiotics
  miscarriage management 311
  pelvic inflammatory disease
    management 149
Bromocriptine
  hyperprolactinaemia treatment
    100
  infertility treatment 372
Bulb of vestibule, vulva 15
Bulbospongiosus muscle 16
Burch's colposuspension operation
  247
Buserelin, infertility treatment 372

CA125, ovarian tumours 253
Cabergoline
  hyperprolactinaemia treatment
    100
  infertility treatment 372
CAH (congenital adrenal
  hyperplasia) 63
Call–Exner bodies, gonadoblastoma
  268

Candida albicans infection 136
Caps, contraception 349
Carbohydrate metabolism,
  menopause 389
Carbon dioxide laser, CIN treatment
  180
Carboplatin
  ovarian tumour treatment
    277, 282
  side effects 282
Carcinoid ovarian tumours 275
Carcinoma, ovarian tumours 264
Carcinosarcoma, uterine sarcoma
  211, 212
Cardinal ligaments 30, 216
Cardiovascular disease, menopause
  see Menopause
Cardiovascular system, hormone
  effects 53
Caruncle, urethra 165
Carunculae myrtiformes 14
CEA, ovarian tumours 253
Cefixime, gonorrhoea treatment 144
Ceftriaxone
  gonorrhoea treatment 144
  pelvic inflammatory disease
    management 149
Central pulmonary embolism 302
Cervical cancer (carcinoma) 178,
  183
  adenocanthoma 184
  adenocarcinoma 184
  atypical epithelium identification
    179
  chemotherapy 189
    surgery *vs.* 193
  clinical findings 183
  diagnosis 186
  differential diagnosis 186
  direct spread 185
  dysplasia 178
  FIGO staging 188
  microinvasive 178
  palliative care 193
  premalignant 178
  prognosis 193
  radiotherapy 189
    advantages 193
    brachytherapy 189
    complications 189
    external beam therapy 189
  screening (cervical smear)
    see Cervical smears
  spread 185
  squamous cell carcinoma 184
  staging 187–188
    magnetic resonance imaging
      188
    stage IA 187
    stage IA1 187
    stage IA2 187

stage IB 187
    stage IB1 187
    stage IB2 187
    stage II 187
    stage IIA 187
    stage IIA1 187
    stage IIA2 187
    stage IIB 187
    stage III 188
    stage IIIa 188
    stage IIIb 188
    stage IV 188
    stage IVa 188
    stage IVb 188
  surgery 190–193
    advantages 193
    chemotherapy *vs.* 193
    complications 192
    exenteration for relapsed
      disease 192
    fertility-sparing surgery 192
    large loop excision of the
      transformation zone 190
    microinvasive 190
    radical hysterectomy and node
      dissection 190–191
    radical surgery 192
  symptoms 183
  see also Cervical intra-epithelial
    neoplasia (CIN)
Cervical intra-epithelial neoplasia
  (CIN) 178
  grade 1 178
    treatment 180
  grade 2 178
    treatment 180
  grade 3 178
    treatment 180
  progression risk 178
  treatment 180–182
    ablation 180–181
    ball diathermy 181
    carbon dioxide laser 180
    cold coagulation 180
    cryosurgery 181
    excisional techniques 181–182
    follow-up 182
    knife cone biopsy 182
    large loop excision of the
      transformation zone 181
    laser cone biopsy 182
    Loop Electrosurgical Excision
      procedure 181
Cervical smears 176
  borderline nuclear changes 177
  colposcopy referral 177
  glandular abnormalities 177
  inflammation 177
  interpretation 177
  mild dyskaryosis 177
  moderate dyskaryosis 177

normal 177
  severe dyskaryosis 177
Cervicitis with ectopy, cervical
  cancer *vs.* 186
Cervix 26, 27
  anatomy 174
  benign squamous metaplasia
    174
  bimanual pelvic examination 79
  cancer *see* Cervical cancer
    (carcinoma)
  diseases 173–193
    see also specific diseases/disorders
  ectocervix 174
  ectopy 148
  endocervix 174
  glands 31
    secretions 132
  histology 31
  normal epithelium 174
  physiological variation 148
  relationship with ureter 28
  trauma, dilatation and curettage
    113
  vaginal discharge 134
  weakness, recurrent miscarriage
    314, 316
Cetrotide, infertility treatment 372
Chancre
  cervical cancer *vs.* 186
  syphilis 145
Chancroid 143
Chaperones, gynaecological
  examination 74
Chemotherapy
  adjuvant, ovarian epithelial
    tumours 277
  cervical cancer 189
  endometrial cancer recurrence
    treatment 210
  mechanisms 281
  ovarian tumours 281
  side effects 282
  sperm production abnormalities
    366
  toxicity 282
  vulval carcinoma 164
  see also specific drugs
Chest x-ray, pulmonary embolism
  303
Chlamydia trachomatis infection 142
  sperm production abnormalities
    366
Choriocarcinoma
  gestational *see* Gestational
    choriocarcinoma
  ovarian tumours 275
Chromosome analysis, genetic
  abnormalities 59
Chronic pelvic inflammatory disease
  150

397

Chronic thromboembolic
   hypertension 305
Ciliated cells, Fallopian tubes 32
Cimetidine, sperm production
   abnormalities 366
CIN *see* Cervical intra-epithelial
   neoplasia (CIN)
Cisplatin, endometrial cancer
   recurrence treatment 210
Clear cell carcinoma
   endometrial cancer 204
   ovarian tumours 263
Clindamycin, bacterial vaginosis 137
Clinical syndromes
   genetic abnormalities 59
   see also specific diseases/disorders
Clitoris 12, 13–14
   embryology 8
Clobetasol propionate, lichen
   sclerosus treatment 157
Clomiphene, infertility treatment
   96, 371
Clotrimazole, *Candida albicans*
   infection 136
Coccygeus muscle 19
   nerve supply 19
COCP *see* Combined oral
   contraceptive pill (COCP)
Coelomic epithelium
   genital ridges 3
   sex cords 3
Coitus
   definition 337
   excitatory phase 332
   orgasm 333
   plateau phase 332
   postcoital (resolution) phase
      333
   problems, vaginal prolapse 220
Cold coagulation, CIN treatment
   180
Colon, surgical injury 291
Colpoperineorrhaphy, posterior 227
Colporrhaphy, anterior *see* Anterior
   colporrhaphy
Colposcopy 179
   definition 179
   referral, cervical smears 177
Combined oral contraceptive pill
   (COCP) 340–341
   amenorrhoea treatment 96
   choice 341
   constituents 341
      drospirenone 341
      ethinyloestradiol 341
      progestogens 341
   contraindications 343
   corpus luteum absence 340
   dysmenorrhoea treatment 121
   endometriosis treatment 127
   failure of 342

heavy uterine bleeding
   management 114
hirsutism treatment 108
low dose 341
mode of action 340
premenstrual syndrome treatment
   130
side effects 342
   endometrium effects 344
   hypertension 343
   neoplasia 344
   ovary 344
   stroke 343
   thromboembolism 343
   vascular disease 343
standard strength 341
venous thromboembolism risk
   341
Common iliac artery 39
Comparative cortical bone
   thicknesses, osteoporosis 388
Complete androgen insensitivity
   62–63
Complete hydatiform mole
   see Hydatiform mole
Complete miscarriage 308
Complete procidentia 217
Compliance, combined oral
   contraceptive pill failure 342
Computed tomography (CT)
   endometrial cancer 206
   hyperprolactinaemia 99
   ovarian tumour diagnosis 255
   pulmonary angiography,
      pulmonary embolism 304
   renogram, ureteric surgical injury
      290
Conception, assisted *see* Assisted
   conception
Concurrent medication, HRT 391
Condoms, contraception 350
Congenital adrenal hyperplasia
   (CAH) 63
Congenital adrenal hyperplasia,
   hirsutism 105
Congenital androgen insensitivity 91
Congenital urinary fistula 293
Conservative management, tubal
   pregnancy treatment 324
Contraception 331–356
   barrier methods 338
   caps 349
   condoms 350
   contraindications 339
   diaphragms 349
   failure rates 339
   history taking 70
   hormonal methods 338, 340–341
   see also Combined oral
      contraceptive pill (COCP)
   implantable chemicals 354

natural methods 338
patient suitability 339
postcoital (morning after) 352
spermicides 338
sponge 350
success rates 338
surgery 338
time of ovulation 351
see also specific methods
Contrast venography, DVT 299
Copper, IUDs 346
Cornual implantation, tubal
   pregnancy 323
Corona radiata 47
Corpus albicans, ovary 37
Corpus luteum 36
   absence, combined oral
      contraceptive pill 340
   FSH 36
   hormones 36, 89
   LH 36
Corpus, uterus *see* Uterus
Cortex, ovary 35, 46
Cortical bone thicknesses,
   osteoporosis 388
Corticosteroids
   congenital adrenal hyperplasia 63
   sperm production abnormalities
      366
Counselling
   infertility 380
   sterilization 353
Cramp, dysmenorrhoea 120
Crinone, infertility treatment 372
Cruciate anastomosis 41
Crush injury, ureteric surgical injury
   290
Cryocautery, genital warts therapy
   141
Cryosurgery, CIN treatment 181
CT *see* Computed tomography (CT)
Cumulus oophorus 47
Curettage
   and dilatation *see* Dilatation and
      curettage
   miscarriage management 312
   placental site trophoblastic
      tumour 196
Cusco's speculum 71
Cyclogest, infertility treatment 372
Cyclophosphamide, sarcoma
   botriodes 171
Cyproterone, hirsutism treatment
   108
Cyst(s)
   Bartholin's glands 158
   uterine retroversion 215
   vagina 168
Cystadenocarcinoma
   mucinous 263, 266
   serous 263, 265

Cystadenoma
   mucinous 263
   serous 263, 265
Cystectomy, ovarian tumours 276
Cystic degeneration, uterine fibroids 199
Cystoceles 218
   anterior colporrhaphy 223–224
Cystometry 236, 242
   abnormal 242
   stress incontinence 242
Cystotomy
   closure 288
   Foley catheter 288
Cyst pedicle torsion, pelvic inflammatory disease vs. 149
Cytogenetics, gestational trophoblastic disease 327
Cytology, ovarian tumours 278

Danazol, endometriosis 128
Deep dyspareunia 73, 334
Deep perineal pouch 17
Deep vein thrombosis (DVT)
   ambulation 300
   clinical features 298
   definition 295
   hydration 300
   investigations 299
   post operative physiotherapy 300
   thromboprophylaxis 300
      graduated elastic compression stocking 300
      low molecular weight heparins 301
      mechanical methods 300
      pneumatic stocking 300
      unfractionated heparin 301
   treatment 301
Defeminisation
   Sertoli–Leydig cell tumour 273
   see also Masculinization
Dehydroepiandrosterone sulphate (DHAS), virilisation 106
Depilatory cream, hirsutism 107
Depilatory waxes, hirsutism 107
Dermatoses, vulva 156–157
Detrusor contraction, micturition 236
Detrusor instability 237
   stress incontinence vs. 241
   symptoms 237
   treatment 249
Dexamethasone, hirsutism treatment 108
DEXA (dual x-ray densitometry), osteoporosis 386
DHAS (dehydroepiandrosterone sulphate), virilisation 106

Diabetes insipidus, incontinence 243
Diabetes mellitus, incontinence 243
Diabetes mellitus type II, polycystic ovarian syndrome 94
Diaphragms, contraception 349
Diathermy, hirsutism 107
Dilatation and curettage 112
   complications 113
   pregnancy termination 319
Dilatation and evacuation, miscarriage management 313
Diverticulitis, pelvic inflammatory disease vs. 149
Doderlein's bacillus 132
   vaginal secretions 15
Donor conception, assisted conception 378
Dopamine agonists, hyperprolactinaemia 98
Double (bicornuate) uterus 65
Doxorubicin, side effects 282
Doxycycline
   Chlamydia trachomatis infection 142
   pelvic inflammatory disease management 149
Drospirenone, combined oral contraceptive pill 341
Drug(s)
   detrusor instability treatment 249
   hirsutism 108
   hyperprolactinaemia 98
   sperm production abnormalities 366
Drug-caused hirsutism 105
Drug interactions, combined oral contraceptive pill failure 342
Dual X-ray densitometry (DEXA), osteoporosis 386
Duplex Doppler leg ultrasound, pulmonary embolism 304
DVT see Deep vein thrombosis (DVT)
Dysfunctional uterine bleeding 110
   blood loss estimation 110
   definition 110
   transvaginal ultrasound 110
Dysgenesis, ovary 64
Dysgerminoma, ovarian tumours 263, 268
Dyskaryosis, severe 177
Dysmenorrhoea 120–121
   aetiology 120
   clinical features 121
   cramp 120
   definition 72
   drug treatment 121
   management 121
   pain 120
   primary 72

   secondary 72
   uterine fibroids 198
Dyspareunia 73, 334
   deep 73, 334
   menopause 385
   superficial 73, 334
   uterine retroversion 215
   vaginal hysterectomy complications 230
Dysplasia, cervical cancer 178
Dysuria, incontinence 239

Early fetal demise 309
Early pregnancy 307–330
   bleeding, gestational trophoblastic disease 327
Early proliferative phase, endometrial cycle 51
Ectocervix 174
Ectopia vesicae, vulva 68
Ectopic deposits, endometriosis 123
Ectopic kidney, ovarian tumours vs. 258
Ectopic pregnancy 320
   aetiology 320
      assisted conception 320
      IUDs 320
      pelvic inflammatory disease 320
      tubal damage 320
   Fallopian tubes see Tubal pregnancy
   ovarian cyst accidents vs. 261
Ectopy, cervix 148
Eflornithine cream, hirsutism treatment 108
EIAs (enzyme immunoassays), syphilis diagnosis 146
Ejaculatory failure 336
Electrocardiogram (ECG), pulmonary embolism 303–304
Electro-cautery, genital warts therapy 141
Electrolysis, hirsutism 107
ELISA (enzyme-linked immunosorbent assay), genital herpes diagnosis 140
Embryo abnormalities, recurrent miscarriage 314
Embryology 1–9
   Bartholin's glands 8
   clitoris 8
   Fallopian tubes see Fallopian tubes
   female external genitalia 7–8
      genital (labial) swelling 8
      genital tubercle 8
      urethral folds 8
   genital ridges 2, 3
   germ cells 2
   labia minor 8

Embryology (Continued)
  male external genitalia 9
    primary urethral groove 9
    scrotum 9
    testes 9
  mesonephric ducts 6
  Müllerian (paramesonephric) duct 5, 6
  Müllerian tubercle 5
  ovary see Ovaries
  para-urethral glands of Skene 8
  rete 3
  urethra 7
  urethral glands 8
  urogenital buds 8
  urogenital sinus 7
  uterus see Uterus
  Wolffian (mesonephric) ridge 5
Embryo transfer, in vitro fertilization 376
Endocervix 174
Endocrine disease
  incontinence 243
  recurrent miscarriage 315, 316
Endometrial cancer 203–204
  aetiology 207
  clear cell carcinoma 204
  computed tomography 206
  diagnosis 203
  grade 1 204
  grade 2 204
  grade 3 204
  histology 204
  magnetic resonance imaging 206
  obesity 207
  polycystic ovarian syndrome 96
  postmenopause 203
  presentation 203
  prognosis 208
    FIGO staging 208
  recurrence 210
    sites 210
    treatment 210
  spread of 206
    local 206
    lymphatic spread 206
  staging 205
    FIGO staging 205
    stage I 205
    stage II 205
    stage III 205
    stage IV 205
  treatment 209
    recurrence 210
Endometrial cycle 51
  early proliferative phase 51
  late proliferative phase 51
  menstruation 51
  secretory phase 51
Endometrial hyperplasia 201–202
  aetiology 202

atypical hyperplasia 201
  classification 201
  clinical findings 201
  complex 201
  investigations 202
  polycystic ovarian syndrome 96
  simple 201
  treatment 202
Endometrioid carcinoma, ovarian tumours 263
Endometrioma, ovarian tumours 263
Endometriosis 123–125
  clinical findings 126
  cyclical activity 125
  differential diagnosis 127
  ectopic deposits 124
  haemorrhage 124
  histogenesis 127
  histology 125
  imaging 127
  laparoscopy 126
  medical treatment 127–128
  menstrual abnormalities 126
  pathology 123
  physical examination 126
  prevalence 126
  secondary pathology 124
  surgical treatment 128
  symptoms 126
  treatment 127–128
  uterine retroversion 215
Endometrium 31
  ablation, heavy uterine bleeding 115
  biopsies 112
    methods 112
    ovulation evidence 362
  cancer see Endometrial cancer
  combined oral contraceptive pill effects 344
  hyperplasia see Endometrial hyperplasia
  investigation 111
  polyps 196
  stromal sarcomas 211, 212
  thickness, transvaginal ultrasound 111
Endoscope, laparoscopy 83, 84
Enterocele 219
  repair of 228
Environmental factors
  recurrent miscarriage 315, 316
  sperm production abnormalities 366
Enzyme immunoassays (EIAs), syphilis diagnosis 146
Enzyme-linked immunosorbent assay (ELISA), genital herpes diagnosis 140

Epithelium
  ovary 46
    tumours see Ovarian tumours
  vagina 24
Epoöphoron 283
  broad ligament 33
Erectile dysfunction 335
  treatment 336
Ethambutol, genital tuberculosis treatment 152
Ethinyloestradiol
  combined oral contraceptive pill 341
  hirsutism treatment 108
Evening primrose oil, premenstrual syndrome treatment 130
Excisional techniques, CIN treatment 181–182
Excitatory phase, coitus 332
Exercise, hypothalamic disorders 101
Explanations to patients, gynaecological examination 74
Expulsion, IUD complications 348
External anal sphincter 16
External beam therapy, cervical cancer 189
External iliac artery 39, 41
External urethral orifice 14
  vulva 14
Extra-amniotic termination, pregnancy termination 319
Extremity elevation, lymphoedema 294

Fainting/collapse, tubal pregnancy 321
Fallopian tubes 33
  abnormalities 64
  carcinoma 285
    clinical staging 285
  ciliated cells 32
  damage, ectopic pregnancy 320
  development 5–6
  diseases/disorders 251–285
    see also specific diseases/disorders
  menopause 385
  patency, infertility see Infertility
  'peg' cells 32
  pregnancy see Tubal pregnancy
  rupture, tubal pregnancy 323
Falloscopy, tubal patency 369
Female external genitalia, embryology see Embryology; specific anatomical features
Femoral artery 41
Ferriman Galway charts, hirsutism 107
Fertility drugs 371–372

Fertility requirements, history taking 70
Fertility-sparing surgery, cervical cancer 192
Fever, surgical complications 294
Fibrin D-dimer assay, DVT 299
Fibroma
    Meig's syndrome 272
    ovarian tumours 263, 272
    vulva 158
FIGO staging
    cervical cancer 188
    endometrial cancer 205
        prognosis 208
    vulval carcinoma 160
Fimbrian cysts 33, 284
Finasteride, hirsutism treatment 108
Fistula formation, surgical complications 292–293
Fitz–Hugh–Curtis syndrome, *Chlamydia trachomatis* infection 142
Flow volume, venous thrombosis 296
Fluid balance chart, incontinence 243
Fluorescent Treponemal antibody tests 146
5-Fluorouracil chemotherapy, vaginal intra-epithelial neoplasia 169
Flutamide, hirsutism treatment 108
Foley's catheter
    cystotomy 288
    Marshall–Marchetti–Krantz urethropexy 246
Folic acid administration, assisted conception 370
Follicle-stimulating hormone (FSH)
    corpus luteum 36
    follicular phase 50
    infertility treatment 372
    luteal phase 50
    menopause 89, 382
    menstruation 50
    ovulation 48, 50
    polycystic ovarian syndrome 94
    premature ovarian failure 93
Follicle tracking, in vitro fertilization 374
Follicular atresia, ovary 37
Follicular phase, hormones 50
Follow-up, CIN treatment 182
Foreign bodies, vaginitis 139
Fornices, vagina 23
Fossa naviculatis 14
Fothergill suture 226
Fourchette 13
Frenulum 13

FSH *see* Follicle-stimulating hormone (FSH)
Full bladder, ovarian tumours *vs.* 255
Funnelling (bladder neck relaxation) 236

Gamete intrafallopian transfer (GIFT) 378
Gartner's duct, broad ligament 33
Gastroenteritis, combined oral contraceptive pill failure 342
GECS (graduated elastic compression stocking), DVT 300
Gemeprost, miscarriage management 312, 313
Genetics
    gestational trophoblastic disease 327
    recurrent miscarriage 314, 316
Genital herpes 140
Genital ridges
    coelomic epithelium 3
    embryology 2, 3
    mesoderm 3
Genital (labial) swelling, embryology 8
Genital tract
    hormone effects 52, 53
    menopausal changes
        see Menopause
Genital tubercle, embryology 8
Genital tuberculosis 151–152
    cervical cancer *vs.* 186
    clinical features 151
    diagnosis 151
    pathology 151
    treatment 152
    urinary fistula formation 293
Genital warts 141
    differential diagnosis 141
Germ cells
    embryology 2
    maturation 58
    see also Meiosis
    tumours *see* Ovarian tumours
Gestational choriocarcinoma 329
    chemotherapy 330
Gestational trophoblastic disease 325
    cytogenetics 327
    genetics 327
    pathology 326
    presentation 327
    treatment 328
    see also Hydatiform mole
Gestational trophoblastic neoplasia 328–329
    malignant 328
    placental site trophoblastic tumour 329

Gestone, infertility treatment 372
GIFT (gamete intrafallopian transfer) 378
Glandular abnormalities, cervical smears 177
Glycosuria, *Candida albicans* infection 136
GnRH *see* Gonadotrophin releasing hormone (GnRH)
GnRHa *see* Gonadotrophin releasing hormone analogues (GnRHa)
Gonadal dysgenesis 92
Gonadal removal, complete androgen insensitivity 62
Gonadoblastoma, ovarian tumours 263, 268
Gonadotrophin(s)
    infertility treatment 372
    in vitro fertilization 374
Gonadotrophin releasing hormone (GnRH)
    ovulation 49, 50
    puberty 54
Gonadotrophin releasing hormone analogues (GnRHa)
    endometriosis treatment 128
    hirsutism treatment 108
    infertility treatment 371, 372
    premenstrual syndrome 129
    premenstrual syndrome treatment 130
    uterine fibroid treatment 200
Gonadotrophin releasing hormone antagonists, infertility treatment 372
Gonorrhoea 144
    diagnosis 144
    examination 144
Goserelin, infertility treatment 372
Graafian follicles 36, 47
    insulin-like growth factor-1 47
    LH 47
Graduated elastic compression stocking (GECS), DVT 300
Granuloma inguinale 143
Granulosa cells 47
    tumour 263
Greene climacteric scale, menopause 384
Gubernaculum, ovary development 4
Gynaecological examination 74
    abdominal examination
        see Abdominal examination
    bimanual pelvic examination 79
    breast examination 83–85
    chaperone 74
    explanations to patients 74
    laparoscopy *see* Laparoscopy
    principles 74
    speculum examination 80–81

Gynaecological examination
  (Continued)
  vulval examination 78
  see also Physical examination
Gynaecological perineum 12
Gynaecomastia, Klinefelter's
  syndrome 61
Gynatresia, vagina 67

Haematoma, vulva 158
Haematometra 90
Haematosalpinx 90
Haemoatocolpos 90
Haemophilus ducreyi infection
  see Chancroid
Haemorrhage
  endometriosis 124
  laparoscopy complications 85
  miscarriage management 311
  uterus see Heavy uterine bleeding
Hairy leukoplakia 153
Heart disease, HRT 390
Heavy uterine bleeding
  management 114–119
  medical management 114
  surgical management 115
    bilateral oophorectomy 118
    endometrial ablation 115
    laparoscopy assisted vaginal
      hysterectomy 119
    microwave endometrial
      ablation 116
    Novasure 116
    subtotal hysterectomy 118
    Thermachoice 116
    total hysterectomy 116–117
    total laparoscopic hysterectomy
      119
    vaginal hysterectomy 119
Heparin
  DVT treatment 301
  pulmonary embolism 305
Hereditary non-polyposis colorectal
  cancer (Lynch II) syndrome 207
Hernia, surgical complications 294
Herpes simplex virus type 1 (HSV1)
  140
  infection see Genital herpes
Herpes simplex virus type 2 (HSV2)
  140
  infection see Genital herpes
HFEA, assisted conception 380
High grade stromal sarcomas,
  uterine sarcoma 212
Hilar cell tumours 263, 274
Hilum, ovary 34, 35
Hirsutism 106
  androgen producing tumours 105
  congenital adrenal hyperplasia
    105
  definition 105

drug-caused 105
Ferriman Galway charts 107
idiopathic 105
management 96, 107–108
  drug treatment 108
  local 107
polycystic ovary disease 105
Histology, endometriosis 125
History taking 69–85, 70–71
  contraceptive requirements 70
  difficult situations 70
  fertility requirements 70
  menstrual abnormalities 109
  menstrual history 71
  obstetric history 70
  parity 70
  smear history 71
HIV infection 153–154
  anti-retroviral drugs 154
  transmission 153
  see also AIDS
Homan's test, DVT 298
Hormonal chemotherapy
  mechanism of action 281
  ovarian tumour treatment 282
Hormonal methods, contraception
  338, 340–341
Hormone-producing tumours,
  ovarian tumours see Ovarian
  tumours
Hormone replacement therapy
  (HRT)
  benefits 390
  breast cancer 390
  breasts, effects on 390
  choice of treatment 392, 393
  concurrent medication 391
  duration 391
  endometrial cancer 203
  heart disease 390
  influencing factors 391
  oestrogen 391
  oral route 392
  osteoporosis 388
  parenteral 392
  percutaneous 392
  quality of life 391
  risks 390
  route of administration 391, 392
  screening 391–392
  stroke 390
  subcutaneous implants 393
  symptoms 391
  transdermal 392
  Turner's syndrome treatment 60
  vaginal preparations 393
  venous thromboembolism 390
  Women Health Initiative 390
  see also Oestrogen replacement
    therapy
Hormones, corpus luteum 36

HRT see Hormone replacement
  therapy (HRT)
Hulka–Clemens clip applicator 355
β-Human chorionic gonadotrophin
  (βHCG), ovarian
  choriocarcinoma 275
Human chorionic gonadotrophin
  (hCG), tubal pregnancy diagnosis
  321
Human papilloma virus(es) (HPVs)
  141
  benign squamous cervical
    metaplasia 174
  genome 175
  infection 175
    cervical disease 175
  see also Genital warts
  vulval intra-epithelial neoplasia
    159
Human papilloma virus 16 (HPV-
  16) 175
Human papilloma virus 18 (HPV-
  18) 175
Hyaline degeneration, uterine
  fibroids 199
Hydatid cyst, ovarian tumours vs.
  257
Hydatids of Morgagni 33, 284
Hydatiform mole 325
  complete 325–326
    genetics 327
  partial 325–326
    genetics 327
  pre-malignant complete 326
Hydration, DVT 300
Hydronephrotic kidney, ovarian
  tumours vs. 257
Hydrosalpinx, chronic pelvic
  inflammatory disease 150
17-Hydroxycorticosteroids, lipoid
  cell tumours 274
21-Hydroxylase deficiency,
  congenital adrenal hyperplasia 63
17-Hydroxyprogesterone (17-OHP),
  virilisation 106
Hymen 12
  development 6, 14
  imperforate 90
  rape 337
Hypercoagulability, venous
  thrombosis 296
Hyperinsulinaemia, polycystic
  ovarian syndrome 96
Hyperplasia, endometrium 201
Hyperprolactinaemia 97–100
  aetiology 98
  amenorrhoea mechanism 99
  diagnosis 99
  recurrent miscarriage 315
  surgery 100
  treatment 100

Hypersplenism, abdominal examination 76
Hypertension, combined oral contraceptive pill 343
Hyperthyroidism, gestational trophoblastic disease 327
Hypogastric plexus 44
Hypogonadotrophic hypogonadism 101
Hypothalamus
  disorders 101
  hormone effects 52, 53
  ovulation 49
Hypothyroidism, hyperprolactinaemia 98
Hysterectomy
  abdominal, urinary fistula formation 292
  endometrial hyperplasia treatment 202
  with pelvic lymphadenectomy, endometrial cancer treatment 209
  placental site trophoblastic tumour 196
  subtotal, heavy uterine bleeding 118
  total see Total hysterectomy
  total abdominal, endometrial cancer treatment 209
  total laparoscopic, heavy uterine bleeding 119
  uterine fibroid treatment 200
  uterine leiomyosarcoma 212
  uterine sarcoma 212
  vaginal see Vaginal hysterectomy
Hysterosalpingo-contrast sonography, tubal patency 369
Hysterosalpingography, tubal patency 368
Hysteroscopy
  endometrial polyps 196
  endometrium investigation 111

ICSI (intracytoplasmic sperm injection) 378
Idiopathic hirsutism 105
IgA (immunoglobulin A) 132
Iliococcygeus muscle 20
Imaging
  DVT 299
  endometriosis 127
  uterine fibroids 199
  see also specific methods
Imipramine, detrusor instability treatment 249
Imiquimod cream, genital warts therapy 141
Immunofluorescence, genital herpes diagnosis 140

Immunoglobulin A (IgA) 132
Immunological problems
  recurrent miscarriage 316
  sperm production abnormalities 366
Immunosuppressive therapy, Candida albicans infection 136
Implantable chemicals, contraception 354
Implantation sites, tubal pregnancy 310
Implants, subcutaneous, HRT 393
Incision, ovarian tumours 278
Incomplete miscarriage 309
Incontinence 74, 239
  bladder function examination 242
  dysuria 239
  endocrine disease 243
  fluid balance chart 243
  frequency 239
  investigation 241
  neurological disease 239, 243
  nocturia 239
  physical examination 241
  urgency 239
  urine bacteriology 243
  urodynamic assessment 243
  vaginal hysterectomy complications 230
  see also Detrusor instability; Stress incontinence; specific types
Inevitable miscarriage 308
Infantile uterus 38
Infections 131–154
  defence mechanisms 132
  IUD complications 348
  laparoscopy complications 85
  recurrent miscarriage 315
  secondary, genital warts 141
  sperm function tests 367
  sperm production abnormalities 366
  tropical 143
  see also specific infections
Infectious morbidity, surgical complications 294
Inferior mesenteric artery 34, 41
Infertility 357–380
  aetiology 358
    endometriosis 126
    female factor causes 359
    genital tuberculosis 152
    male factor causes 359
    pregnancy termination complications 319
  definitions 358
  examination, laparoscopy 85
  investigations 360
    primary setting 360
    secondary setting 360
    see also specific investigations

ovulation evidence 361–363
  basal body temperature changes 361
  clinical symptoms and signs 361
  endometrial biopsies 362
  serial ultrasound 363
  serum progesterone 362
  tests 362–363
prevalence 358
primary 358
secondary 358
sperm function tests 367
  antisperm antibodies 367
  post coital test 367
  in vitro assessment 367
sperm production tests 364
  abnormalities 366
  microscopy 365
  samples 365
  semen analysis 364
treatment 96
  counselling 380
  fertility drugs 371–372
  surgery 373
  see also Assisted conception
tubal patency 368–369
  assessment contraindications 369
  assessment requirements 369
  falloscopy 369
  hysterosalpingo-contrast sonography 369
  hysterosalpingography 368
  laparoscopic hydrotubation 368
Inflammation 132
  Bartholin's gland obstruction 133
  cervical smears 177
Infundibulopelvic ligament 29, 231
Inguinal glands, superficial 42
Inguinal lymph node, genital herpes diagnosis 140
Inhibin, ovulation 50
Inspection, ovarian tumours 278
Insulin-like growth factor-1, Graafian follicles 47
Insulin sensitizing agents, hirsutism treatment 108
Intermenstrual bleeding
  definition 71
  endometrial polyps 196
  placental site trophoblastic tumour 196
Interna; iliac artery 39
Intracytoplasmic sperm injection (ICSI) 378
Intra-epithelial neoplasia (AIN) 159
Intra-urethral pressure, micturition 234

Intra-uterine devices (IUDs) 338, 346
    complications 348
    copper 346
    ectopic pregnancy 320
    insertion 347
        local anaesthetic 347
        tenaculum forceps 347
    Mirena 346
    mode of action 346
    pelvic infections 346
    post-coital contraception 338–339
    progestin 346
Intrauterine insemination (IUI) 378–379
Intravenous urography, ureteric surgical injury 290
Intravesical pressure, micturition 234
In vitro assessment, sperm function tests 367
In vitro fertilization 374–376
    efficacy 377
    egg collection 375
    egg supply 374
    embryo transfer 376
    fertilization 375
    follicle tracking 374
    gonadotrophins 374
    indications 374
    natural cycle suppression 374
    risks of 376–377
    treatment schedule 374–376
In vitro maturation, assisted conception 379
Ipsilateral lymphadenectomy, vulval carcinoma treatment 163
Irregular bleeding, definition 71
Irritation, vaginal discharge 134
Ischial tuberosity 12, 18
Ischiocavernous muscle 16
Ischiococcygeus muscle 20
Ischiorectal fossa 18
Isoniazid, genital tuberculosis treatment 152
Isthmus uteri 26
IUDs see Intra-uterine devices (IUDs)
IUI (intrauterine insemination) 378–379

Kallmann's syndrome 101
Kaposi sarcoma 153
Karyotype analysis, gonadal dysgenesis 92
Ketoconazole, sperm production abnormalities 366
17-Ketosteroids, lipoid cell tumours 274
Kidney palpation, abdominal examination 76

Klebsiella infection see Granuloma inguinale
Klinefelter's syndrome 61
Knife cone biopsy, CIN treatment 182
Kobelt's tubules 33
    cysts 284
Krükenberg tumours 263, 270

Labial (genital) swelling, embryology 8
Labia majora 12, 13
    menopause 385
Labia minora 12, 13–14
    embryology 8
    menopause 385
Laboratory studies, genetic abnormalities 59
Lactate dehydrogenase (LDH), dysgerminoma 268
Laparoscopy 83–85
    complications 85
    endometriosis 126
    endoscope 83, 84
    hydrotubation, tubal patency 368
    indications 85
    ovarian cyst accidents 259
    ovarian tumours 276
    salpingostomy, infertility treatment 373
    sterilization 355
    technique 83–84
    trochar 83
Laparoscopy assisted vaginal hysterectomy (LAVH), heavy uterine bleeding 119
Laparotomy, ovarian cyst accidents 259
Large loop excision of the transformation zone (LLETZ) cervical cancer 186, 190
    CIN treatment 181
Laser ablation
    genital warts therapy 141
    ‹ vaginal intra-epithelial neoplasia 169
Laser cone biopsy, CIN treatment 182
Laser vaporisation, vulval intra-epithelial neoplasia treatment 159
Last menstrual period (LMP) 71
Late proliferative phase, endometrial cycle 51
Lateral fornices, vagina 23
LAVH (laparoscopy assisted vaginal hysterectomy), heavy uterine bleeding 119
LDH (lactate dehydrogenase), dysgerminoma 268

LEEP (Loop Electrosurgical Excision procedure), CIN treatment 181
Left renal vein 34
Leg wraps, lymphoedema 294
Leiomyosarcoma, uterine sarcoma 211, 212
Leucorrhoea, vaginal discharge 135
Levator ani muscle 19, 216
Levator (anal) fascia 18
Levonorgestrel
    endometrial hyperplasia treatment 202
    post-coital contraception 352
Levonorgestrel Intrauterine System (LNG-IUS)
    dysmenorrhoea treatment 121
    heavy uterine bleeding management 114
LGV (lymphogranuloma venereum) 143
LH see Luteinizing hormone (LH)
Libido, loss of 333
Lice, vulval inflammation 133
Lichen sclerosus 157
    differential diagnosis 157
    malignancies 157
    vulval examination 78–79
Ligaments, uterus 29–30
Ligation, ureteric surgical injury 290
Lipid metabolism, menopause 389
Lipoid cell tumours 263, 274
Lipoma, vulva 158
Liquid-based cytology, cervical cancer screening 176
Liver enlargement, abdominal examination 76
LLETZ see Large loop excision of the transformation zone (LLETZ)
LMP (last menstrual period) 71
LMWHs see Low molecular weight heparins (LMWHs)
LNG-IUS see Levonorgestrel Intrauterine System (LNG-IUS)
Local anaesthetic, IUD insertion 347
Local excision, vulval intra-epithelial neoplasia treatment 159
Local spread, endometrial cancer 206
Loop Electrosurgical Excision procedure (LEEP), CIN treatment 181
Lower genital tract disorders, menstrual abnormalities 90–91
Low grade stromal sarcomas, uterine sarcoma 212
Low molecular weight heparins (LMWHs)
    DVT 301
    pulmonary embolism 305

LUF (luteinised unruptured follicle syndrome) 363
Lumen, ureter 233
Luteal phase, hormones 50
Luteinised unruptured follicle syndrome (LUF) 363
Luteinizing hormone (LH)
  corpus luteum 36
  follicular phase 50
  Graafian follicles 47
  infertility treatment 372
  luteal phase 50
  menopause 382
  menstruation 50
  ovulation 50
  polycystic ovarian syndrome 94
  recurrent miscarriage 315
Lymphadenectomy
  pelvic, uterine sarcoma 212
  vaginal carcinoma treatment 171
Lymphatics 42–43
  cancer metastases 42–43
  cervical cancer (carcinoma) spread 185
  endometrial cancer spread 206
  ovarian tumour spread 277
  vulval carcinoma spread 161
Lymphocysts, surgical complications 294
Lymphoedema
  surgical complications 294
  vulval carcinoma surgery 164
Lymphogranuloma venereum (LGV) 143
Lymphomas, AIDS 153
Lynch syndrome, ovarian tumours 264

Mackenrodt's ligaments 30
Magnetic resonance imaging (MRI)
  cervical cancer staging 188
  endometrial cancer 206
  hyperprolactinaemia 99
  ovarian tumour diagnosis 255
  uterine fibroids 199
  vaginal carcinoma 170
Male external genitalia, embryology see Embryology
Malignancies
  lichen sclerosus 157
  vagina 169
Manchester repair, prolapse 223, 225–226
Marshall–Marchetti–Krantz urethropexy 246
Marsupialization, vulval inflammation treatment 133
Masculinization
  Sertoli–Leydig cell tumour 273
  see also Defeminisation
Masculinovoblastoma 274

Maternal age, recurrent miscarriage 314
Maternal diabetes, recurrent miscarriage 315
Mature cystic teratoma, ovarian tumours 269
Mayer–Rokitansky–Kuster–Hauser syndrome 91
Mayer–Rokitansky syndrome 65, 67
MEA (microwave endometrial ablation), heavy uterine bleeding 116
Mechanical devices, stress incontinence treatment 244
Median sacral artery 41
Medical termination of pregnancy 318, 319
Medico-legal problems 337
Medroxyprogesterone acetate, endometrial cancer recurrence treatment 210
Meig's syndrome, fibroma 272
Meiosis 58
Melanoma, vaginal carcinoma 171
Menarche 88
  definition 71
Menopause 55, 381–393
  anti-Müllerian hormone 382
  cardiovascular disease 389–390
    blood flow 389
    carbohydrate metabolism 389
    lipid metabolism 389
    mortality rate 389
    risks 389
  causes 382
  conception possibility 393
  contraception 393
  definition 71, 382
  differential diagnosis 382
  FSH 89, 382
  genital tract changes 385
    dyspareunia 385
    Fallopian tubes 385
    labia majora 385
    labia minora 385
    ovaries 385
    uterus 385
    vagina 385
    vaginal dryness 385
    vulva 385
  Greene climacteric scale 384
  LH 382
  menstruation changes 55
  oestrogen 89, 382
  osteoporosis 386–388
    bisphosphonates 388
    comparative cortical bone thicknesses 388
    HRT 388
    oestrogens 388
    raloxifene 388

risk factors 389–390
  physiological amenorrhoea 89
  premature 2, 382
  signs and symptoms 383
    psychological symptoms 383
    severity and duration 383
    urogenital atrophy 383
    vasomotor symptoms 383
Menorrhagia
  definition 71
  placental site trophoblastic tumour 196
Menstrual abnormalities 87–130, 109
  amenorrhoea see Amenorrhoea
  causes 109
  dysfunctional uterine bleeding see Dysfunctional uterine bleeding
  endometriosis 126
  history taking 109
  hypothalamic disorders 101
  lower genital tract disorders 90–91
  ovarian disorders 92–96
    see also Ovaries
  pituitary disorders 97–100
  uterine disorders 90–91
    see also specific diseases/disorders
Menstruation
  abnormalities see Menstrual abnormalities
  blood loss, IUD complications 348
  changes, menopause 55
  endometrial cycle 51
  FSH 50
  history taking 71
  LH 50
  normal cycle 88
  prostaglandin F2-α 51
Mesenteric cyst, ovarian tumours vs. 257
Mesentery, ovary development 3
Mesoderm, genital ridges 3
Mesonephric ducts, embryology 6
Mesonephric (Wolffian) ridge, embryology 5
Mesovarium, ovary 34
Metastases, lymphatic system 42–43
Metformin, infertility treatment 371
Methotrexate, tubal pregnancy treatment 324
Metronidazole
  bacterial vaginosis 137
  Trichomonas vaginalis 138
Microinvasive cervical carcinoma 178
Microinvasive surgery, cervical cancer 190

Microscopy
  adenomyosis 122
  Chlamydia trachomatis infection
    142
  sperm production tests 365
Microwave endometrial ablation
  (MEA), heavy uterine bleeding
  116
Micturition 234–235
  detrusor contraction 236
  frequency
    incontinence 239
    vaginal prolapse 220
  intra-urethral pressure 234
  intravesical pressure 234
  voiding mechanism 236
Mifepristone
  miscarriage management 312, 313
  pregnancy termination 318, 319
Mild dyskaryosis, cervical smears
  177
Mirena, IUDs 346
Miscarriage 308–309
  complete 308
  incomplete 309
  inevitable 308
  management 310, 310–312
    anti-D immunoglobulin 312
    complications 311
    curettage 312
    dilatation and evacuation 313
    expectant management 312
    less than 12 week gestation
      310–312
    medical management 312, 313
    more than 12 week gestation
      313
    surgery 310, 313
  missed 309
  recurrent *see* Recurrent
    miscarriage
  threatened 308
Misoprostol, miscarriage
  management 312, 313
Missed miscarriage 309
Mittelschmerz 72
Moderate dyskaryosis, cervical
  smears 177
Mons pubis 12, 13
Montgomery's tubercles 82
Motivation, contraception failure
  rates 339
MRI *see* Magnetic resonance
  imaging (MRI)
Mucinous cystadenocarcinoma,
  ovarian tumours 263, 266
Mucinous cystadenoma, ovarian
  tumours *see* Ovarian tumours
Mucoid degeneration, uterine
  fibroids 199
Mucosal prolapse, urethra 165

Mucous cervical polyps, cervical
  cancer *vs.* 186
Mullerian agnesis 91
Müllerian (paramesonephric) duct,
  embryology 5, 6
Müllerian tubercle, embryology 5
Multiple births, in vitro fertilization
  376
Muscles
  pelvis 19
  see also specific muscles
Muscularis, ureter 233
Myoma, vulva 158
Myomectomy
  disadvantages 200
  uterine fibroid treatment 200
Myometrium, uterine fibroids 197

Nafarelin, infertility treatment 372
Natural cycle suppression, in vitro
  fertilization 374
Natural methods, contraception
  338
Nausea and vomiting, gestational
  trophoblastic disease 327
Necrobiosis, uterine fibroids 199
Neoplasia, combined oral
  contraceptive pill 344
Nephrostomy, percutaneous 291
Nerve supply
  coccygeus muscle 19
  pelvis 43–44
Neurological disease, incontinence
  239, 243
Nitrofurantoin, sperm production
  abnormalities 366
Nocturia, incontinence 239
Novasure, heavy uterine bleeding
  116
Nucleic acid amplification tests
  (NAATs)
  Chlamydia trachomatis infection
    142
  gonorrhoea diagnosis 144
Nucleic acid hybridization tests,
  gonorrhoea diagnosis 144
Nulliparous adults, vagina 23

Obesity
  abdominal examination 77
  abdominal ultrasound 77
  endometrial cancer 207
  ovarian tumours *vs.* 257
  vulval inflammation 133
Obstetric history taking 70
Obturator fascia 18
Obturator internus muscles 19, 20
Oestradiol tablets, pessaries 222
Oestriol cream, pessaries 222
Oestrogen(s)
  actions of 52

benign squamous cervical
  metaplasia 174
  cyclical changes 51
  detrusor instability treatment 249
  endometrial hyperplasia 202
  high-dose, Asherman's
    syndrome 91
  HRT 391
  menopause 89, 382
  osteoporosis 388
  ovulation 48
  pregnancy 89
  premenstrual syndrome treatment
    130
Oestrogen-producing ovarian
  tumours 272
Oestrogen receptors 52
Oestrogen replacement therapy
  complete androgen insensitivity 62
  premature ovarian failure 93
Ofloxacin, pelvic inflammatory
  disease management 149
Oil of evening primrose,
  premenstrual syndrome treatment
  130
Oligoamenorrhoea
  definition 71
  polycystic ovarian syndrome 95
Oophorectomy, bilateral, heavy
  uterine bleeding 118
Operative hysteroscopy, placental
  site trophoblastic tumour 196
Ophthalmia neonatorum, *Chlamydia
  trachomatis* infection 142
Oral route, HRT 392
Orgalytran, infertility treatment
  372
Organ removal, ovarian tumours
  278
Organ systems, pelvic pain 72
Orgasm
  coitus 333
  failure to achieve 333
Osteoporosis
  bone mineral density 386
  menopause *see* Menopause
  ultrasonic densitometry 386,
    387–388
Ova/ovum
  blighted 309
  collection 375
  supply 374
Ovarian arteries 34, 41
  ureter 233
Ovarian hyperstimulation syndrome,
  in vitro fertilization 377
Ovarian tumours 262–263
  BRCA 1 264
  BRCA 2 264
  carcinoma 264
  chemotherapy 281

Ovarian tumours (Continued)
clinical features 252–254, 262
large 253
palpation 254
pedicles 254
pressure symptoms 252–254
size 252
small 253
upper pole 254
complications 259
differential diagnosis 259
pedicle torsion 259
differential diagnosis 255–258
ascites 255
broad ligament cysts 258
computed tomography 255
ectopic kidney 258
full bladder 255
hydatid cyst 257
hydronephrotic kidney 257
mesenteric cyst 257
MRI 255
obesity 257
pancreatic cyst 257
pelvic inflammation 257
pregnancy 255
pyosalpinx 257
rectus sheath haematoma 257
retroperitoneal tumours 258
transplanted kidney 258
ultrasound 255, 256
uterine fibroids 256
epithelial tumours 263, 265–266
adjuvant chemotherapy 277
prognosis 425
staging 277
surgical debulking 277
see also specific tumours
germ cell tumours 263, 267–271
Brenner tumour 271
clinical features 267
dysgerminoma 268
fibroma 272
gonadoblastoma 268
Krukenberg tumours 270
mature cystic teratoma 269
solid teratoma 269
staging 267
teratomas 269–270
see also specific types
treatment 267
undifferentiated 268
yolk sac tumours 270
histology 263
hormone-producing tumours 272
androgen-producing 273–274
carcinoid (serotonin-producing
tumour) 275
choriocarcinoma 275
hilar cell tumours 274
lipoid cell tumours 274

non-functioning tumours 275
oestrogen-producing 272
Sertoli–Leydig cell tumour
273–274
struma ovarii (thyroid type
tumour) 275
investigations 262
Lynch syndrome 264
mucinous cystadenocarcinoma
266
mucinous cystadenoma 266
pseudomyxoma peritonei 266
risk factors 264
risk of malignancy index 262
serous cystadenocarcinoma 265
serous cystadenoma 265
sex cord stromal tumours 263
spread of 277–278
blood stream 277
direct 277
lymphatics 277
transcoelomic 277
staging 279–280
stage I 279
stage II 279
stage III 280
stage IIIa 280
stage IIIb 280
stage IIIc 280
stage IV 280
stromatous tumours 263
surgery 276, 277–278
cystectomy 276
cytology 278
incision 278
inspection 278
laparoscopy 276
organ removal 278
ovariotomy 276
tumour markers 253
Ovaries 34–37
abnormalities 64
age-related changes 38
blood supply 34
combined oral contraceptive pill
344
corpus albicans 37
corpus luteum see Corpus luteum
cortex 35, 46
cyclical hormonal changes 51
see also specific hormone
cysts 259–261
abdominal examination
75, 77
differential diagnosis 261
rupture of 260–261
development 2–4
descent 4
gubernaculum 4
mesentery 3
diseases/disorders 251–285

menstrual abnormalities 92–96
see also specific diseases/disorders
dysgenesis 64
epithelium 46
follicular atresia 37
hilum 34, 35
histology 35–37
menopause 385
mesovarium 34
premature failure 93
primordial follicle 46
tumours see Ovarian tumours
tunica albuginea 35
Ovariotomy, ovarian tumours 276
Overflow incontinence 239
Ovoblastoma 274
Ovulation 46–50
bleeding vs. ovarian cyst accidents
261
evidence, infertility see Infertility
FSH 48, 50
GnRH 49, 50
hypothalamus 49
inhibin 50
LH 50
oestrogen 48
Ovulation method (Billings'
method) 351

Paclitaxel
ovarian tumour treatment 282
side effects 282
Paediatric AIDS 154
Paediatric vulvo-vaginitis 139
Paget's disease of the vulva 159
Pain
dysmenorrhoea 120
endometriosis 126
tubal pregnancy 321
PAIN (perianal intra-epithelial
neoplasia) 159
Palliative care, cervical cancer 193
Palpation
abdominal examination 76
ovarian tumours 254
Pancreatic cyst, ovarian tumours vs.
257
Papanicolaou staining, cervical
cancer screening 176
Papaverine, erectile dysfunction
treatment 336
Paramesonephric (Müllerian) duct,
embryology 5, 6
Parasympathetic nerves
bladder/urethra 235
pelvis 44
Para-urethral glands of Skene 8
Parenteral route, HRT 392
Parietal layer, pelvic fascia 21
Parity, history taking 70
Paroöphoron, broad ligament 33

Paroöphoron tubules, hilum 35
Parovarian cysts *see* Broad ligament
Partial hydatiform mole
    see Hydatiform mole
Partial vaginectomy, vaginal intra-
    epithelial neoplasia 169
Patient documentation, sterilization
    354
Patient selection, vaginal
    hysterectomy complications 230
Patients, explanations to 74
PCOS *see* Polycystic ovarian
    syndrome (PCOS)
Pedicles
    ovarian tumours 254
    torsion, ovarian tumour
        complications 259
'Peg' cells, Fallopian tubes 32
Pelvic diaphragm 20
    functions of 20
Pelvic fascia 21
    parietal layer 21
    relations of 21
    visceral layer 21
Pelvic floor exercises, stress
    incontinence treatment 244
Pelvic inflammatory disease (PID)
    149
    acute 149
    bacteriology 149
    chronic 150
    differential diagnosis 149
    ectopic pregnancy 320
    management 149
Pelvic lymphadenectomy, uterine
    sarcoma 212
Pelvis
    bimanual examination
        see Bimanual pelvic
        examination
    blood supply 39–41
        collateral blood supply 41
        see also specific blood vessels
    infections, IUDs 346
    inflammation
        ovarian cyst accidents *vs.* 261
        ovarian tumours *vs.* 257
    models, bimanual pelvic
        examination 79–80
    muscles of 19
        see also specific muscles
    nerve supply 43–44
        autonomic nerves 44
        parasympathetic nerves 44
        see also specific nerves
    pain 72–73
        organ systems 72
        severity of 73
        tubal pregnancy 321
        see also Dyspareunia
Penicillin, syphilis treatment 147

Percutaneous antegrade stents,
    urinary fistula therapy 293
Percutaneous nephrostomy, ureteric
    surgical injury 291
Percutaneous route, HRT 392
Perforation, laparoscopy
    complications 85
Perianal intra-epithelial neoplasia
    (PAIN) 159
Perihepatitis, *Chlamydia trachomatis*
    infection 142
Perimenopause 71
Perineal body 16
Perineal muscles 17
Perineum 12
    anatomical 12
    gynaecological 12
    muscles of 17
        see also specific muscles
    true 12
Periosteitis,
    Marshall–Marchetti–Krantz
    urethropexy 246
Peripheral pulmonary embolism 302
Peritoneal cavity rupture, tubal
    pregnancy 323
Periurethral injections, stress
    incontinence treatment
    244
pH, vagina 24
Physical examination 69–85
    amenorrhoea 102
    incontinence 241
    see also Gynaecological
        examination
Physiological amenorrhoea
    see Amenorrhoea
Physiology 45–55
Physiotherapy, stress incontinence
    treatment 244
PID *see* Pelvic inflammatory disease
    (PID)
Pipelle de Cornier, endometrial
    biopsy 112
Piriformis muscle 19, 20
Pituitary
    disorders, menstrual
        abnormalities 97–100
    tumours, hyperprolactinaemia 98
Pituitary antagonists, infertility
    treatment 372
Placenta, hormone production 89
Placental site trophoblastic tumour
    196, 329
Plant chemotherapeutics,
    mechanism of action 281
Plastic surgery, vagina 172
Plateau phase, coitus 332
Plexus of Frankenhauser 44
PLS (post thrombotic leg syndrome)
    295

PMS *see* Premenstrual syndrome
    (PMS)
PMT (premenstrual tension) 53
Pneumatic stocking, DVT 300
Podophyllotoxin, genital warts
    therapy 141
Polycystic ovarian syndrome
    (PCOS) 94–96
    clinical features 94
    diabetes mellitus type II 94
    diagnosis 95
    FSH 94
    hirsutism 105
    LH 94
    long-term effects 96
    recurrent miscarriage 315
    sex hormone binding globulin 94
    treatment 96
        amenorrhoea 96
        hirsutism 96
        infertility treatment 96
Polyps
    uterine fibroids *vs.* 197
    uterus 196
POP (progesterone only pill) 344
Post-coital bleeding, definition 71
Postcoital (morning after)
    contraception 352
Postcoital (resolution) phase, coitus
    333
Post coital test, sperm function tests
    367
Posterior colpoperineorrhaphy,
    vaginal prolapse 227
Posterior fornix, vagina 23
Posterior wall vaginal prolapse
    219
Postmenopause
    bleeding 203
    endometrial cancer 203
    superficial dyspareunia 334
    uterus 38
Post molar gestational trophoblastic
    neoplasia 328
Post operative physiotherapy, DVT
    300
Post thrombotic leg syndrome (PLS)
    295
Pouch of Douglas 23
Pratt's sign, DVT 298
Pregnancy
    abdominal examination 75
    Candida albicans infection 136
    early *see* Early pregnancy
    ectopic *see* Ectopic pregnancy
    Fallopian tubes *see* Tubal
        pregnancy
    IUD complications 348
    oestrogen 89
    ovarian tumours *vs.* 255
    physiological amenorrhoea 89

Pregnancy termination 317–319
  complications 319
    immediate 319
    late 319
  first trimester 317–318
    medical termination of
      pregnancy 318
    surgical termination of
      pregnancy 317
  second trimester 319
    dilatation and curettage 319
    extra-amniotic termination 319
    medical termination 319
Pre-implantation genetic diagnosis
  (PIGD), assisted conception 379
Pre-malignant complete hydatiform
  mole 326
Pre-malignant disease, vagina 169
Premature ejaculation 335
Premature menopause 2, 382
Premature ovarian failure, FSH 93
Premenstrual syndrome (PMS) 53,
  74, 129
  clinical features 129
  investigations 129
  treatment 130
Premenstrual tension (PMT) 53
Pre-pregnancy infection screening,
  assisted conception 370
Prepuce 13
Presacral nerves 44
Pressure symptoms
  ovarian tumours 252–254
  uterine fibroids 198
Previous miscarriage, recurrent
  miscarriage 314
Primary amenorrhoea 71
Primary dysmenorrhoea 72
Primary infertility 358
Primary syphilis 145
Primary urethral groove,
  embryology 9
Primordial follicle, ovary 46
Progesterone
  actions of 52
  cyclical changes 51
  endometriosis treatment 127
  heavy uterine bleeding
    management 114
  infertility treatment 372
  ovulation evidence 362
  pregnancy 89
  premenstrual syndrome treatment
    130
Progesterone challenge test,
  amenorrhoea 102
Progesterone only pill (POP) 344
Progestin
  endometrial hyperplasia treatment
    202
  IUDs 346

Progestogen(s)
  combined oral contraceptive pill
    341
  endometrial cancer recurrence
    treatment 210
  endometrial cancer treatment 209
  endometrial hyperplasia treatment
    202
  implants 345
  injectable 344
  premature ovarian failure 93
Progynova, infertility treatment 372
Prolactin
  amenorrhoea 102
  lactation 89
Prostaglandin(s)
  dysmenorrhoea 120
  pregnancy termination 319
Prostaglandin analogues, miscarriage
  management 312, 313
Prostaglandin E2, pregnancy
  termination 319
Prostaglandin F2-α, menstruation 51
Prostaglandin synthetase inhibitors
  dysmenorrhoea treatment 121
  heavy uterine bleeding
    management 114
Protein C deficiency, recurrent
  miscarriage 316
Protein C resistance, recurrent
  miscarriage 315
Protein S deficiency, recurrent
  miscarriage 316
Pseudomyxoma peritonei 266
Psychological symptoms
  hormone effects 53
  menopause 383
Psychosexual counselling 333
  erectile dysfunction treatment 336
  vaginismus treatment 334
Pubertal uterus 38
Puberty 54
  absent/late 88
  definition 54
  GnRH 54
Pubococcygeus muscle 20
Pudendal artery 40, 43
Pudendal nerve 18, 43
Pudendal vessels 18
Pulmonary embolism 302–304
  central 302
  investigations 303
    arterial blood gases 303
    chest x-ray 303
    computed tomographic
      pulmonary angiography 304
    duplex Doppler leg ultrasound
      304
    ECG 303–304
    ventilation/perfusion (V/Q)
      scans 304

  management 303
  mortality 306
  peripheral 302
  treatment 305
Pulmonary thromboembolism (PT)
  295
Pyelography, antegrade 291
Pyometra, cervical cancer
  (carcinoma) 185
Pyosalpinx
  chronic pelvic inflammatory
    disease 150
  ovarian tumours vs. 257
Pyridoxine (vitamin B6),
  premenstrual syndrome treatment
  130

Quality of life, HRT 391
Quinagolide, hyperprolactinaemia
  treatment 100

Radiation burns, urinary fistula
  formation 293
Radical hysterectomy
  and node dissection, cervical
    cancer 190–191
  urinary fistula formation 292
  vaginal carcinoma treatment
    171
Radical surgery, cervical cancer
  192
Radical vulvectomy, vulval
  carcinoma treatment 162, 163
Radiotherapy
  cervical cancer see Cervical cancer
    (carcinoma)
  endometrial cancer treatment
    209
  vulval carcinoma 164
Raloxifene, osteoporosis 388
Rape 337
  definition 337
  general examination 337
  hymen 337
  record keeping 337
  skin swabs 337
  vulval examination 337
Record keeping, rape 337
Rectocele 219
  anterior colporrhaphy 223
  posterior colpoperineorrhaphy
    227
Rectovaginal examination, bimanual
  pelvic examination 79
Rectus sheath haematoma, ovarian
  tumours vs. 257
Recurrent miscarriage 314–316
  causes 314–315
    autoimmune factors 315
    cervical weakness 314, 316
    embryonic abnormalities 314

409

Recurrent miscarriage *(Continued)*
    endocrine factors 315, 316
    environmental factors 315, 316
    genetics 314, 316
    hyperprolactinaemia 315
    immunological problems 316
    infections 315
    maternal age 314
    maternal diabetes 315
    polycystic ovarian syndrome
        315
    previous miscarriage 314
    thrombophilias 315, 316
    thyroid disease 315
    uterine abnormalities 314, 316
    definitions 314
    investigation 316
    treatment 316
Reiter's syndrome, *Chlamydia
    trachomatis* infection 142
Renal artery, ureter 233
Renogram, ureteric surgical injury
    290
Reproductive immunology, assisted
    conception 379
Resistant ovary syndrome 93
Rete, embryology 3
Retroflexion, uterus retroversion
    214
Retroperitoneal tumours, ovarian
    tumours *vs.* 258
Rhesus immunization, miscarriage
    management 311
Rhythm method (safe period) 351
Rifampicin, genital tuberculosis
    treatment 152
Right ovarian vein 34
Ring pessaries 222
Risk of malignancy index (RMI),
    ovarian tumours 262
Route of administration, HRT 391,
    392
Rudimentary uterus 65
Rupture into lumen, tubal
    pregnancy 323

Sacral nerves 18
Sacrotuberous ligament 12, 18
Salpingectomy, tubal pregnancy
    treatment 324
Salpingo-oophorectomy, bilateral
    see Bilateral salpingo-
    oophorectomy
Salpingostomy, tubal pregnancy
    treatment 324
Samples, sperm production tests
    365
Sarcoma botriodes 171, 211
Sarcoma, ovarian tumours 263
Sarcomatous change, uterine
    fibroids 199

Scabies, vulval inflammation 133
SCC *see* Squamous cell carcinoma
    (SCC)
Scrotum, embryology 9
Sebaceous cysts, vulva 158
Secondary amenorrhoea 71
Secondary dysmenorrhoea 72
Secondary infections, genital warts
    141
Secondary infertility 358
Secretory phase, endometrial
    cycle 51
Selective serotonin uptake inhibitors,
    premenstrual syndrome treatment
    130
Semen analysis 364
Septated uterus 66
Serial ultrasound, ovulation evidence
    363
Serotonin-producing ovarian
    tumours 275
Serous cystadenocarcinoma, ovarian
    tumours 263, 265
Serous cystadenoma, ovarian
    tumours 263, 265
Sertoli–Leydig cell tumours 263,
    273–274
Serum human chorionic
    gonadotrophin (hCG), tubal
    pregnancy diagnosis 321
Serum progesterone, ovulation
    evidence 362
Severe dyskaryosis, cervical smears
    177
Sex chromosome acquisition X
    (super-female) 61
Sex cords
    coelomic epithelium 3
    stromal tumours 263
Sex development disorders
    57–68
    congenital abnormalities 62–63
        cloacal origin 68
    genetic abnormalities 59–61
        chromosome analysis 59
        clinical syndromes 59
        investigations 59
        laboratory studies 59
    see also specific diseases/disorders
Sex hormone binding globulin
    (SHBG)
    hirsutism 105
    polycystic ovarian syndrome 94
Sex hormones
    erectile dysfunction treatment
        336
    see also specific hormones
Sexual history 332
Sexuality 331–356
Sexual problems 333
    libido, loss of 333

    male 335
    orgasm, failure to achieve 333
    see also specific problems
Sexual transmission, *Candida
    albicans* infection 136
Shaving, hirsutism 107
SHBG *see* Sex hormone binding
    globulin (SHBG)
Shelf pessaries 222
Sidenasil (Viagra), erectile
    dysfunction treatment 336
Sims' speculum 81
Skeleton, hormone effects 53
Skene's ducts 14
Skin conditions, vulval examination
    78–79
Skin swabs, rape 337
Smear history, history taking 71
Soap substitutes, lichen sclerosus
    treatment 157
Solid teratoma, ovarian tumours 269
Specimens, vaginal discharge 135
Speculum examination 80–81
Sperm function tests *see* Infertility
Spermicides, contraception 338
Sperm production, infertility
    see Infertility
Sphincter ani 18
Sphincter urethrae 17
Spironolactone, sperm production
    abnormalities 366
Sponge, contraception 350
Squamous cell carcinoma (SCC)
    cervical cancer 184
    vaginal carcinoma 170
Squamous epithelium, vagina 132
Staging
    cervical cancer *see* Cervical cancer
        (carcinoma)
    endometrial cancer
        see Endometrial cancer
    Fallopian tube carcinoma 285
    ovarian epithelial tumours 277
    ovarian germ cell tumours 267
    ovarian tumours *see* Ovarian
        tumours
Stamey needle suspension procedure
    247
'Stein Leventhal' syndrome 94
Sterilization 353–354
    counselling 353
    laparoscopic 355
    patient documentation 354
    success rates 353
Steroids, lichen sclerosus treatment
    157
STOP (surgical termination of
    pregnancy) 317
Stress incontinence 74, 238
    cystometry 242
    demonstration of 241

Stress incontinence *(Continued)*
   detrusor instability *vs.* 241
   surgery 244
   treatment 244
   vaginal prolapse 220
Stroke
   combined oral contraceptive pill
      343
   HRT 390
Stromatous ovarian tumours 263
Struma ovarii, ovarian tumours 275
Subcutaneous implants, HRT 393
Subtotal hysterectomy, heavy uterine
   bleeding 118
Sulfasalazine, sperm production
   abnormalities 366
Super-female (sex chromosome
   acquisition X) 61
Superficial dyspareunia 73, 334
Superficial inguinal glands 42
Superficial transverse perineal
   muscle 16
Support hosiery, lymphoedema 294
Surgery
   cervical cancer *see* Cervical cancer
      (carcinoma)
   complications *see* Surgical
      complications
   contraception 338
   endometrial cancer treatment
      209
   genital tuberculosis treatment 152
   infertility treatment 373
   miscarriage management 310, 313
   ovarian tumours *see* Ovarian
      tumours
   pulmonary embolism 305
   stress incontinence 244
   uterine fibroid treatment 200
   vaginal intra-epithelial neoplasia
      169
Surgical complications 287–306
   adhesions 293
   bladder injuries 288
   bowel injury 291
   fever 294
   fistula formation 292–293
      see also specific types
   hernia 294
   infectious morbidity 294
   lymphocysts 294
   lymphoedema 294
   ureter injuries *see* Ureteric surgical
      injury
   urinary fistula 292–293
   urinary tract injuries 288
   venous thrombosis *see* Deep vein
      thrombosis (DVT); Venous
      thrombosis
Surgical debulking, ovarian epithelial
   tumours 277

Surgical termination of pregnancy
   (STOP) 317
Sympathetic nerves, bladder/urethra
   235
Syphilis 145–147
   chancre 145
   diagnosis 145, 146
   primary 145
   signs and symptoms 147
   treatment 147
   urinary fistula formation
      293
Syphilitic condylomata, genital warts
   vs. 141

Tamoxifen, endometrial cancer 203
Taxanes, ovarian tumours 277
TCRE (trans-cervical resection of
   endometrium) 115
Tenaculum forceps, IUD insertion
   347
Teratomas, ovarian tumours 263,
   269–270
Testes, embryology 9
Testosterone
   complete androgen
      insensitivity 62
   measurement, polycystic ovarian
      syndrome 95
   physiology 105
   Sertoli–Leydig cell tumour 274
   virilisation 106
Theca interna 47
Thecoma, ovarian tumours 263
Thermachoice, heavy uterine
   bleeding 116
Threadworm, paediatric vulvo-
   vaginitis 139
Threatened miscarriage 308
Thromboembolism
   combined oral contraceptive pill
      343
   venous *see* Venous
      thromboembolism
Thrombophilias, recurrent
   miscarriage 315, 316
Thromboprophylaxis, DVT *see* Deep
   vein thrombosis (DVT)
Thrombosis, venous *see* Venous
   thromboembolism
Thrush *see Candida albicans* infection
Thyroid disease, recurrent
   miscarriage 315
Thyroid stimulating hormone
   (TSH), amenorrhoea 102
Thyroid tumour choriosarcoma,
   ovarian tumours 263
Time of ovulation, contraception
   351
Torsion of the pedicle, uterine
   fibroids 199

Total abdominal hysterectomy,
   endometrial cancer treatment 209
Total hysterectomy
   Fallopian tubes carcinoma 285
   heavy uterine bleeding 116–117
   laparoscopic, heavy uterine
      bleeding 119
Total laparoscopic hysterectomy,
   heavy uterine bleeding 119
Total vaginectomy, vaginal intra-
   epithelial neoplasia 169
Toxicity, chemotherapy 282
Toxic shock syndrome 147
TPHA (Treponema pallidum
   haemagglutination), syphilis
   diagnosis 146
Tranexamic acid, dysfunctional
   uterine bleeding management 114
Transabdominal scanning,
   endometrium investigation 111
Trans-cervical resection of
   endometrium (TCRE) 115
Transcoelomic spread, ovarian
   tumours 277
Transdermal route, HRT 392
Translocation, IUD complications
   348
Transnasal surgery,
   hyperprolactinaemia 100
Transplanted kidney, ovarian
   tumours *vs.* 258
Transvaginal ultrasound
   dysfunctional uterine bleeding
      110
   endometrium investigation 111
   tubal pregnancy 322
Transverse cervical (Mackenrodt's;
   cardinal) ligaments 30
Transverse septum, vagina 67
Traumatic epithelial cysts, vagina
   168
Treponema pallidum
   haemagglutination (TPHA),
   syphilis diagnosis 146
Treponema pallidum infection
   see Syphilis
Trichomonas vaginalis infection
   vaginal discharge 137–138
   vaginal pH 138
Tricyclic antidepressants, detrusor
   instability treatment 249
Trochar, laparoscopy 83
Trophectoderm biopsy 379
True perineum 12
TSH (thyroid stimulating hormone),
   amenorrhoea 102
Tubal abortion 323
Tubal pregnancy 321–322
   diagnosis 321–322
      serum hCG 321
      ultrasound 321

Tubal pregnancy *(Continued)*
implantation sites 310
pelvic inflammatory disease *vs.* 149
peritoneal cavity rupture 323
rupture into lumen 323
signs 321–322
symptoms 321
treatment 324
conservative management 324
methotrexate 324
salpingectomy 324
salpingostomy 324
tubal abortion 323
tube rupture 323
Tuberculosis, genital *see* Genital tuberculosis
Tumour markers
ovarian tumours 253
see also specific markers
Tunica albuginea, ovary 35
Turner's syndrome 60
gonadal dysgenesis 92
premature ovarian failure 93

UFH (unfractionated heparin), DVT 301
Ultrasonic densitometry, osteoporosis 386, 387–388
Ultrasound
abdominal 77
duplex Doppler leg ultrasound 304
DVT 299
endometrial cancer 203
IUD translocation 348
obesity 77
ovarian tumour differential diagnosis 255, 256
polycystic ovarian syndrome 95
pulmonary embolism 304
transvaginal *see* Transvaginal ultrasound
tubal pregnancy diagnosis 321
ureteric surgical injury 290
uterine fibroids 199
Undifferentiated germ cell tumours 268
Unfractionated heparin (UFH), DVT 301
Unicornis uterus 66
Unilateral salpino-oöphorectomy, germ cell ovarian tumours 267
Upper pole, ovarian tumours 254
Ureter 231–232
blood supply 233
course of 289
histology 233
relationship with cervix 28
relationship with uterus 28

Ureteric surgical injury 289
clinical features 290
crush injury 290
investigations 290–291
ligation 290
management 290–291
treatment 291
Urethra
caruncle 165
closure 235
diseases 165
see also specific diseases/disorders
embryology 7
glands, embryology 8
innervation 235
meatus, vulval examination 78
mucosal prolapse 165
orifice 12, 14
sphincter incompetence 238
urethrocele 165
Urethral folds, embryology 8
Urethral slings, stress incontinence 245, 248
Urethral syndrome 240
Urethroceles 165, 218
Urethropexy, stress incontinence 245
Urgency, incontinence 239
Urinary catheters 230
Urinary fistula, surgical complications 292–293
Urinary incontinence
see Incontinence
Urinary sphincters, artificial 244
Urinary tract
anatomy 231–232
infections 240
injuries, surgical complications 288
symptoms 74
Urination *see* Micturition
Urine bacteriology, incontinence 243
Urodynamic assessment, incontinence 243
Urogenital angle 12
Urogenital atrophy, menopause 383
Urogenital buds, embryology 8
Urogenital diaphragm 17, 18
Urogenital sinus, embryology 7
Urography, intravenous 290
Urogynaecology 213–249
Uterine artery embolisation, uterine fibroid treatment 200
Uterine fibroids 197
complications 199
diagnosis 199
dysmenorrhoea 198
investigations 199
myometrium 197
ovarian tumours *vs.* 256

polyps *vs.* 197
pressure symptoms 198
prevalence 198
symptoms and signs 199
torsion, ovarian cyst accidents *vs.* 261
transvaginal ultrasound 111
treatment 200
uterine retroversion 215
Uterine sarcoma 211–212
carcinosarcoma 211, 212
clinical features 211
endometrial stromal sarcomas 211, 212
high grade stromal sarcomas 212
histology 211
leiomyosarcoma 211, 212
low grade stromal sarcomas 212
Utero-sacral ligaments 30, 216
Uterovaginal prolapse 216
causes 216
first degree 217
incidence 216
second degree 217
third degree 217
Uterus 25–31
abnormalities 65–66
absence 65
with accessory horn 65
arcuate 66
double (bicornuate) 65
menstrual abnormalities 90–91
recurrent miscarriage 314, 316
rudimentary 65
septated 66
unicornis 66
uterus bicornis 65
uterus bicornis bicollis 65
uterus bicornis unicollis 65
uterus didelphys 65
adult 38
age-related changes 38
bimanual pelvic examination 79
blood supply 39–40
corpus 26
cavity 27
development 5–6
diseases 195–212
dysfunctional bleeding
see Dysfunctional uterine bleeding
endometrial polyps 196
fibroids *see* Uterine fibroids
heavy bleeding *see* Heavy uterine bleeding
placental site trophoblastic tumour 196
polyps 196

Uterus *(Continued)*
  prolapse 213–249
  retroversion *see below*
  see also specific diseases
  endometrium *see* Endometrium
  enlargement, abdominal
    examination 75
  glands 31
  histology 31
  infantile 38
  isthmus uteri 26
  ligaments 29–30
    see also specific ligaments
  measurements 25
  menopause 385
  outlet obstruction, cervical cancer
    (carcinoma) 185
  post-menopause 38
  pubertal 38
  relationship with ureter 28
  retroversion 214–215
    anteverted 214
    causes 215
    diagnosis 215
    retroflexion 214
    symptoms 215
    treatment 215
  septated 66
  synechiae, dilatation and
    curettage 113
  trauma, dilatation and curettage
    113
  uterine glands 31
Uterus bicornis bicollis 65
Uterus bicornis unicollis 65
Uterus bicornis uterus 65
Uterus didelphys 65

Vabra Curettage, endometrial biopsy
  112
Vagina 22
  abnormalities 67
    absence 67
    gynatresia 67
    transverse septum 67
    vertical septum 67
  acidity 132
  age-related changes 38
  anterior fornix 23
  bimanual pelvic examination
    79
  bleeding
    cervical cancer (carcinoma)
      183
    tubal pregnancy 321
  blood supply 39–40
  carcinoma 170–171
    clinical features 170
    clinical staging 171
    magnetic resonance imaging
      170

melanoma 171
prognosis 171
sarcoma botriodes 171
site 171
spread 171
squamous cell carcinomas 170
treatment 171
cysts 168
  superficial dyspareunia 334
development 6, 14
discharge 74, 134
  bacterial vaginosis 137
  Candida albicans see Candida
    albicans infection
  cervical cancer (carcinoma)
    183
  clinical features 134
  composition 134
  examination 135
  leucorrhoea 135
  source of 134
  Trichomonas vaginalis 137–138
diseases 167–172
  benign disease 168
  bleeding *see above*
  carcinoma *see above*
  cysts *see above*
  malignant disease 169
  pre-malignant disease 169
  prolapse *see below*
dryness, menopause 385
epithelium 24
fistulae, cervical cancer
  (carcinoma) 185
fornices 23
histology 24
menopause 385
nulliparous adults 23
orifice 12, 14
pH 24
  Trichomonas vaginalis 138
plastic surgery 172
prolapse 74, 218
  anterior 218
  anterior colporrhaphy 223–224
  clinical features 220
  differential diagnosis 221
  pessary treatment 222
  posterior colpoperineorrhaphy
    227
  posterior wall 219
  stress incontinence 220
secretions 24
squamous epithelium 132
transverse septum 90
traumatic epithelial cysts 168
Vaginal dilators, vaginismus
  treatment 334
Vaginal hysterectomy 229–230
  heavy uterine bleeding 119
  late complications 230

operative complications 230
post-operative complications 230
prolapse 223
Vaginal intra-epithelial neoplasia
  (VAIN) 159, 169
Vaginal preparations, HRT 393
Vaginal rings 344
Vaginal ultrasound, uterus
  dimensions 25
Vaginectomy
  partial 169
  total, vaginal intra-epithelial
    neoplasia 169
  vaginal carcinoma treatment 171
Vaginismus 73, 334
  treatment 334
Vaginitis 139
  atrophic 139
  foreign bodies 139
  paediatric vulvo-vaginitis 139
  secondary causes 139
Vaginosis, bacterial 137
VAIN (vaginal intra-epithelial
  neoplasia) 159, 169
Vascular disease, combined oral
  contraceptive pill 343
Vasectomy 356
Vasomotor symptoms, menopause
  383
Vault haematoma, vaginal
  hysterectomy complications 230
Vault prolapse 219
Venography, contrast 299
Venous thromboembolism
  HRT 390
  risk, combined oral contraceptive
    pill 341
Venous thrombosis 295–297
  pathology 296
  prophylaxis 295
  risk factors 295
  sites 297
  see also Deep vein thrombosis
    (DVT)
Ventilation/perfusion (V/Q) scans,
  pulmonary embolism 304
Vermiculation 231
Verrucous carcinoma, genital warts
  vs. 141
Vertical septum, vagina 67
Vestibule 12, 14
Viagra (sidenasil), erectile
  dysfunction treatment 336
VIN (vulval intra-epithelial
  neoplasia) 159
Vincristine, sarcoma botriodes 171
Viral infections, sperm production
  abnormalities 366
Virchow's triad, venous thrombosis
  296–297
Virilisation 106

413

Visceral layer, pelvic fascia 21
Visual inspection, vulval
    examination 78–79
Vitamin B6 (pyridoxine),
    premenstrual syndrome treatment
    130
Voiding mechanism, micturition 236
Volume, vaginal discharge 134
V/Q (ventilation/perfusion) scans,
    pulmonary embolism 304
Vulva 12, 13–14
    abnormalities 68
        absence 68
        ectopia vesicae 68
    age-related changes 38
    bulb of vestibule 15
    carcinoma 160–164
        aetiology 160
        chemotherapy 164
        clinical features 160
        FIGO staging 160
        histology 160
        incidence 160

lymphatic spread 161
        prognosis 164
        radiotherapy 164
        surgical treatment 162, 164
    diseases 155–165
        benign tumours 158
        carcinoma *see above*
        dermatoses 156–157
        fibroma 158
        haematoma 158
        inflammation 132
        lipoma 158
        myoma 158
        Paget's disease 159
        sebaceous cysts 158
        see also specific diseases/disorders
    examination 78
        rape 337
    external urethral
        orifice 14
    menopause 385
    vaginal discharge 134
    vestibule 14

Vulval intra-epithelial neoplasia
    (VIN) 159
Vulvectomy, radical 162, 163
Vulvovaginitis, superficial
    dyspareunia 334

Warfarin, DVT treatment 301
Warts, genital *see* Genital warts
Wolffian (mesonephric) ridge,
    embryology 5
Women Health Initiative, HRT trials
    390

X-rays
    chest, pulmonary embolism 303
    IUD translocation 348
    mammography 82

Yolk sac tumours 263, 270
Yoon ring applicator 355

Zidovudine, AIDS transmission 154
Zona pellucida 46

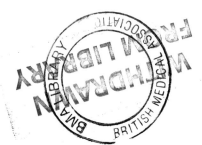